HERBAL HEALING SECRETS
of the
Orient

Darlena L'Orange, L.Ac.

PRENTICE HALL
Paramus, New Jersey 07652

Library of Congress Cataloging-in-Publication Data

L'Orange, Darlena
    Herbal healing secrets of the Orient   /   by Darlena L'Orange.
        p.   cm.
        Includes bibliographical references and index.
        ISBN 0-13-849324-3 (cloth). — 0-13-849316-2 (pbk.)
        1. Herbs—Therapeutic use—Encyclopedias.   2. Medicine, Oriental—Encyclopedias.
    I. Title.
    RM666.H33L26   1998
    615'.321'095—dc21   97-41799
                                                                                          CIP

Acquistions Editor: *Doug Corcoran*
Production Editor: *Eve Mossman*
Formatting/Interior Design: *Robyn Beckerman*

© *1998 by Prentice Hall*

Printed in the United States of America

10 9 8 7 6 5 4 3 2 1

ISBN 0-13-849324-3 (cloth)   ISBN 0-13-849316-2 (pbk.)

PRENTICE HALL
Paramus, NJ 07652

A Simon & Schuster Company

On the World Wide Web at http://www.phdirect.com

Prentice Hall International (UK) Limited, *London*
Prentice Hall of Australia Pty. Limited, *Sydney*
Prentice Hall Canada, Inc., *Toronto*
Prentice Hall Hispanoamericana, S.A., *Mexico*
Prentice Hall of India Private Limited, *New Delhi*
Prentice Hall of Japan, Inc., *Tokyo*
Simon & Schuster Asia Pte. Ltd., *Singapore*
Editora Prentice Hall do Brasil, Ltda., *Rio de Janeiro*

Dedicated to My Loved Ones

Lona LaOrange
Earl and Joan LaOrange
Lara and Kili Cubilla
Teresita Perez
Thelma Barrett-Walker
George

and especially
to Terry, whose incredible love, support,
and understanding made it all possible

Acknowledgments

Special thanks to Gary Dolowich, MD, L.Ac., an inspiring healer and teacher, who gave me the gift of 5 Elements—the Heart and Spirit of Traditional Chinese Medicine.

Thanks to the work of wonderful healers, teachers, and friends such as Miriam Lee; Michael, Lesley and Shasta Tierra; Christopher Hobbs; Roy Upton; Martha Benedict; Holly Guzman; Lela Carney; Lara Grasso-Cubilla; dedicated members of the American Herbalists' Guild and herbalists worldwide, our rich herbal past is being preserved.

Exceptional teachers and professors along life's path have made all the difference. Thank you Baba Hari Dass, Bernardino Ducci, Rob Edwards, Diane Gifford-Gonzalez, Dorothy Holloway, Carole Kelley, Vasant Lad, Diane Lewis, Triloki Pandey, Adrienne Zihlman.

Doug Corcoran, senior editor, Prentice Hall, thank you for your confidence in me; your patience, guidance, and expert editing skills.

Foreword

Who knows who the first person was who decided to chew some plantain leaf (a common wayside weed found growing around the world) and apply it for relief of a venomous bite, cut, or injury? . . . or the first human to dig up a ginseng root to discover its healing properties? The fact that it worked and has continued to work (probably for millennia) forms the foundation for our respect and use of these time-honored herbs. The unspoken thesis of this book is that first and foremost herbal medicine emanates from and is continually renewed by the experiences of the lay people, nonherbalists, possibly even more so than by that of professionals.

Perhaps no people have had a more lively interest in the health-giving medicinal properties of plants than have the Chinese people. Yet, as Traditional Chinese Medicine (in the form of both acupuncture and Chinese herbal medicine) finds its way into the mainstream of health care in the West, it is too often belabored in a philosophical thought system that is inaccessible to most Western people.

The danger is to think that herbs used in Chinese medicine (even though many grow in areas throughout the world) can be prescribed and used only by a professional class of Traditional Chinese Medical Doctors who have been trained in their proper use. In fact, I know many practitioners who firmly believe this. It is my opinion, and undoubtedly the opinion of the author of this book, that such an attitude invites a kind of stagnation of experience and knowledge that is vital to the further evolution of herbal medicine that could ultimately lead to the exclusive use of herbs by a professional class. This defies the use of herbs as the people's birthright and can ultimately threaten the existence of herbalism, if that same professional class, for any reason, ceases to exist.

In China, all herbs and medicine are freely available. It is the common experience of all traditional Chinese households to know and use a wide number of herbs for a variety of common ailments, as well as for tonics cooked with food. It is time that people of the West (who have learned to integrate the use of various vitamins and other health supplements) also learn to integrate the even greater health benefits of Chinese herbs as part of their regular health program. These are all appropriately described in this book.

Darlena, my former student (who has for some time been regarded as a respected herbalist and acupuncturist in her community), has made an important contribution to the mainstream appreciation and use of Chinese herbs. I am proud of her ability to convey the inner meaning and spirit of Chinese herbal medicine so that larger numbers of people will feel confident in their use. This book should prove to be a considerable help to the understanding of patients of Traditional Chinese Medical practitioners who use herbs in their practice and to all other health practitioners and herbalists who are seeking a better understanding of Traditional Chinese Herbal Medicine.

As we embark into the twenty-first century, we bear witness to the paradox of phenomenal technical and scientific achievements contrasted with the incremental growth of interest in all aspects of traditional and natural healing. The reasons for this are found in the realization by many of the shortcomings in the dominant technological medicine of our time. Increasing numbers of people are turning to traditional herbs and healing as a result of their dissatisfaction with the too frequent inability of Western medicine to provide more than mere symptomatic relief of diseases—often resulting in uncalculated and disastrous side effects.

Whatever the reasons, our interest in herbs will always be an expression of at least some part of us that will always belong to earth as Gaia, our mother. It attests to the inevitability that whatever we may accomplish, wherever we may traverse, in order to remain healthy and whole, vital aspects of earth and nature must, in some way, accompany us even unto the stars . . . for we need and depend on the air we breathe, the water we drink, and the plants that embody the very essence of life to serve as our food and our medicine.

Dr. Michael Tierra
OMD, L.Ac., Herbalist AHG

Introduction

Long before supermarkets and fast-food restaurants, prior to living in cities and towns, our ancient ancestors roamed the earth hunting, gathering, and sharing the bounty of the hunt or harvest in small bands of 25 to 30 people. Our forefathers and mothers, through taste, instinct, and experimentation, relied on healing substances from plants, minerals, and animals that were not a part of their everyday diet. In 1960, archaeologists discovered evidence of human beings using herbal remedies in the burial site of a Neanderthal man dating back some 60,000 years ago. Soil analysis revealed extraordinary amounts of plant pollen from eight species of medicinal plants that had been consciously placed around the body of the dead man. Today, herbalists around the world are still using seven of the those eight healing plants.

It is truly a remarkable experience to be one of the growing number of herbalists dedicated to renewing our interest in age-old, time-tested remedies that link us to an ancient past when herbs were a regular part of the human diet. Somewhere along our journey, folk wisdom and natural healing were almost completely forgotten as technological advances thrust us into the industrial revolution and twentieth-century life as we know it. Today, many dedicated herbalists are ensuring that our rich herbal past is being preserved and passed on to yet another generation who seems increasingly eager to bridge the chasm between the worlds of traditional healing systems and Western scientific medical practice. The two systems can work together harmoniously, as is witnessed in Chinese hospitals where acupuncture and herbalism are given their own wing in a completely modern medical setting.

It's time to invite you into my world—the world of a practicing herbalist/acupuncturist/anthropologist. The field of anthropology taught me some valuable lessons regarding the great importance of communicating to you personal experiences that have colored the way I see the world. You have the right to know the unique events that shaped my life and, therefore, the way I think. Since no culture, group, or person has a corner on the truth, it's important that you understand my biases before making up your mind regarding how to foster and build health and well-being into your own life. The same holds true for any health practitioner with whom you might have contact. Don't give away your power to a "perceived" authority figure. Always ask questions. To flow smoothly through life's changes, it's important for us to remain open to receive new (or perhaps old) truths—but keep a discerning mind.

For me, that path of herbs is a way of life. I haven't taken an aspirin in 25 years, though antibiotics proved essential on a 1994 trip to India. In our family, we regularly use herbs to effectively cure everyday complaints, from sore throats to upset tummies. We have a large herb garden and healing herbs always manage to find their way into our meals. Later, you'll get some of those recipes.

Having grown up on a small farm in Pratt, Kansas, I was introduced to the use of some "country remedies" as a child. I'll never forget the prickly-pear-cactus cough syrup my mother and Mrs. McDaniels, the neighbor lady, cooked up when I had whooping cough. It worked pretty well and didn't taste bad at all—wish I had the recipe! Often, I sat with my sister, Lona, on the front porch swing, dreaming of faraway places, especially the wide-open pampas of Argentina.

Given my incredible curiosity about other cultures and my love of music, it seems only natural that the years 1972 to 1977 found me attending the National University of Music in Mendoza, Argentina. This is where my first formal introduction to herbalism took place. I had been plagued with bleeding duodenal ulcers for more than eight years. The Argentine doctors wanted to operate. Hearing this, my clarinet professor literally threw me in his car and took me to Juancito, a local herbal healer. Juancito gave me a few interesting bags of twigs, leaves, and bark with instructions for their preparation and advised me about diet. Suffice to say that X-rays taken six weeks later confirmed that the ulcers had finally healed, and I haven't been troubled since. After that, I started studying herbs in earnest. In 1977, we moved to Santa Cruz, California, where I was employed at Fmali, a local herb company.

When our daughter, Lara, was 14 years old, she became very ill and could not keep food or water down. She was admitted to our community hospital for observation and testing. Our doctor said the tests were inconclusive and the next logical step would be exploratory surgery. Desperate at the thought of surgery, I took Lara to our acupuncturist, Michael Tierra. When Michael pressed a specific acupuncture point just below the knee, Lara expressed great discomfort. This point is used in Traditional Oriental Medicine to diagnose appendicitis (appendectomies are performed only in extreme cases, and the appendix is saved approximately 95 percent of the time in China). Instead of exploratory surgery, Michael inserted six acupuncture needles for 20 to 30 minutes and then sent us home with herbs and instructions regarding diet. That evening, for the first time in two weeks, Lara was able to eat a very light dinner.

In my own case, alternative healing methods had cured ulcers, large ovarian cysts, and severe allergies. Our daughter's experience was the clincher. I knew I had to practice Oriental Medicine. I entered a three-year program at East/West Clinic with Michael Tierra in 1985 to study acupuncture and herbs (including Western, East Indian Ayurvedic, and Chinese).

The great news is that Lara, now 27, finished a B.S. degree in Sports Medicine at San Diego State University and has completed a three-year Masters program at Pacific College of Oriental Medicine in San Diego, California. She is joining me so we can practice together—a mother/daughter team. Currently, I am a faculty member at the American School of Herbalism in Santa Cruz, California, and have an active practice in Soquel.

Now that you've heard our story, I want to introduce you to simple, basic Oriental health concepts and 108 healing herbs commonly used in Traditional Oriental Medicine. You'll meet a number of my patients who have benefited from their use. The therapeutic application of healing herbs and foods shouldn't be considered a "secret" and need not remain a great mystery. Too frequently in my practice, I am confronted with patients who are taking the current "herbal fad," such as ginseng or royal jelly to increase stamina, or ephedra to lose weight. The truth is that all herbs are not for all people all of the time. In this book, you learn ways to determine which healing flavors, foods, and herbs are good for you and your loved ones. You are given some of my favorite herbal prescriptions that are time-tested and have worked wonders for people suffering from various diseases that seemed to elude the standard medical approach. One of the main purposes of this book is to pass on to you some basic skills in treating common conditions that you currently diagnose yourself and for which you purchase medications at a drugstore without prescription—conditions such as that nagging cough, cold, or flu; headache; PMS; or indigestion after a night on the town. Please always consult a licensed health care practitioner for serious problems, however. Although herbs can work wonders, and I sincerely feel that they are often a more effective means for treating chronic diseases, it's important to remember that herbal therapy cannot make up for poor nutrition, lack of exercise, overwork, or other practices that conflict with good health. It is also important not to overromanticize any approach to health as being superior to another. As we move into the twenty-first century, somehow we need to integrate traditional herbal medical wisdom with modern twentieth-century scientific advances.

Contents

Chapter 4
COMMON AILMENTS AND THEIR
SIMPLE HERBAL HOME REMEDIES **221**

Chapter 5
DELICIOUS RECIPES TO INCORPORATE HEALING HERBS AND FOODS INTO YOUR DAILY DIET 259

Chapter 6
SIMPLE WAYS TO UNDERSTAND THE NATURE OF YOUR DISEASE 323

Chapter 7
EASY WAYS TO DECIDE WHICH HERBS/FOODS WILL HEAL YOU AND YOUR FAMILY　**339**

Chapter 1

Natural Healing with Herbs and Foods

The healer of disease is Nature.

—Hippocrates

Cultivating Health in Our Human Garden

Is the human body a garden or a machine? Traditional healing systems view human beings as a part of nature while Western science is based on the idea that humankind is separate from nature. Here in the West, disease is thought of as an attacking entity, the cause of which must be discovered. Once that cause is determined, a powerful antibiotic may be taken to destroy the germ. To the contrary, Oriental medical thought is not interested so much in the *cause* of the disease but, instead, asks *why* the person's immune system was so weak as to succumb to the bacteria, virus, or other unwanted visitor in the first place.

In the West we have grown up with the body as machine metaphor—you know, the heart is a pump, the bladder and kidneys are plumbing, the brain is a computer, and our joints are hinges that become rusty with old age. Try as we might to remove ourselves from this mechanistic viewpoint, we are a part of our culture; this is symbolism we learned at a very early age. It's extremely important to be aware of our thinking process and how it makes us relate to our world, its myriad and marvelous other creatures, and our fellow human beings! Shortly, I'm going to ask you to take a different type of

1

journey with me, one rich in metaphors that relate to the human body as a part of nature. Both viewpoints, body as machine and body as a garden, are equally valid and should be used at the appropriate time and place.

Herbal medicine gives us herbal antibiotics to fight off minor infections and adaptogenic herbs such as astragalus, ginseng, and codonopsis to help build immunity; Western medicine gives us antibiotics to kill germs that are out of control. It is extremely important to recognize when the body is not strong enough to fight off the invader, so that appropriate Western medical intervention can take place. However, as an herbalist, I consider a healthy lifestyle along with adaptogenic herbs to be the ultimate answer to true health and well-being once the immediate crisis has been resolved.

Now it's time to consider the miracle of your human body from a more naturalistic point of view. Come with me—we'll take that long overdue journey into the ever-changing human garden. Let's start our venture into traditional Oriental healing with herbs and foods by considering some sage advice from Hippocrates, the Father of Western Medicine:

Whoever wishes to investigate medicine should proceed thus:
In the first place, consider the seasons of the year
and what effect each of them produces.

—HIPPOCRATES

FIVE SEASONS TO VIBRANT HEALTH AND WELL-BEING

Hippocrates and the ancient Chinese actually had a lot more in common than we might realize! Together, let's try to bridge worlds. Modern humankind, in moving from the farm to the city, severed its roots from Nature and the seasonal cycles throughout the year that signaled the need for lifestyle changes. Let's begin our quest for health by taking the advice of Hippocrates and investigate the effects seasonal changes have upon our health from the Oriental medical view. You'll be amazed at how much this sounds like the good common-sense advice we once received from our grandmothers. You're going to run into a few words in Chinese, don't let that intimidate you. By the end of Chapter 3, they'll be old friends. For now, just get a feel for the Oriental view of the human body as a garden and how the seasonal changes affect our health and well-being.

Spring: Nature's Time of Rebirth

Tiny tendrils spiral upward toward the sun,
   while roots sink deeply into the rich soil.

Waking from winter's slumber to life's call,
   new life stirs as each seed seeks the sun.
All of creation reaches outward toward the light.
In this season of opening, expansion,
   and growth that comes in myriad colors,
   hear nature's many sweet, yet different refrains.
Each of them rings true as the new seed,
   in harmony with its vision,
   grows to flower and fruit.

—DARLENA

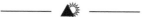

Welcome to the world of ancient Chinese farmers who depended upon the earth for their livelihood and on seasonal cues as to when to till, sow, tend, and harvest their crops. The center of the Chinese world was, literally and figuratively, the earth. Like other traditional cultures engaged in farming, the Chinese depended upon the fruits of the land for survival. They experienced the vast power of nature and sought to be in harmony with its seasons, rhythms, and patterns that connected all things to each other. Chinese art, philosophy, and medicine were all nourished by the same naturalistic thought process and represent the essence of nature as seen by the artist/poet/healer—in balance and in flux.

In Traditional Oriental Medicine, Spring, nature's time of rebirth and sudden growth, is the season associated with the Wood Element that governs the Liver and Gall Bladder Acupuncture Meridians (sometimes referred to as energy channels). As the life process reawakens after its winter slumber, movement surges to the surface. Just as spring initiates the rising of sap in the trees, the Liver (or Wood Element) lifts the body's *Blood* and *Qi* (refers to vital energy and is pronounced *"chee"*). Patients will often complain of neck and shoulder tension in the springtime, and I tell them that their sap is rising too—just like all of nature. The Gallbladder Channel runs up through the shoulders and neck.

Think of the new growth that comes in Spring—willows, maples, roses—all of our green friends send forth leafy arms to touch the sun. For this reason "wood" is the element associated with springtime. The Wood Element refers to the growing structure—roots, trunk, and branches of trees—the spine, limbs, and joints in a human being. In the Oriental medical system, arthritis (of the "wind" type, which is characterized by pains that come and go suddenly or that shift locations) is viewed as a Wood imbalance.

Beginning, or creation, is the nature of spring, and the Wood Element instigates movement and arouses the intellect by allowing tension and pressure to build. Mentally, the Wood Element is responsible for clarity and your ability to focus, plan, and make decisions. A Wood imbalance could manifest as poor planning, organization, or judgment. A very strong Wood Element could result in excessive mentality, and such a person could be prone to headaches as well as to neck and back tensions.

The color associated with Wood is the green of young plants or the green of verdant hillsides in springtime. Someone who is strongly attracted to this color or has a great dislike for it may be exhibiting a Wood imbalance. The climate for spring is characterized by wind—just think of those March winds that blow in the April showers. Wind nourishes Wood; however, too much wind can be harmful and results in migratory or moving pains in the human bodyscape. If our Wood Element is injured by overexposure to extreme winds, symptoms might include allergic sensitivities, sinus or skin problems, or irritated, watery eyes.

Western science recognizes well over 150 liver functions and views the liver as the body's master laboratory. Basically, the liver stores and distributes nourishment to the entire body; is involved in the formation and breakdown of blood cells; filters toxins from the blood; and creates bile that is stored in the gallbladder to break down fats.

According to Oriental medicine, the Wood Element, or Liver, regulates the flow of blood and Qi (vital energy) throughout the body; stores blood and nourishes the eyes; and harmonizes digestion, emotions, sexuality, and reproduction (PMS is associated with Liver qi stagnation or congestion). The Wood Element is also responsible for the smooth movement of ligaments and tendons.

In Traditional Oriental Medicine, mind and body are not separated. Mood swings are the first indicator that something is amiss in our human garden. Anger is the emotion attributed to a stressed Wood Element, and the shouting voice that accompanies anger could signal that someone is suffering from a Wood imbalance. Much can be said about the liver's function in harmonizing emotions. A smoothly functioning liver creates an even, flowing disposition and the ability to take confident, decisive action based on clear judgment. When the liver is overtaxed by coffee, alcohol, drugs, stress, rich foods, or imbalanced hormones, the resulting impatience and irritability is the first sign that our Wood Element needs some tending.

According to Oriental thought, when our Liver/Gallbladder Organ System functions well, we are able to set appropriate boundaries. Do you know anyone who would say, "I'm sorry," to someone who steps on his or her foot? Or in contrast, do you know a person who gets angry and yells at the person whose foot he or she stepped on? The first person probably suffers from Deficient Liver function—he or she is apologetic for "being in the way" and does not have the self-esteem necessary to defend his or her own boundaries. The overactive Wood Element results in the opposite scenario, however, with an inappropriate extension of the person's boundaries, "How dare you get in my way?"

One of modern society's greatest insults to our mistreated Wood Element was the invention of margarine and other solid vegetable oils. The liver cannot process hydrogenated oils; though not saturated, they are foreign substances to the human body. Hydrogenation is a chemical process combining vegetable oils with hydrogen to make them solid and spreadable at room temperature. Recognized by the American Heart Association as having detrimental effects on our health, hydrogenated oils do not elevate cholesterol; however, they do lower immunity, cause cell membrane irregularities, and have negative effects on our nervous system. (Note: See the recipe for "Better Ghee" in Chapter 5—a healthful and delightfully delicious alternative for margarine.)

But, now it's springtime. A time of new beginnings—nature bursting forth all around us. It's time to get moving with new plans, daily exercise, appropriate rest and relaxation, and a light, lively, slightly sour diet to clear the liver, mind, and emotions.

Yes, you read that right. Sour is the flavor attributed to springtime in Traditional Oriental Medicine. It is a taste too often missing from the average American diet. In nature, the sour flavor is abundant in springtime in the form of sour berries, fruits, and greens. Sour substances are astringent, detoxifying, and show antibacterial and antiviral activity. In small amounts, the sour flavor tonifies our Wood Element and can help the liver throw off toxins. In Chapters 5, 6, and 7, you learn more about the healing qualities of the sour flavor, considered to be one of the Five Healing Flavors in the Orient. But for now, we have to move on quickly because the seasons are changing. Can't you feel the energy shift as we start to move into summer, the season of greatest light, considered the most yang time of year. (Note: *Yang* is pronounced yong as in *"song."*)

Simple Home Helpers for Wood Element Imbalances

Disharmony	Foods and Herbs that Can Help	Avoid
Allergies	Bamboo shoots, beets, beet tops, carrots, cabbage, garlic, ginger, leafy greens, tea, yams	Chocolate, citrus, corn, eggs, wheat
Arthritis (Wind type) Characterized by migrating pains that shift locations, occasional dizziness	Black beans, green leafy veggies, grapes, most whole grains, scallions	Red meat, sugar, alcohol, cigarettes
Cataracts	Black beans, chrysanthemum, cilantro, cloves, lycii berries, water chestnuts, sesame seeds, spinach, walnuts, yams	Salt, spices, garlic
Hepatitis	Apple, aduki beans, barley, beet greens, cabbage, carrot, celery, corn silk, cucumber, dandelion greens, grapefruit, lotus root, millet, orange, pears, pineapple, rice, squash, watermelon	Alcohol, coffee, chocolate, sugar, fatty and fried foods
Hives	Black beans, black sesame, chrysanthemum, cornsilk, ginger, mung beans, mint, pearl barley, shiitake mushrooms	All food items listed above
High Blood Pressure	Apples, bamboo shoots, bananas, celery, chrysanthemum, corn, eggplant, garlic, hawthorn berries, lemons, lotus root, mung beans, mushrooms, peas, plums, seaweed, sunflower seeds, tofu	Alcohol, cigarettes, coffee, caffeine, fatty or fried foods, overeating, stimulants, stress
Neck and Shoulder Tension	Kudzu root is phenomenal	
PMS	Black pepper, cinnamon, dang gui, fennel, ginger, green onions, hawthorn berries, jujube dates, orange peel, spinach, walnuts	Cold foods, coffee, cigarettes, sugar, shellfish, stimulants, vinegar

Summer: Nature's Time of Expansion

See how the peach tree
              bends with ripened fruit.

Daily, heaven's golden orb
shares more of its power with us
as fruits ripen on the vine.
During this fire phase of luxurious growth,
nature's springborn creatures frolic
in summer sunlight.
This is the season to explore the
potential of our outer bounds, while
basking in the strength and quiet
of our tranquil inner core.

—DARLENA

———— ☀ ————

According to ancient Chinese medical texts, the energies of summer create "heat in the Heavens and fire on Earth." The summer season is characterized by luxurious growth, brightness, creativity, lightness, and increased outward activity. Summer is the time to play—to arise early, walk barefoot in the morning dew, and gather nourishment from the sun—especially in the early morning and late afternoon.

The Fire Element pertains to the Summer Season, as does the red color. Just think of the brilliant flame colors of a desert sunset or a bright red rose. Also associated with the summer season is the emotion of joy (or, in its absence, sorrow) and a voice filled with happiness or the sound of laughter like that of children at play. If our Fire Element is in balance, we are able to integrate and express our thoughts, feelings, and sensations and experience love in all its forms. Imbalance in this element can be signaled by such symptoms as palpitations, chest pain, confusion, anxiety, panic attacks, or ceaseless chatter. In Traditional Oriental Medicine, the Heart/Small Intestine and Pericardium/Triple Warmer are the organ systems associated with the Fire Element. The human heart not only propels red blood through the vessels, according to Oriental thought, it houses the *shen* (translated as both Mind and Spirit). The presence of shen is that remarkable sparkle you see in the eyes of a wise, kind, compassionate soul.

Also associated with the Fire Element is the scorched smell (think of the fragrance of burning wood), the southerly direction, and the sense of taste. See Diagram No. 1 for a list of all the Five Elements and their correspondences. It has taken me years to get a true feel for the relationships the ancient Chinese described in this chart. Every day is a new learning experience as I see a patient and perhaps hear a shouting sound in his or her voice (Wood Element imbalance) or smell a body fragrance that could be described as a scorched smell (Fire Element imbalance). But it's summertime and the energy is high. We need to get moving.

The great news is that summer's abundant supply of fresh fruits and vegetables require that we spend less time in the kitchen cooking. These foods need less heat and shorter cooking times. Steam or simmer foods as quickly as possible to guarantee very little depletion of natural vitamins, minerals, and enzymes. Add spices such as ginger and cayenne to stimulate perspiration— the body's natural mechanism to eliminate stored toxins and summer heat. However, minerals are lost through perspiration, stress, and consumption of refined foods. They need to be replaced by eating the widest variety of organic produce available—be sure to check your local farmers' market.

Persons with reduced digestive fire may find that the consumption of raw food results in loose stools filled with undigested food particles. To remedy the situation, the bitter flavor comes to the rescue. Bitter is the healing flavor associated with the Fire Element (guess that's the bad news!). Lightly steam bitter greens such as endive, arugula, or dandelion greens to stimulate digestion; also, lightly cook all foods and consume smaller amounts. The bitter flavor is relatively unfamiliar in American cuisine. It serves an incredibly important function: Bitters aid digestion as well as having anti-inflammatory, antispasmodic, and antibacterial effects. Many traditional cultures start their meals with a salad made from bitter greens. So boost your immune system this summer by eating plenty of nature's green germ fighters.

It is tempting to use cold, congesting foods (such as iced drinks and ice cream) to cool off. According to Traditional Oriental Medical thought, eating these foods introduces coldness into the system. Our digestion is weakened when summer heat is combined with too much cold food. Coldness creates contraction, which stops perspiration and traps the heat inside. This process interferes with good digestion—it is like throwing water on a fire— and that's exactly what happens to our "digestive fire."

Wonderful light refreshing foods that are perfect for summer consumption include organically grown local fresh fruits and veggies—baby greens, mung bean sprouts, tofu, fish and other lean meats, and herb teas such as chamomile, mint, and chrysanthemum. Lemons and limes cool summer heat as well as offer a good dose of Vitamin C—use them in your summer dressings. Moderation should be observed, however, since eating too many foods that disperse heat also disperses our yang energy, which can make it more difficult for us to stay warm in cooler seasons. Eating heavy foods (especially those high in refined flours, sugars, and saturated fats) on a hot, sunny day creates sluggishness. It's a good idea to save larger servings of nuts, seeds, grains, and red meats for foggy coastal areas during summer weather.

Summer is the time to increase activity, to start engaging in short walks or other exercise programs if this has been an unfulfilled goal. Take advantage of the longer daylight hours. Most important—take time to smell the roses . . . and don't forget to call that old friend you haven't talked to for a while! Nothing warms the heart and nourishes the soul more than meaningful relationships.

SIMPLE HOME HELPERS FOR FIRE ELEMENT IMBALANCES

Disharmony	Foods and Herbs that Can Help	Avoid
Anorexia	Barley, beans, bell pepper, cilantro, cinnamon, corn, garlic, ginger, green onions, mustard greens, persimmons, potatoes, pumpkin, rice, yam	
Anxiety	Corn, kamut (Egyptian) wheat, gardenia, longan berries, zizyphus seeds	Coffee, stimulants
Arthritis (Heat type) Characterized by sudden onset, red, swollen, hot, painful joints	Abundant fresh fruit and veggies, cabbage, dandelion, mung beans, soybean sprouts. Apply poultices of crushed dandelion greens—change every two hours.	Alcohol, cigarettes, green onion, spicy foods, stress
Coronary Heart Disease	Bananas, black sesame seeds, celery, chrysanthemum, garlic, ginger, green tea, hawthorn berries, kamut wheat, lotus root, lotus seeds, mung bean sprouts, mung beans, pearl barley, persimmons, seaweed, shiitake mushrooms, soy sprouts, sunflower seeds, water chestnuts, watermelon, wheat bran	Alcohol, cigarettes, coffee, fatty foods, spicy foods, highly refined foods. stress, lack of sleep

Disharmony	Foods and Herbs that Can Help	Avoid
Indigestion Due to lack of digestive enzymes	Dandelion greens, hawthorn berries, papaya, pineapple, figs, bitter greens (dandelion, endive, arugula) daikon radish, orange, apple, lemon	Rich foods, fatty foods, and stress while eating

Doyo: Nature's Seasonal Transitions

Nature seems to halt . . . while earth's

cycles pause . . .

. . . then slowly start to shift.

Strangely still, yet animated,
  hummingbird hovers suspended over
  a fragrant honeysuckle blossom.
Late summer—nature's harvest-time.
Warm, moisture-laden air carries sweet
  scents of over-ripened fruits.
Fields of golden grains drenched in sunshine
  must be gathered, stored, and shared.

—DARLENA

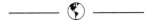

This is it—the fifth season! Bet you've been curious. The word *doyo,* when translated from Chinese, means "transition." Often, late summer or "Indian summer" is the time of year most often associated with the Earth Element. However, doyo actually relates to the time just before all seasonal changes. It occurs for two to three weeks before the two solstices and the two equinoxes—or roughly speaking, doyo is from:

> March 1 until the first day of spring, or March 20;
> June 1 until the first day of summer, or June 21;
> September 1 until the first day of autumn, or September 22;
> and December 1 until the first day of winter, or December 21.

Have you noticed how, for two to three weeks before seasonal changes, there's something in the air—you can't quite put your finger on it, yet it could be described as an "electrical" stillness. You might feel more emotional, less balanced. The weather is changeable, as if nature were trying to shift gears. (There—they just slipped out—"electrical" and "shift gears" are perfect examples of how machine metaphors permeate our Western thought process.) Often, we find ourselves coming down with a cold/flu or body aches and pains during these times of transition. Watch it! Better yet, keep a little journal noting the date you experience certain symptoms. You will begin to see a pattern. Frequently that nagging pain in the shoulder joint will visit you every year in September, the neck and upper-shoulder tension sometime in March, or perhaps low back pain in December. In the clinic this year, I saw about 23 cases of shoulder pain over the three-week period leading to autumn. Chinese medical wisdom never ceases to amaze me. The lung and colon acupuncture meridians run up the arm and through the shoulder joint—these are the organ systems associated with the fall season in Traditional Oriental Medicine. However, this discomfort could appear any time of year if you are experiencing a Metal Element imbalance; it is just seen more frequently in the fall. Remember that those minor aches and pains are your body's friendly reminders that something is not quite right in your human garden. Don't simply mask the symptoms with pain relievers. Now is the time to address the imbalance before chronic disease sets in. Do you remember one of Benjamin Franklin's sayings, "An ounce of prevention is worth a pound of cure"? The Chinese have a similar saying, "It's too late to start digging a well when you're already thirsty."

But back to the Earth Element. The earth represents the center of the world for agriculturists who depend upon it for nurturance and support. Our human body is truly composed of earth—transformed through the miracle of sunlight by our green friends to produce all the foods we consume in one form or another.

In Traditional Oriental Medicine, the Earth Element is associated with the stomach and spleen and pancreas, our organs of digestion, located in the center of the body. The Earth Element has a natural cadence—just think of nature's rhythmic cycles—the day-to-night 24-hour cycle, the 28-day moon cycle, and of course, seasonal changes. Do you have a tendency to skip meals? Our personal Earth Element needs to be nourished in a rhythmic way at regular intervals to avoid drops in blood sugar and resulting feelings of hunger, fatigue, and lack of mental clarity.

Life is truly amazing. Each of us is caretaker to trillions of tiny life forms, our cells, that have miraculously grouped together to form "us"—each a unique and totally different individual. Every one of those cells requires certain quantities of proteins, fats, and carbohydrates on a regular basis, to repair cell walls and to reproduce. On a cellular level, messenger enzymes are released by cells in need of food or oxygen. If their messages are not answered, even more enzymes are released, which we may experience as feelings of worry, anxiety, or mood swings. Too often, we'll reach for a caffeine or sugar fix instead of stopping for a regular meal, adding injury to insult on a cellular level. Unfortunately, in our Western race to "go/see/do/and accomplish," we have gotten far away from the idea of truly nourishing ourselves at a deep fundamental level with simple, fresh, life-giving home cooked whole foods, the ones you find around the edges of your supermarket, including all sorts of fresh leafy and root vegetables, fruits, cuts of lean meat and fish, dairy products, and whole grains and beans. It is the full sweet flavor associated with the Earth Element in Oriental Medicine that gives the required nourishment for building muscles and all body tissues requiring protein to rebuild and glucose to use as their fuel. For true health and well-being to occur, we need to nourish our Earth Element on a regular basis.

While sweetness is the flavor associated with the Earth Element, it is important not to confuse the empty sweet flavor of candy, refined white flour and sugar products, and carbonated soda drinks with the full sweet flavor of wholesome vitamin- and mineral-packed fresh produce. Special treats certainly have their place to sweeten our existence, but sweet cravings often indicate your body is desperately in need of nurturing full-sweet foods. Many immune-enhancing tonic herbs are found in this category, including astragalus, codonopsis, dioscorea, ginseng, jujube date, and licorice.

One important note about nutrition before we move on. You remember the old adage, "One person's food is another person's poison?" Believe me, dietary requirements regarding the quantity and ratio of carbohydrates, proteins, and fats we each require varies incredibly. Currently accepted dietary doctrine regarding high intake of complex carbohydrates and low intake of protein and fat can be dead wrong for some people while it is totally right for others. I speak from firsthand experience regarding this matter. Since 1985, I consumed what today is considered a nearly perfect diet—only whole grains, veggies, very little meat protein, and about 15% fat while watching calories—only to gain some 70 pounds over a ten-year period. I tried many different approaches to lose weight, with no success, until I ran into a book called "The Zone" by Barry Sears, Ph.D. I decided to try his plan for a week to disprove what I thought was a ridiculous approach to weight loss: Three meals and two snacks a day composed of 40% carbohydrates/30% protein/30% fat. Suffice to say that by the end of eight months, 70 pounds had dropped off effortlessly. I've never eaten so much food in my life. While the amount of fat I eat has risen from 15 to 30%, my cholesterol level dropped 50 points. If you, or someone in your family has a chronic weight problem, please consider looking into Sears' approach. According to Sears, about 25% of the population has a serious problem in dealing with carbohydrates that rank high on what is known as the glycemic index. Regardless of the number of calories they take in, weight loss is nearly impossible if certain complex carbohydrates, like those found in rice, corn, wheat, and potatoes, are ingested in more than very minor quantities. These carbohydrates cause a rapid release of insulin in carbohydrate-sensitive individuals. Simply put, you can't burn fat with high levels of insulin in your blood stream no matter how much calories are restricted. This certainly proved to be the answer to my problem and I was force to discard a lot of today's dietary dogma. After trying the diet for six months myself (with a number of modifications based on good nutritional practices of including only whole, organic foods, herbs, and sea veggies) I felt secure in recommending it to some of my overweight patients. Sears' "block method" uses lean body mass and physical activity factors as a means of arriving at the quantity of food to be consumed daily. These calculations are to be used as a starting point for the minimum amount of protein and, therefore, calories to be consumed daily. I have found, however, unless someone has a small frame, these calculations tend to be too conservative. In general, my patients and I consume 1 to 3 more blocks per day than recommended by Sears (depending upon size of bone structure), and are experiencing great results. For persons who can't bear the thought of calculating blocks, researchers Drs. Rachael and Richard Heller offer another approach to controlling insulin release in a wonderfully informative book entitled, "The Carbohydrate Addict's Diet." To determine if you might be carbohydrate sensitive, please take Hellers' "Carbohydrate Sensitivity Test" found in Chapter 5. While Sears' approach fits my personal lifestyle better, some of my patients have had great results with the Heller and Heller method (which does not impose any caloric restrictions). Also, there is a lot of interesting new research out showing that blood type can be an indicator of which foods we best assimilate. Recommended readings can be found in the Resources Section of this book, please see page 357.

It's gratifying to see that scientific research is proving what Oriental medical wisdom has long held, that each of us requires different foods and herbs in order to achieve true balance. *In the same way that different plants require totally different soils, fertilizers, sunshine, moisture, and other growing conditions, human beings require different diets, amounts of exercise, climates, and herbal treatment.* Please remember this important bit of Oriental wisdom before offering the herb that worked wonders for you to a person with a completely different body type.

In Traditional Oriental Medicine, the Earth Element gives us our ability to assimilate both food and information. If you are overwhelmed by too much food or information you can suffer from physical or mental indigestion. A balanced Earth Element grants us the capacity to be nurturing, poised, and sympathetic. Signals of an Earth Element imbalance can include muddled thinking, feelings of being scattered and overwhelmed by details, worry, lethargy, mood swings, water retention, difficult weight loss, easy bruising, tender muscles, and varicose veins (to mention a few).

The sound associated with the Earth Element is that of singing. You can often hear a singing quality in the voice of a person with a strong Earth Element. The color associated with Earth is the golden color of ripe grains or the rich orange color of pumpkin and butternut squash. Our sense of taste is attributed to the Earth Element as is the sweet fragrance and damp climate. But let's move on. If the Earth is too damp we can get stuck in the mud. We hope the harvest has been gathered before the rains set in.

SIMPLE HOME HELPERS
FOR EARTH ELEMENT IMBALANCES

Disharmony	*Foods and Herbs that Can Help*	*Avoid*
Arthritis (Damp type) Characterized by swelling, stiffness, dull, aching pain, sluggishness	Aduki beans, barley, coix, cornsilk tea, mung beans, mustard greens	Cold foods, sugar, highly refined foods made with white flour, fatty foods, cheese
Diarrhea	Banana, basil, black pepper, blueberries, burnt rice or toast, cinnamon, garlic, ginger, lotus seeds, peas, pearl barley, raspberry leaves, yams	Cold or raw foods, most fruits, juices, overeating
Edema	Aduki beans, apples, bamboo shoots, beef, black beans, celery, cornsilk, fish, garlic, ginger skin tea, green onions, mulberries, oats, peaches, pearl barley, poria cocos, seaweed, tangerines, water chestnuts, watermelon, zhu ling	Rich or fatty foods, salty foods, wine, lamb, shellfish
Hypoglycemia	Almonds, barley, chicken, fish, fresh whole fruits, oatmeal, rye, soybeans, tofu, vegetables, walnuts	Sweeteners, coffee, chocolate, white-flour products.

Disharmony	Foods and Herbs that Can Help	Avoid
		Eat 4 to 5 small meals daily; include protein and a small amount of fat with all meals or snacks.
Indigestion	Dandelion greens, hawthorn berries, papaya, pineapple, figs, bitter greens (dandelion, endive, arugula), daikon radish, fenugreek, mint, orange, apple, lemon (Dry and age organic orange peel for one month. Brew tea of peels and drink after each meal).	Rich foods, fatty foods, and stress while eating
Morning Sickness	Bamboo shavings, carp, cardamom, ginger, grapefruit peel, lentils, millet, orange peel, persimmon calyx (cap). Drink ginger and cardamom tea or ginger and grapefruit or orange peel tea (add a touch of honey or maple syrup). Discontinue remedies once morning sickness stops.	Fatty meats or cold cuts, overeating

If you find yourself suffering from any of the above discomforts, simply increase your daily intake of the foods and herbs recommended. You can create a delicious soup, stew, or herbal tea by combining some of the items.

Autumn: Nature's Time of Release

Autumn-touched leaves flutter to the ground
    as nature enters this phase of letting go.

Days shorten while sap, the life
    blood of our green friends, sinks
    to the roots once again.
Fall's first white frost shimmers
    opalescent in the morning light.
Spring and summer's outward
    surge of growth complete,
    it's now time to journey inward
    as nature's balance shifts.

—DARLENA

The autumn equinox, September 22, marks the birth of the dark, *yin* cycle of the year when daylight lasts less than 12 hours. During the fall season, nature's energy is moving downward and inward. As leaves drift to the ground and sap sinks back into the roots, we should finish up those projects started in the spring and summer seasons and prepare for winter's resting time.

In Traditional Oriental Medicine, autumn, nature's time of pulling in and letting go, is the season associated with the Metal Element, which governs the lung- and large-intestine acupuncture meridians (sometimes referred to as energy channels). The balance of *intake,* through eating nourishing food and breathing in oxygen, and *output,* through breathing out, elimination of waste, and exercise are essential for good health. Both the lung and large intestine organ systems have important functions related to letting go, or elimination. Imbalance sets the stage for colds and flu, lung infections, bowel irregularities, and constipation. Autumn is the season to let go of the old by clearing out the waste of what has already been used on all levels. This might be the time of year for you to clean your closet, toss out those old magazines, and/or undertake a light, cleansing fast (check with your health practitioner).

Feeling resigned or stuck? It is important to remember that only by letting go do we make room for the new to enter our lives.

The color associated with Metal is white, like the first frost glistening on blades of grass. Someone who is strongly attracted to this color or has a great dislike for it may be exhibiting a Metal imbalance. The climate for autumn is characterized by *dryness,* which nourishes Metal (just picture the dry, brown grass and leaves of fall). In Oriental medical thought, the dry climate helps eliminate mucous discharges characteristic of colds and flu. Too much dryness can be harmful, however, and results in constipation and dry skin. If you are experiencing dryness, please remember to balance with foods that moisten. Full, sweet foods of the Earth Element increase moisture in the human body; they include grains (particularly millet), beans, lean cuts of meat and fish, dairy products, and orange veggies such as yams, winter squash, and carrots.

The flavor associated with the Metal Element is described as spicy, acrid, or pungent. The spicy flavor is utilized in Traditional Oriental Medicine to disperse congestion and stagnation. It contains essential oils and resins that irritate the mucosa, increasing blood and lymph flow while counteracting mucous production. During autumn, it is important to increase your immunity by consuming more spicy foods such as onion and garlic.

Both of these foods are sources rich in sulfur, a natural antibiotic. Other spicy foods include leek, scallion, horseradish, radish, ginger, celery and mustard seed, parsnip, black and cayenne pepper, and aromatic spices such as cinnamon, nutmeg, clove, cardamom, thyme, sage, rosemary, fennel, and mint.

The nose opens into the lungs, and smell is the sense associated with the Metal Element. Mucus is the body fluid associated with autumn and the Metal Element in Chinese medicine. Don't fall into autumn. Prevent sore throats, as well as nasal and sinus infections, by gargling with one teaspoon of sea salt to a pint of water two to three times per week. You can also gently breathe some of this saltwater into the nostrils and then blow your nose. Also cooking your grains, beans, and soups with a slice of astragalus root can help build immunity. Western studies have shown this herb improves the action of the thymus and spleen and builds immunity by reducing the generation of T-suppressor cells and increasing the activity of killer T-cells.

The emotion attributed to autumn in Oriental thought is grief. An imbalanced Metal Element can manifest itself in the form of depression and unhappiness, fatigue, indecision, or confusion with a strong need for reliance on addictive substances for an energy boost, particularly coffee and cigarettes. Autumn is also a time when we are tempted to overindulge. Watch out for cold, congesting foods such as ice cream. Halloween and Thanksgiving are just around the corner with their array of extremely tempting, empty sweets. Remember that excess refined sugar and flour are converted into mucus by the body. Mucus creates a wonderful growing environment for unfriendly bacteria.

The Metal Element, in balance, is associated with communication and clear thinking, openness to new ideas, a positive self-image, and ability to relax, let go, and be happy. Autumn is the time to consolidate our energy, get more rest, and take quiet walks. It is the ideal time for study, introspection, and a hot, spicy cup of ginger tea to warm the nose and toes.

SIMPLE HOME HELPERS FOR METAL ELEMENT IMBALANCES

Disharmony	*Foods and Herbs that Can Help*	*Avoid*
Acne	Alfalfa sprouts, aloe vera, beet tops, cabbage, carrot tops, carrots, celery, cherries, cucumbers, dandelion greens, lettuce, mung beans, papaya, pear, persimmon, raspberries, squash, water (plenty of it!), watermelon	Fatty, oily, or spicy foods, coffee, alcohol, cigarettes, sugar, chocolate, red meat, shellfish

Disharmony	*Foods and Herbs that Can Help*	*Avoid*
Anal Itch	Apple-cider vinegar: Wash anal area thoroughly with clear water (no soap). Saturate a cotton ball with vinegar and bath the area 2 times daily until it clears, which is usually quite fast. If the area is irritated you may experience slight stinging.	Canned and fresh citrus juice, dried fruit, corn syrup
Asthma	Almonds, apricot kernels, basil, carrots, daikon radish, figs, loquats, molasses, mustard greens, pumpkin, sesame seeds, sunflower seeds, tangerines, walnuts	Cold food, fruit juices, shellfish, bananas, mung beans, ice cream, watermelon
Bronchitis (Chronic)	Apricot kernels, chrysanthemum, daikon radish, ginger, ginkgo nuts, lily bulb, lotus roots, papaya, pears, persimmons, pine nuts, pumpkins, red or black jujube dates, seaweed, walnuts, water chestnuts, white pepper, yams	Alcohol, caffeine, cold drinks, cigarettes, spicy foods, getting chilled, overwork
Cold (Common)	*Wind cold type: Chills, fever, no sweating, stiff neck and shoulders, clear mucus, body aches* Basil, cilantro, cinnamon, ginger, garlic, mustard greens, parsnip, scallions, soupy rice porridge	Heavy foods, meats, vinegar shellfish
	Wind heat type: High fever, some chills, sore throat, cough, headache, cough, sweating, yellow mucus apples, burdock root, cabbage, cilantro chrysanthemum flowers, dandelion, pears, drink plenty of water and mint/chrysanthemum/dandelion tea	Hot foods, foods mentioned above re: wind cold
Constipation	Alfalfa sprouts, almonds, apples, bananas, beets, bok choy, cabbage, cauliflower, figs, peaches, pears, pine nuts, sesame seeds, walnuts, yams, yogurt	Red meats, spicy and fried foods, stress
Sinusitis (Chronic)	Chrysanthemum, garlic, ginger, green onions, magnolia flower	Cigarettes, coffee, stress, smog

Winter: Nature's Time of Inward Gathering

Bare branches silhouetted against gray skies—
> tiny seeds slumber, dreaming of spring's awakening.

> *The peach tree stands bare and brittle*
> *now, leaves fallen from its limbs.*
> *Deep down, under earth's frozen crust,*
> *life's mystery pulses in its roots.*
> *Our sun's power wanes in this*
> *season of nature's outer death,*
> *while we gather strength from silent*
> *depths of the spirit's inner core.*

—DARLENA

———— ● ————

In Traditional Oriental Medicine, the Water Element is said to pertain to the Winter Season, as are dark-blue or black colors, the emotion of fear, the northerly direction, the salty flavor, cold climate, sense organ of hearing (or the ears), Kidney and Urinary Bladder Organ Systems, putrid smell, time of day—from 3 P.M. to 7 P.M., body fluid—urine, and body tissue—bones. The groaning sound is characteristic of a Water Element imbalance. Have you heard the low creaking sound of tree limbs rubbing together during a winter storm? You can hear that same groaning in the voice of a person experiencing a Water imbalance.

While the Kidney is linked to the Water Element in Oriental Medicine, it also has a Fire component. That Fire (known as Kidney Yang) is related to functions of the adrenal cortex and reproductive and hormonal processes. Emotions are generally reflected in the Water Element, but fear is the emotion most closely connected with Water. When we are experiencing low Kidney energy (adrenal fatigue), fear can become a year-round problem that intensifies in wintertime. With an imbalanced Water Element we can become reticent, blunt, suspicious, detached, sarcastic, absentminded, or pessimistic. Physical manifestations of an imbalanced Water Element include headaches above the eyes, hypertension, kidney stones, osteoporosis, bony tumors, ringing in the ears, constipation, stiffness in the spine and joints, weakness in the knees, frequent urination, and hardening of the arteries (to mention a few). Deep wisdom and quiet, reflective gentleness characterizes a Water Element in balance.

Cold actually nourishes our Kidney and Urinary Bladder Systems by causing energy to contract back into the organs, giving them a chance to clear, rebuild, and rejuvenate. Extreme cold or wetness insults or injures our Kidney Fire. The Kidney and Urinary Bladder System needs to be kept warm and dry and requires extra rest. The inward-moving energy of winter season can also become stagnant, however, manifesting as depression. Therefore, it is important to keep moving with light exercises, but at the same time, not to exhaust all reserves in the holiday whirl.

Traditional Oriental wisdom tells us that it is always important to protect sensitive parts of the body from wind and cold, but even more so in the winter season. For example, wear jackets and scarves to protect "wind points" on the back of the neck, shoulders, upper chest, and throat. The waist and low back areas must also be kept warm and protected—this is the site of that all-important Kidney Fire or Life Gate *(Ming Men)*. Believe it or not, simply wearing a woolen garment around the waist can help alleviate soreness and stiffness of the lower back.

Cold, congesting foods (raw salads, tropical fruits, iced drinks) are best avoided during the winter season. Eating these foods introduces coldness into the system. Your body has to work extra hard to bring these foods up to body temperature for the digestion process to take place, while combating outside chill as well (a double insult). The result can be an increase in winter "colds" and flu.

In winter, it is best to bake, broil, or boil foods. Soups are particularly supportive of the digestive organs during this season, adding needed warmth from the inside out. Warming, kidney-nourishing foods include shiitake mushrooms, aduki beans, roasted buckwheat, millet, brown rice, miso, root veggies, winter squashes and yams, and lean cuts of pork, fish, or poultry. Warming herbs include basil, marjoram, cumin, fennel, cardamom, ginger, garlic, and cinnamon. Parsley and nettles support the Water Element by eliminating dampness and contributing needed mineral salts to build and maintain a strong skeletal system (remember "Bones" are the body tissue linked to the Kidney System). The salty flavor, in small amounts, supports the Kidney and Urinary Bladder function. If you do not cook with sea veggies, now is the time to start. The human body is composed of over 70 percent water; the human brain over 90 percent. The chemical composition of the water in our bodies is almost exactly like ocean water, only slightly diluted. Many cultures with a sea coast have the tradition of eating seaweed, including the Chinese, Japanese, Russians, Northern Europeans, Egyptians, Scandinavians, British, Aztec, Maori, and Icelandic people (to mention a few). What better way to get mineral salts in the exact proportion our human cells inherently understand than in the sea veggies growing out there in the oceanic environment? You'll find some great recipes using sea vegetables in Chapter 5.

Winter is a good time to stop smoking or drinking coffee. Smoking greatly restricts circulation, promoting coldness in the extremities. Coffee "highs" tap into valuable energy stores of the adrenal glands, which exhausts Kidney Yang, causing you to run on empty. (From a mechanistic point of view, the adrenals are our human battery pack.) If you truly love the flavor of coffee, however, treat yourself to a cup or two a week, but make it a special experience where you go to a wonderful coffee shop and sit down to slowly sip and savor every last drop.

Winter is the season of rest—a time to rebuild, renew, and replenish our deeply burning Kidney Fire that will blossom forth in spring with creative energy for new adventures, projects, and friendships. Cuddle up by the fireplace with that good book you've been wanting to read and a cup of ginger tea or warm, spicy apple cider.

Actually, winter is a good time to begin your herbal studies. People often ask, "Why herbs?" Herbs are our direct link to draw nourishment from nature in a fundamental way. Research shows that lactating cows and pregnant giraffes search out scarce plants that are high in valuable stores of calcium and phosphorus. Unfortunately, we human beings seem to have lost that natural instinct. But I sometimes wonder if that instinct is completely gone. Have you ever taken off down a lush, overgrown country trail on a warm spring day and before long found yourself chewing on a sweet stem of grass, nibbling on a wild sorrel leaf, or harvesting fresh berries?

SIMPLE HOME HELPERS FOR WATER ELEMENT IMBALANCES

Disharmony	*Foods and Herbs that Can Help*	*Avoid*
Arthritis (Cold type) Characterized by coldness in the joints and sharp, stabbing pain. Heat brings relief.	Black beans, chicken, garlic, ginger, grapes, green onions, mustard greens, sesame seeds (especially black), parsnip, pepper, spicy foods. Rub ginger on the painful areas.	Cold, raw foods, cold weather
Bladder Infections (chronic)	Black beans, chrysanthemum, cilantro, cloves, lycii berries, water chestnuts, sesame seeds, spinach, yams, walnuts	Spices, salt, garlic
Kidney Stones	Beet tops, celery, cornsilk, green tea powder, parsley, pearl barley, seaweed, walnuts, water chestnuts, watercress, watermelon	Spicy, fried foods, spinach, tomatoes, citrus, hard water

Disharmony	Foods and Herbs that Can Help	Avoid
Prostate Enlargement	Anise, cherries, figs, mangos, pumpkin seeds, seaweed, sunflower seeds	Rich, fatty foods, alcohol, caffeine, cigarettes, stimulants
Tinnitus (Ear Ringing)	Aduki beans, black beans, black sesame seeds, black jujube dates, celery, chestnuts, chrysanthemum, grapes, lotus seeds, oyster shell, pearl barley, walnuts, yams	Loud noise, spicy foods, alcohol, coffee, stress

Simply increase your daily intake of the foods and herbs recommended. You can create a delicious soup, stew, or herbal tea by combining some of the items.

HERBS—OUR VITAL LINK TO NATURE

Healing herbs were once an important part of our ancestors' everyday diet—a direct link to nature that provided essential nutrients, vitamins, and minerals in the way the human body evolved to understand. They still resonate to our ancient genetic code, regulating the body according to the unique needs of the individual. Many herbs have the ability to perform many different functions, stimulating the body's self-healing capabilities while addressing specific imbalances. Garlic, for example, can raise or lower blood pressure.

The fundamental difference between treating disease with herbs versus treating it with Western drugs can be summed up simply by saying that herbs possess the unique ability to enhance health, while many pharmaceuticals kill disease. Prevention is strongly emphasized in the natural healing arts. Herbs are taken not only to ease the pain that accompanies disease, but to eliminate the underlying condition responsible for creating that annoying pain in the first place. Herbs have the unique ability to stimulate the body's self-healing capabilities. True healing can take place only when the causes of disease are addressed at the root of the emotional or physical imbalance.

Our hunting and gathering ancestors consumed a very different diet from the one the average person does in modern America today. They ate according to what was available in their particular locale, and this changed seasonally. Natural healing teaches us that nature offers us exactly the right nutrients, at the right time, to prepare the human body for coming seasonal

5-Element Correspondences in Traditional Chinese Medicine

	Wood	Fire*	Earth	Metal	Water
Season	Spring	Summer	Late summer	Fall	Winter
Color	Green	Red	Yellow	White	Dark Blue or Black
Yin Organ	Liver	Heart	Spleen	Lungs	Kidneys
Yin Organ Time	1 A.M. to 3 A.M.	11 A.M. to 1 P.M.	9 A.M. to 11 A.M.	3 A.M. to 5 A.M.	5 P.M. to 7 P.M.
Yang Organ	Gall Bladder	Small Intestine	Stomach	Large Intestine	Bladder
Yang Organ Time	11 P.M. to 1 A.M.	1 P.M. to 3 P.M.	7 A.M. to 9 A.M.	5 A.M. to 7 A.M.	3 P.M. to 5 P.M.
Emotion	Anger	Joy/Sorrow	Sympathy/Worry	Grief/Depression	Fear
Climate	Wind	Heat	Humidity	Dryness	Cold
Direction	East	South	Center	West	North
Sense Organ	Eyes/Sight	Tongue/Speech	Mouth/Taste	Nose/Smell	Ears/Hearing
Fluid	Tears	Sweat	Saliva/Lymph	Mucus	Urine
Tissue Fortified	Tendons	Blood/Vessels	Flesh/Muscles	Skin/Hair	Bones
Sound	Shouting	Laughing	Singing	Crying	Groaning
Smell	Rancid	Scorched	Fragrant	Rotten	Putrid
Taste	Sour	Bitter	Sweet	Pungent	Salty
Quality	Growth	Ripening	Transition	Harvest	Storage
Indicator	Nails	Complexion	Lips	Body Hair	Hair on Head
Controls	Earth	Metal	Water	Wood	Fire
Injured By	Wind	Heat	Damp	Dry	Cold
Activity	Seeing	Walking	Sitting	Reclining	Standing

5-Element Correspondences in Traditional Chinese Medicine, *continued*

	Wood	Fire*	Earth	Metal	Water
Planet	Jupiter	Mars	Saturn	Venus	Mercury
Cooking	Steam	Raw	Stew	Bake	Saute
Grain	Wheat	Corn	Millet	Rice	Bean
Animal	Chicken	Lamb	Cow	Horse	Pig
Fruit	Plum	Apricot	Date	Peach	Black Cherry
Mother/Son	Son of Water	Son of Wood	Son of Fire	Son of Earth	Son of Metal
Relationships	Mother of Fire	Mother of Earth	Mother of Metal	Mother of Water	Mother of Wood
Positive Aspect	Enthusiasm	Love	Thoughtfulness	Spirituality	Courage
Task	Creativity	Compassion	Caring	Find Meaning	Find Inner Strength
Resolve Emotional Imbalance	Forgiveness	Surrender (Ego)	Service	Companionship	Faith
Spiritual Quality	Soul	Spirit	Thought	Instinct	Will

*The Fire Element has two paired sets of organ systems—the Heart/Small Intestine and Pericardium/Triple Warmer.

Yin Organ	Pericardium	
Yin Organ Time	7 P.M. to 9 P.M.	
Yang Organ	Triple Warmer	
Yang Organ Time	9 P.M. TO 11 P.M.	

changes. In contrast, anthropological studies show that almost exactly 20 years after refined convenience foods are introduced to a traditional society, the first cases of chronic disease start to surface in the form of cancer, heart disease, diabetes, arthritis, and many other devastating illnesses. It takes thousands upon thousands of years for a life form to adapt to changes in its environment or diet. Simply speaking, our "advances" in industrializing foodstuffs and chemically compounding pharmaceutical drugs over the past 75 years have far surpassed our genetic ability to adapt to those changes. Basically, we are still walking around in bodies almost exactly like those of our ancestors who lived 30,000 years ago. We need the same natural herbs and foods.

It's interesting to construct a list of all the foods you eat on a regular basis—give it a try. You will be amazed at how truly short that list is. You will come up with a few ingredients that are combined and recombined in many different ways, many of them are highly refined, nutrient-poor food items with an incredibly long shelf life such as white sugar and white flour.

Convenience Foods: Nature's Enemies

Leave your drugs in the chemist's
pot if you can heal the patient with food.

—HIPPOCRATES

Back on the farm, when I ran out of glue while constructing a kite or a Mayday basket, I always relied on mixing some white flour together with a little water—this makes an effective glue substitute. Try it! The bad news is that this is exactly what happens inside the human body! Autopsies show that the average American is carrying around 12 pounds of fecal matter encrusted—glued—pasted on the walls of his or her intestines. This fecal matter not only increases autotoxicity, it obstructs our body's ability to absorb important life-giving nutrients. Highly refined convenience foods coat the intestinal lining, creating an acidic environment that kills off our friendly bacteria. Most health practitioners (Oriental or Western) will agree that much ill health or disease is a direct result of too much acidity. This is where fresh green and orange veggies, nonacidic fruits, and herbs come to the rescue—many of them have alkalinizing qualities. Often, I won't even give herbs to new patients but will recommend they make some dietary shifts the first week or two. (I've also been known to take patients, on their first visit, to a health-food store.) You would be amazed at how many minor aches, pains, and discomforts vanish once the patient simply incorporates more of nature's gentle green healers into his or her diet. The big plus is that the high fiber in fresh, whole foods gently starts scrubbing down the walls of those intestines.

As you change your diet for the better, acid-loving, unfriendly bacteria start to die off. This is one of the major reasons you might experience some increased gas for a while—the death of many unwanted micro-organisms creates flatulence or gas (evil wind in Oriental medicine). As your system becomes more alkaline, healthy bacteria that aid digestion and assimilation will begin to proliferate. Be sure to eat at least one to two tablespoons of yogurt daily (or take an acidophilus/bifidus supplement) to increase the number of those friendly bacteria in your intestinal tract.

Discovering Your Pathway to Great Health

In my workshops, I tell participants there are five "white," or highly processed foods detrimental to our health and well-being that came to us with modern advances. They include (1) White flour, (2) White sugar, (3) White salt (highly processed salt), (4) White oil (oil whose chemical composition has been changed due to the high heat of processing), and (5) White addictions (those substances that can be detrimental to our health and well-being such as coffee, alcohol, or tobacco, in excess, that are accepted and expected to be taken when offered in social gatherings).

All five substances are found in enormous quantities in those center aisles of your supermarket. They have a shelf life of "forever." I'll often ask patients why they would want to eat something that can sit on a shelf for months at a time and not be attacked by ravenous little creatures like molds, bacteria, or fungus? If these food items are not appetizing to other one-celled life forms why does anyone think our tiny little cells would find the nutrients appetizing or life giving? Think about it.

It is important to make changes slowly and take one step at a time—that way they will last. Don't get overwhelmed; simply start wherever you can. That might mean simply increasing your veggie or fruit consumption on a daily basis. Then you might scrutinize the number of white flour products that make their way into your diet. Perhaps you could start purchasing breads made with whole grains, or better still, cook a pot of brown rice or barley for dinner and rolled oats in the morning for breakfast (not instant, but the kind that takes about seven minutes to cook).

Next, you might want to move on to the issue of white sugar; try other natural sweeteners such as sucanat, maple or rice syrup, or unprocessed honey. Sugar cravings can indicate you need more of the full, sweet flavor. Remember that the most healthful full, sweet flavor comes from whole foods that were described in the section on "Doyo" under seasonal changes; they include fruits, veggies, lean meats and low-fat dairy products, whole grains, and beans.

Processed white salt can be replaced by natural, unprocessed sea or earth salt, miso, sea veggies, gomasio, or mixtures of herbal condiments.

Good oils are essential for good health. Each one of our tiny cells constructs its walls, double-layered membranes, from phospholipids—phosphates and fatty acids. The fatty acids cells use for their walls come from the oils we ingest. The topic of "white" oils is a little more difficult to deal with; they show up in virtually all products down the center aisles of the supermarket. Cottonseed oil is often used in the food-manufacturing industry because it's cheap and can be labeled "vegetable oil." It has the highest content of pesticide residues and contains a fatty acid called cyclopropene that has a toxic effect on the gallbladder and liver. One rule to keep in mind is that any fat that is solid or semisolid at room temperature is not good for you. However, let's summarize this section by recommending the oils that are good for you. Purchase unrefined "cold" or "expeller-pressed" oils such as olive or canola. The best sources of good oils include fresh nuts or seeds such as almonds, sunflower or pumpkin seeds, and avocados. Oils need to be stored in a cool, dark cupboard and refrigerated after opening. Please see the bibliography for informative books on fats—I feel that your health depends on it.

We're down to the last of the five substances that are best left on supermarket shelves. This category included "White Addictions" such as smoking or drinking too much alcohol. Addictions are best addressed when you are ready to deal them. Often, addictive substances are simply crutches to help us get by. It's probably wise not to remove the crutch until we thoroughly understand the problem and are prepared to change our lifestyle. Too often we make resolutions only to disappoint ourselves that we "failed." However, it's extremely important to recognize if an addiction is jeopardizing our health and happiness or the well-being of our loved ones. Please seek professional help if the problem is serious.

Remember, take your time and be kind to yourself in making changes. Most important, I tell my patients never to feel guilty. Be gentle with yourself and leave a place in your life for that special treat that brings you joy—it just might be a piece of a chocolate bar! Also, be sure to experiment with a few herbal teas—nerve-soothing chamomile; tummy-settling peppermint, or mineral-packed, adrenal-supporting nettles might be good starters.

Chapter 2

EASY WAYS TO STORE AND PREPARE ORIENTAL HERBS

ADVANTAGES OF ORIENTAL HERBS

A number of the healing herbs presented in Chapter 3 will be familiar to you. Some of them, like dandelion, might be considered "weeds" that grow nearby. The logical question is, "What's so Oriental about Oriental herbs, and why are we importing them if they're growing in our own backyard?"

Of first concern before pulling up that knotweed plant growing alongside the highway is the importance of identifying it as the *medicinal species* that is used to treat a specific condition. Many related species treat different ailments; some species could be of no medicinal value at all, while others may actually be harmful. Before gathering herbs on your own, you will need to expand your knowledge by learning plant identification. Recommended resources are listed on page 357.

Second, even if the plant is the correct species, you need to consider its growing environment and, therefore, its possible unique characteristics. If it's growing alongside the highway, has it absorbed contaminants from the asphalt and passing cars, not to mention possible pesticides and weed killers?

Which brings us to the third consideration and answer to our original question: What's so Oriental about Oriental herbs? Herbs have been cultivated, used medicinally based on a unique system of energetics, and have had their healing effects recorded in the Orient for thousands of years. We have much to learn from the Oriental herbal tradition. Remember, the unique flavor of a food or herb tells you everything about its healing properties. Astragalus, for example, is considered a sweet, slightly warm herb. Herb enthusiasts in the United States have been trying to grow astragalus for a number of years. Only recently are domestically grown astragalus roots beginning to take on the characteristic "sweet" flavor needed for the root to be truly effective.

As an herbalist, I feel that, ideally, our herbal aids should come from nearby. Here in the West, however, many of our healing plants have been plowed under over the past 75 years as we commercially prepared and chemically fertilized our soils to yield a hybrid crop of wheat, maize, or potatoes. We need to learn the proper growing environment for many healing herbs before they are going to be of therapeutic value. In contrast, ageless tradition in the Orient has preserved its rich herbal legacy and growing secrets. Specific soil compositions and natural soil enrichers and growing conditions are known to create herbs of a specific healing quality. Until we learn how to naturally and organically produce sufficient quantities of codonopsis and astragalus roots that are truly sweet, or peony root that is bitter and sour, we will have to depend upon our friends in the Orient. As mentioned, a growing number of conscientious domestic cultivators are now selling some species of quality organic "Oriental" herbs—they are listed in the Resources section (please see page 357).

In this chapter you are given simple ways to incorporate the healing properties of Oriental herbs in your everyday life—ways to store and prepare herbs in various forms. Many herbs can be purchased at your local health-food store or ordered through one of the growing number of suppliers in the United States (also listed in the Resources section of this book). Bulk herbs are prepared in diverse ways for internal consumption or external application. Each preparation has its unique advantages and disadvantages. Internally, herbs are taken in the form of teas, tablets, pastes, pills, capsules, extracts, or syrups. Externally, the healing power of herbs is captured through the use of herbal compresses, baths, gargles, liniments, oils and salves, or plasters.

STORING HERBS

If you wish to experience healing Oriental herbs as they have been prepared since antiquity, you might want to purchase them in the most natural state possible, that is, dried. Dried herbs come in various forms—whole, cut and sifted (to remove any hard parts such as twigs), sliced, or powdered. Herbs in this natural form need to be stored in dry, airtight containers, preferably glass or earthenware, and kept in the cupboard or dark closet, protected from light, excessive heat, and moisture, which causes them to break down and oxidize. You can discourage the advances of hungry little bugs by adding a few bay leaves or peppercorns to each jar.

Because herbs are natural substances, they do not have a shelf life of forever like many items in the modern supermarket. Dried leaves and flowers will lose considerable potency in about six months. Nonaromatic barks and roots generally last from one to two years. Bulk herbs are frequently available in powdered form; they usually last from one to six months. However, powders can be adulterated. Therefore, it's important for an herbalist to become familiar with the "true flavor" of an herb by purchasing it in its whole form at first. Once you've developed your "taste," any additives or fillers can be easily detected by sampling the powder. Powdered herbal extracts are now also available; their use will be discussed in the upcoming section. Needless to say, it's important to purchase your herbs from reputable sources.

SIMPLE HERBAL PREPARATIONS

Herbal Teas

With each culture, we find distinct preferences regarding ways to administer herbs. The East Indian Ayurvedic practitioners frequently give herbal pills, mixed with a sweetening agent such as honey; clarified butter (called ghee) is often added to the mix. Throughout Europe and Australia, where herbs are legally prescribed in medical clinics, you find herbal extracts the most common means of administering herbs. In the Orient, however, it is believed that the most healing properties are derived from herbs when they are simmered slowly for a long period of time and ingested in tea form. My own preference for administering herbs is usually through their addition to food, or in tea form. In the upcoming chapters you find many ways to cook with wonderful herbal tonifiers, so, for now, let's talk about ways to prepare teas, as well as their advantages and disadvantages.

If you visit the herbal wing in a Chinese hospital, you find hundreds of small pots of smelly roots and barks gently simmering away—a different concoction for each patient. Depending upon flavors that have been missing from your life (often *sour* and more frequently *bitter* for many Americans), you might be in for a surprise upon sampling your first herbal brew. Frequently, after a few cups, the fragrance and flavor actually become tolerable if not downright welcomed. (If not, don't despair—there are alternatives discussed in the upcoming sections.) Some herbal blends are actually quite delicious, so keep your fingers crossed—you may be in for a treat.

Preparing Herbal Teas (Decoctions)

Once you get the procedure down, cooking up a pot of herbal tea is one of the least expensive and simplest ways to introduce healing herbal allies into your life. You can make up two or three days' worth of tea at a time and store it in a glass container in the refrigerator. Warm up each cup as needed or carry it in a thermos to work.

In Chapter 3 you are given gram and ounce measurements for each herb; these represent recommended *daily dosages* for a 150-pound adult. If you want to make up a three days' supply, multiply by three, including the amount of water given in the cooking instructions that follow, which represent amounts for a one-day supply (usually, approximately three cups of liquid are remaining after the cooking process).

COOKING INSTRUCTIONS FOR HERBAL TEAS

It is extremely important to cook your herbs in a glass, stainless steel, or earthenware cooking container. No aluminum pans, please! You will need approximately 4 to 6 cups of spring water (no chlorinated tap water). The amount of water depends on cooking time required as indicated below.

If your formula contains oyster shell, dragon bone, or other minerals, these need to be simmered approximately 30 minutes before adding heavy roots and barks, so first bring your water to a boil, then turn the heat down to low, just high enough to maintain a simmer. Keep your pot covered throughout cooking and steeping time.

- Add mineral substances to 6 cups of boiling water: Simmer 30 minutes. (If there are no minerals in your formula, bring 4 to 5 cups of water to a boil and proceed with the following instructions. If there were minerals in your formula, simply proceed as directed.)
- Add heavy roots and bark: Continue simmering 20 to 30 minutes
- Add lighter twigs, fruits, leaves: Simmer an additional 10 to 15 minutes
- Remove from heat and add aromatic leaves and flowers (such as mint): Cover and let steep for 10 to 20 minutes
- Strain the herbs out of your formula. Pick out edible herbs like codonopsis, ginseng, and jujube dates and enjoy them as a treat when desired.

Some herbalists may recommend that you add 3 cups of water to the strained herbs and bring the formula to a simmer for an additional 20 minutes. This practice would work well with a very hard substance like reishi mushroom. However, in general, overcooking an herbal formula can create too much acidity. I recommend only one cooking for almost all herbal formulas.

While the preceding instructions may sound a bit complicated, after one or two times through it, you'll have the method down pat. Simply store the remaining strained liquid in the refrigerator and warm (don't boil) as required. An immense amount of satisfaction comes from participating in creating your own cure in this age-old tradition.

Let's talk about the advantages and disadvantages of purchasing whole, cut, and sifted or sliced bulk herbs. You are assured of obtaining the whole herb with all its healing characteristics intact as long as you are purchasing from a reputable company or individual. Once you have the herbs, you can formulate many different healing prescriptions, as needed, in the most natural way possible. You will not be ingesting unwanted binders, additives, capsules, sweet syrups, or alcohol. You will, however, need to take care in storing your herbs properly. And, if you want to use your herbs, you will have to take the time to prepare them.

Capsules, Pastes, and Pills

As herbs have gained in popularity over the past 25 years, we are seeing many commercially prepared tablets, pills, and capsules in the marketplace, even in pharmacies and supermarkets. In this section, you are given standard dosages, as well as instructions for making your own healing herbal pastes, pills, and capsules.

If you have bulk herbs and a heavy-duty grinder, you can powder them to prepare your own pills or capsules. Or you can purchase herbs in a powdered state. Powdered herbs are generally not used to brew teas because of their inability to dissolve, which creates a gritty texture.

ALL ABOUT CAPSULES   Powdered herbs, in capsulated form, are an alternative to herbal teas. Capsules come in three standard sizes: "0" are the smallest capsules; they are easy to swallow, making them the ideal size for children and adults who have difficulty swallowing medications; "00" is the standard size capsule—each one holds approximately 1/2 teaspoon (or 650 mg) of herbal powder; "000" is the largest-size capsule and works well for larger adults who do not have trouble swallowing. Following is a chart to help you calculate the quantity of each size capsule you would be required to take daily, based on your approximate body weight. *The standard dosage is considered to be two size "00" capsules, three times daily for the average 150-pound adult. In other words, two tightly packed size "00" capsules contain approximately 1 teaspoon of powdered herbs; and 1 teaspoon of powdered herbs equals 1 cup of herbal tea in potency.*

STANDARD CAPSULE
MEASUREMENTS AND DOSAGES

Body Weight	DOSAGE Number of Capsules	Times Daily	Capsule Size	Approximate Teaspoons per dosage	Mg
55 lbs	1	3	"0"	3/8	500
110 lbs	2	3	"0"	3/4	1000
165 lbs	3	3	"0"	1-1/8	1500
220 lbs.	4	3	"0"	1-1/2	2000

Note: For persons weighing over 220 pounds, add approximately 1 capsule per day for each additional 18 pounds of body weight.

OR

75 lbs.	1	3	"00"	1/2	650
150 lbs	2	3	"00"	1	1300
225 lbs.	3	3	"00"	1-1/2	1950

Note: For persons weighing over 225 pounds, add approximately 1 capsule per day for each additional 25 pounds of body weight.

OR

*90 lbs.	1	3	"000"	2/3	800
185 lbs.	2	3	"000"	1-1/3	1600

Note: For persons weighing over 185 pounds, add approximately 1 capsule per day for each additional 30 pounds of body weight.

*A 90-pound person would probably find it difficult to swallow such a large capsule.

You can usually obtain empty capsules at your health-food store. While most capsules are made of animal gelatin, those made of vegetable gelatin are available as well. Some people with digestive weakness find it difficult to digest capsules. For them, another possible alternative is the use of rice papers. Sprinkle 1/4 to 1/2 teaspoon of your powdered herbal formula in the center of the paper, then fold or roll the paper to create the smallest capsule-like form possible.

For persons wishing to pack their own capsules, fill a small, but deep bowl approximately 1/4 to 1/2 full of your powdered herbal formula. Separate the capsule, then use both sides of it to scoop up powder. Tap them against the side of the bowl and then scoop up more powder. Repeat this procedure until both halves of the capsule are well packed; once filled, carefully close capsule ends together and place the filled capsule in another container.

PREPARING YOUR OWN POWDERED HERBAL FORMULA

Let's say you now have powdered herbs and capsules at hand and are ready to prepare your own formula. You're concerned about how to measure out quantities of herbs. It's really simple! In Chapter 4, you are given some classical Oriental healing formulas, so let's take one of them as an example:

PUERARIA (KUDZU) COMBINATION   Treats the common cold accompanied by severe chills, congestion, diarrhea, neck and upper-back stiffness, and extreme muscle aches or spasms.

Kudzu root	8.0 grams *or* approximately 1/5 ounce	
Ephedra	4.0	1/7 ounce
Jujube dates	4.0	1/7 ounce
Cinnamon twigs	3.0	1/10 ounce
Peony root (white)	3.0	1/10 ounce
Licorice	2.0	2 to 4 slices
Ginger (dried)	1.0	3 to 5 small slices

Since this is a formula for acute cold and flu symptoms, you will probably want to make enough for only three or four days. When working with powdered herbs you do not have to worry *at all* about measuring grams or ounces. Using the number given in the grams column, take 8 teaspoons of kudzu root, 4 teaspoons each of ephedra and jujube dates, 3 teaspoons each of cinnamon twigs and white peony root, 2 teaspoons of licorice, and 1 teaspoon of ginger. Mix the herbs very thoroughly. This method of measuring creates perfect proportions of the herbs called for in the herbal prescription. If you want to make a larger quantity for chronic conditions, use a larger measuring unit like a tablespoon or a 1/4-cup-size measuring device.

Now, if you add up the numbers of teaspoons of herbs you used in making up your formula, you would come up with a total of 25 teaspoons. Remember that two tightly packed, size "00" capsules contain approximately 1 teaspoon of powdered herbs, and 1 teaspoon of powdered herbs equals 1 cup of herbal tea in potency. You have just created the equivalent of 25 cups of herbal tea. If you are a 150-pound adult, you will want to take about six capsules a day—so your formula will last four days. If you want to make this formula for a 75-pound child, use a 1/2-teaspoon measuring unit instead of a full-teaspoon size, since the child would require only one half the dosage. A 37-pound child would require one quarter the amount (37 pounds is approximately one quarter of 150 pounds), so use a 1/4-teaspoon measuring unit. Just remember, in making up powdered herbal formulas, it is the *proportion of herbs* to each other that is important. If you are preparing an herbal formula with only three or four herbs, you might want to double or triple the quantities in order to create a larger amount of powdered formula.

While herbs tend to deteriorate once they've been powdered, encapsulated herbs will keep for about a year if stored in a tightly sealed glass jar in a dark, dry, cool place. If you find that capsules are your preferred means of ingesting herbs, you may want to purchase one of several types of capping machines that can usually be ordered through a natural-foods store.

PREPARING HERBAL PASTES AND PILLS

What if you're feeling pretty puny and just cannot deal with making up capsules? It's even more simple to prepare pastes and pills. Decide on the herbal formula that best describes your disease; measure out the powdered herbs as described earlier, and add just a touch of glycerin, barley, or rice syrup to create a thick paste (only enough to hold the powdered herbs together). *You can also use honey, but never give it to children who are under two years of age—it can be quite harmful to them.* It's that simple! You have just created a healing paste that can last for up to three years in a tightly covered glass container that is kept in a cool, dry, dark place. Children weighing about 35 pounds will take 1/4 teaspoon, 3 times daily; a 75-pound child will take 1/2 teaspoon, 3 times daily; and a 150-pound adult will take 1 full teaspoon, 3 times daily.

For the sake of argument, let's say you really want to make pills. Measure out 1 level teaspoon of your healing herbal concoction, cut it up into 4, 6, or 8 equal chunks, then roll the herbal dough into little balls. Place the pills on a cookie sheet in a clean, dry location; it will take them 10 to 12 hours to dry. If you want, you could place them in a very low oven (170° to 220°) for an hour or so, until they dry out. Keep a watchful eye over your healing creation, however, so the pills don't burn.

Be sure to remember how many pills make up a teaspoon of pill dough—1 teaspoon still equals 1 cup of herbal tea. If you made six herbal balls per teaspoon and you weigh approximately 150 pounds, you will want to take approximately 18 pills per day (or 6 pills, 3 times daily); a 75-pound child will take 9 pills daily (or 3 pills, 3 times daily); a 40-pound child should be given 5 pills (2 pills, 2 times daily, and 1 pill, 1 time).

You have even a *second option* for preparing pills that are sweetener-free. Powdered licorice root or slippery-elm powder are both sweet and make excellent binders. Approximately 10 percent of your herbal concoction needs to be a binder to help hold the pill together. So for each 10 teaspoons (or 10 measuring units) of herbal powder you are preparing, add 1 teaspoon (or 1 measuring unit) of licorice or slippery-elm powder. If your formula already has licorice in it, you might need to add only a little more to get up to the 10 percent ratio of licorice to herbs. Now slowly add spring water and mix thoroughly to form a very stiff dough. Follow the instructions given earlier to formulate herbal pills. *(Note: If you suffer from edema or high blood pressure, do not use licorice as a binder—slippery elm is a better choice for you.)*

Store herbal pills in a tightly covered glass container, in a cool, dark, dry place for up to a year.

Let's talk about the advantages and disadvantages of ingesting powdered herbs in the form of capsules, pastes, and pills. Powdered herbal remedies are made of the entire herb—all of its medicinal parts are present. Ideally, you would powder your own herbs shortly before use; if not, powdered herbs should be purchased from a reputable source to ensure they have not been adulterated with fillers or other low-quality herbal substitutes. The unpleasant flavor of some herbs doesn't matter if encapsulated—you won't taste them. Herbal pastes and pills are normally sweeter than herbal teas and can be quite palatable. Capsules may be difficult for some people to digest, whereas herbal pastes and pills are tasted and partially digested in the mouth, thus preparing the body for its herbal cure. Many herbalists feel that our human garden is better able to assimilate herbs that have been tasted and not simply dumped in an encapsulated form in an unsuspecting stomach. Also, powdered herbs have not been cooked, so our digestive system has to break through cellulose walls in order to extract the healing nutrients. Herbal capsules, pastes, and pills are all convenient; they travel well; they're easy to take, and unlike tinctures, no alcohol need be ingested.

Note: As a die-hard herbalist in the Oriental tradition, I generally prefer to prepare and ingest herbal teas. If time is of the essence, however, I will often forgo the formalities of making capsules, pastes, or pills by placing a teaspoon of powdered herbs on my tongue and chasing it down with a swig of spring water. If you're brave enough to attempt this method, be sure not to breathe in through the mouth when you have powdered herbs on your tongue. There's a minor chance that you could inhale some of the powder into your lungs. The coughing and sputtering that follows is not a pleasant experience.

TABLETS

Herbal tablets are popular these days. There are two distinct manufacturing processes used to create tablets. The first, or standard process, involves the use of powdered herbs, a binding substance (or something that holds them together), and a moisturizing agent (a substance that contains water). Tablets also normally contain actisol (a wood-pulp fiber) that soaks up water and enables the tablet to crumble once it hits the stomach. Vegetable oil is usually sprayed on the surface of the tablet to facilitate swallowing (by smoothing the surface). Various binding agents are used—slippery elm, acacia bark, guar gum from the guar plant, or dicalcium phosphate (a substance that comes from mineral calcium). Another neutral substance, magnesium sterate, is usually added to the herbal dough in order to keep the mix moving smoothly through the tabulating machines, otherwise they tend to clog up. Approximately 5 to 15 percent of each tablet created by this process consists of additives.

The second process, representative of the way many Chinese pills are created, results in only 1 to 3 percent additives. *Wet-granulation* is the name of this method in which herbs are first soaked in water and then spun dry. Small granules are the end result of this procedure; they are then pressed together to form a tablet. While this method is not commonly used, employees at natural-food stores can determine which process is employed by manufacturing companies; it's as simple as a phone call.

Under normal circumstances, one typical tablet is roughly equal to half a cup of tea or one "00" capsule. The normal dosage for a 150-pound adult is two tablets, three times daily (just like "00" capsules). To determine typical tablet dosages based on body weight, see the following chart:

STANDARD TABLET MEASUREMENTS AND DOSAGES

Body Weight	*DOSAGE* Number of Tablets	Times Daily	Approximate Teaspoons per Dosage	Mg
50 lbs.	1	2	1/2	650
75 lbs.	1	3	1/2	650
150 lbs.	2	3	1	1300
225 lbs.	3	3	1-1/2	1950

Note: For persons weighing over 225 pounds, add approximately 1 tablet per day for each additional 25 pounds of body weight.

Tablets are more expensive than bulk herbs. They are generally slower acting and less potent than tinctures, but they do not contain alcohol. Although tablets do contain binders, they usually do not have undesired additives such as corn, soy, wheat, sugar, starch, yeast, salt, dairy products, preservatives, artificial colors, or fragrances. However, it's always important to read each company's label to see what ingredients are actually in the product you are purchasing. Some persons with weak digestive systems find it difficult to break down tablets. Another difficulty with purchasing herbs in tablet form is that it's not easy for the average consumer to determine the quality of the product he or she is purchasing. Some of the herbs used in the manufacturing process could be old, or of poor quality. As a conscientious consumer you can examine the contents of a capsule by opening it, or you can mash a tablet with the back of a spoon or a rolling pin. Taste and smell the herbs inside—they should have the same taste, fragrance, and color of the original plant.

HERBAL EXTRACTS

Herbal extracts are a practical means of ingesting herbs for some people. Consumers can find the topic of herbal extracts confusing since there are a number of extract variations: (1) Tincture; (2) Concentrated Liquid Extracts; (3) Double Extractions; (4) USP Standardized and (5) Standardized or Guaranteed Extract; and (6) Powdered Extracts. Let's look at the manufacturing process behind each type so you'll know what you're preparing or purchasing.

Simple Directions for Formulating Tinctures

Tinctures, sometimes also called herbal extracts, are made by soaking fresh or dried herbs in a solvent (called *menstruum* in herbal lingo), most frequently alcohol and water; however, sometimes vinegar or glycerin are used. A good-quality vodka is the best alcohol to use because of its lack of taste and color. Tinctures are an incredibly practical means of preserving the healing qualities of herbs for years to come (three years or more). If you have some herbs that you fear won't be used promptly, you can capture their healing essence by making a tincture. It's possible to tincture individual herbs or whole herbal formulas. The advantage of tincturing individual herbs is that later you can mix them, in the desired proportions, to create your own herbal formulas.

Let's talk dosages. The average dose is 30 drops (which is 1/4 teaspoon or 1/2 dropperful—based on a 1-ounce dropper that is most commonly used for commercially prepared tinctures). *In other words, 1/4 teaspoon of herbal tincture roughly equals 1 cup of herbal tea, or 1 teaspoon of powdered herbs, or two "00" capsules, or 2 standard-sized herbal tablets.* A 150-pound adult would normally take 30 drops of tincture, three times daily.

Tinctures are extremely concentrated, so it's frequently better to add them to a liquid (water or juice) for ingestion. Some people are mildly allergic to alcohol; also, it can be a minor irritant to delicate mucous membranes. In truth, however, the actual amount of alcohol you are consuming is minimal; 2 droppersful of liquid extract taken three times daily for seven days equals the amount of alcohol in one beer. Since the average 150-pound adult would take only 1 dropperful three times daily as his or her dosage, it would take 14 days of tincture taking to reach the amount of alcohol in one beer. However, if desired, almost all the alcohol can easily be removed by simply adding 1/2 dropperful of tincture (or your required dosage) to 1/2 cup of boiling water; immediately turn the heat down to a very low simmer for 5 to 10 minutes. The alcohol will evaporate. (Note: You can prepare two or three cups of tea ahead of time and refrigerate. However, once the alcohol has been evaporated, the herbal tea should be used within a couple of days.)

Tinctures made from alcohol may not be for persons having religious or other objections to their consumption, or for persons with health considerations such as allergic reactions, liver disease, or alcoholism. However, most persons need not be concerned. More and more scientific studies are demonstrating that minor amounts of alcoholic beverages (such as wine or beer) can enhance health and aid digestion. Studies also confirm, however, that more than one drink a day actually increases the risk of cardiovascular disease, liver disease, and other degenerative disorders. Moderation is the secret to success in this regard.

Are you ready to make a tincture of some of those herbs you have stored away in that dark closet? It's an extremely simple process.

Concentrated Liquid Extracts

Almost all the moisture and alcohol have been removed from this type of tincture, resulting in a thick, semisolid liquid. The extract can later be made into pills or reconstituted into a liquid form with the addition of alcohol or glycerin. Concentrated extracts of this type are usually found only in clinics.

PREPARING AN HERBAL TINCTURE

- Place 4 ounces of dry, powdered herbs in a glass jar. (To make fresh herbal tinctures, use 8 ounces of fresh herbs.)
- Pour 1 pint (or 2 cups) of good-quality vodka over the herbs.

  (Note: The herbs should be covered by approximately 1 inch of alcohol; if not, add enough vodka for all herbs to be submerged.)
- Cover the jar tightly and shake well; store in a cool, dark place.
- Every day, for the next two weeks, remember to shake the jar well to mix the herbs and alcohol.
- After two weeks, your can strain the mixture by tightly tying a piece of cheesecloth over the mouth of the jar, or by laying a piece of cheesecloth in your kitchen colander. Pour the liquid into a bowl. Wring out the herbs in the cheesecloth to get the last drops of tincture.
- Store your tincture in a tightly covered glass container or pour into eyedropper bottles. Keep in a cool, dark location.

Double Extractions

This procedure requires twice the time, work, and herbs of the ordinary tincture described earlier. First, a regular tincture is made. Then, a fresh batch of dried or fresh herbs is added to the strained liquid. The procedure is then repeated. Very few herb companies use this method.

USP Standardized

Prior to World War I and the advent of synthetic drugs, pharmacies actually sold tinctures according to proportions established in the pharmacist's guidebook known as the *U.S. pharmacopoeia* (USP). Some companies still use the standards outlined in this book, but few herb companies can afford the expense of a pharmaceutical license. Although herbal medicine is regularly prescribed by doctors in Europe, herbs in the United States usually cannot be legally advertised or sold as medicines. Standardization is also difficult because herb qualities and manufacturing methods differ.

Standardized or Guaranteed Extract

Although many laboratory scientists prefer standardized or guaranteed extracts, some herbalists refuse to use this type of herbal compound. Herbal extracts, usually in tincture or pill form, are guaranteed to contain a certain amount of the herb's main active ingredient. If the extract falls short of this quantity, then a purified amount of the "active" constituent is added back in to increase potency to the guaranteed level. (For example, one sees milk thistle products standardized to 80 percent silymarin, or ginseng products guaranteed to contain 10 percent ginsenosides.) However, plants have many ingredients that all work together, or synergistically, to create a healing effect. Some plants contain well over 500 different compounds. It is extremely difficult to isolate each one of those compounds and conduct extensive testing on each in order to establish which one is truly the "active ingredient." By isolating only one of those ingredients and labeling it as "the active ingredient," we are disregarding nature's inherent wisdom and discarding the rest of the herb's wonderful healing compounds. To quote experts on the subject, "Nature is still mankind's greatest chemist, and many compounds that remain undiscovered in plants are beyond the imagination of even our best scientists." (Botanist Walter Lewis, Ph.D., and microbiologist Memory Elvin-Lewis, Ph.D., in their book *Medical Botany*.)

Powdered Extracts

Powdered herbal extracts are made by first preparing a decoction (tea prepared with water) or tincture (alcoholic), then removing the liquid by a drying process. Ideally, very little heat is used. One popular method involves spraying the herbal liquid through a fine nozzle in a vacuum chamber onto a "carrier" such as vegetable gum, pure cellulose, lactose, or calcium carbonate. Warm air is blown through the liquid. This rapid drying process preserves delicate plant constituents. The standard daily dosage of highly concentrated herbal powders is 1/4 teaspoon per 20 pounds of body weight. Powdered extracts are excellent for persons who suffer from weak digestion and poor assimilation.

GLYCERITES AND SYRUPS

A glycerite is an herbal extract using glycerin instead of alcohol, and herbal syrups are made with natural sweeteners, such as honey or sugar. A glycerite is a sweet, syrupy liquid, but it does not alter blood sugar like other sweeteners (molasses, rice or barley syrup, honey, or sugar). There are three types of glycerin on the market: The first type is derived from animal fat and is a by-product of the soap-making process (although soap is not edible, the glycerin is); the second type of glycerin is vegetable in origin; the third type (which is becoming popular) is a synthetic form of glycerin that comes from petroleum. You can purchase vegetable glycerin through natural-food stores, and glycerin made from animal fat is generally sold in pharmacies.

Like other extracts, glycerites are also quite concentrated; *the average dosage is the same as an alcohol tincture, or about 30 drops equal 1/4 teaspoon, which roughly equals 1/4 teaspoon of herbal tincture, or 1 cup of herbal tea, or 1 teaspoon of powdered herbs, or two "00" capsules, or 2 standard-sized herbal tablets.*

Like alcohol, a glycerite has the potential of irritating the mucous membranes and should be diluted in water or juice before ingestion. The sweet flavor of a glycerite makes it quite acceptable to most children, and no alcohol is ingested. However, while glycerin's molecular structure is similar to that of alcohol, it is not as good a solvent. It doesn't carry active ingredients into the blood as effectively, and important constituents can be lost.

Healing homemade syrups and glycerite formulas are easy to make and kids love them.

MAKING AN HERBAL SYRUP OR GLYCERITE

- Slowly simmer 2 ounces of herbs in 1 quart of spring water until only one half of the liquid remains (or about a pint).

- Strain liquid through a tea strainer or cheesecloth.

- While still warm, add 2 ounces of sweetener (rice or barley syrup, molasses, glycerin, or honey) and stir until dissolved. *Note: Never give honey to children under two years of age—it can harm them.*

- Store syrup in a tightly covered glass container in the refrigerator— it will last about a month.

You can create a soothing cough syrup using this recipe!

QUICK AND EASY HERBAL PREPARATIONS FOR EXTERNAL USE

Externally, the healing power of herbs is captured through the use of herbal compresses, baths, gargles, liniments, oils and salves, or plasters. Like all the previous recipes, the following herbal tips represent simple ways to bring the healing power of herbs into your everyday life.

Herbal Compresses

Herbal compresses (sometimes called a fomentation) are effective in treating a variety of discomforts—from muscle cramps to headaches, sore throats to bruises. They are also used almost any time you need to increase circulation by alternating hot and cold therapies. Simply make up a strong herbal tea with fresh, bulk, or powdered herbs, a tincture, or glycerite formula. Dip a soft cloth in the warm formula and wring it out. Fold the cloth and lay it on the skin. Cover the cloth with a towel and then place a hot-water bottle over the towel and leave it in place for approximately 20 minutes. Afterwards, if you want to increase circulation to the area, apply a cold compress for 5 to 10 minutes and follow up with another hot compress. Repeat as needed.

Baths

Create your own healing herbal bath blend. The combinations are limitless. Herbs can be used individually or in combination to stimulate circulation, lower fevers, calm the nerves, help heal infections or treat various skin problems, and eliminate everyday aches, pains, or muscle cramps. Simply make a good, strong herbal tea as directed at the beginning of the chapter and add it to hot bath water. Nothing relaxes the spirit like a wonderful warm bath. Since stress is a major contributing factor in most of our diseases, a soothing bath might prove to be one of your most potent herbal treatments.

Do you suffer from cold feet? Simmer 4 or 5 large slices of fresh ginger root in a quart of water for 20 to 30 minutes. Add enough cool water to create a warm, soothing foot bath and soak away. Ginger is a stimulating herb that will help increase circulation.

Gargles

Herbal teas can be used as gargles to stimulate circulation and heal red, inflamed throat tissue. Remember, many herbs have strong antibiotic characteristics (such as scutellaria, honeysuckle, and forsythia); they also possess analgesic, anti-inflammatory, demulcent, and antiseptic qualities. You can gargle once an hour for acute cases, or as needed. Store the liquid in your refrigerator for up to three days. See Chapter 4, the section on "Sore Throats, etc." for herbal recommendations.

Healing Herbal Liniments, Oils, and Salves

Liniments are actually tinctures or herbal extracts that are gently rubbed onto the skin to increase circulation and ease the discomfort of arthritis, rheumatism, or strained muscles and ligaments. Liniments will frequently contain stimulating herbs such as cayenne, ginger, cinnamon, or mint and antispasmodic herbs to relax muscles and tendons such as eucommia, gastrodia, ligusticum, salvia, angelica, mugwort, or achyranthes.

You can follow the instructions on page 41 for making a tincture. Liniments can be made with vodka or gin; however, rubbing alcohol, sesame or olive oil, or vinegar can be cheaper and effective substitutes for the vodka. Vinegar can be diluted by adding 50 percent water.

Since powdered herbs will make oils gritty, it's preferable to use sliced or cut and sifted herbs. When making healing oils, always add a touch of Vitamin E oil as a preservative. To create a thick salve that will adhere to the skin, melt beeswax and gently mix it into your herbal oil.

Note: If rubbing alcohol is used as the solvent, mark your container clearly; it is poisonous if accidentally taken internally.

Store your healing oils, salves, and liniments in tightly capped jars in a cool, dark place for up to a year.

Chapter 3

HARNESSING THE HEALING POWER
OF HERBS

You're ready to start experimenting with some gentle herbal healers to enhance your health and well-being.

This chapter gives you a few helpful pointers: first, how to calculate dosages for children; second, you are given a few herbal rules of thumb regarding length of time to take various herbal formulas; third, you learn the basics regarding how to create an herbal formula. Be sure to utilize the all-important upcoming chapters. Chapter 4 lists symptoms from A to Z, along with possible herbal remedies to help resolve the disharmony; Chapter 5 is full of recipes to help you incorporate healing herbs and foods into your everyday diet. Chapters 6 and 7 take you even deeper into the world of the Oriental herbal healer and give you simple, yet powerful tips that form the very foundation of Oriental medicine.

In the upcoming section on herbs, you see that many of the maximum daily dosages range from about 3 grams up to 15 grams. If we translate these amounts into ounces, 3 grams equals about 1/10 of an ounce and 15 grams equals roughly 1/2 an ounce. Needless to say, it would be difficult to accurately weigh 1/10 of an ounce on a pound scale. If you have a sensitive postage scale, however, you could weigh out 1 ounce and then divide that amount (by eye) into two piles weighing 1/2 ounce each. You could further divide the 1/2-ounce pile again to arrive at 1/4 ounce, and so forth. These are really small quantities, weightwise, but you'll be surprised at their bulky volume since leaves and flowers can be quite light. Though not essential, you might find it helpful to purchase a small, inexpensive gram scale.

CALCULATING DOSAGES FOR CHILDREN

Children respond wonderfully to herbal therapy. A standard formula for calculating correct dosages for little ones is called "Clark's Rule." It is assumed that the average adult weighs 150 pounds. If a child weighs 75 pounds, then the proper dosage would be one half of the adult amount since 75 is one half of 150. If the adult dosage is 1 cup of herbal tea, then the child would be given 1/2 cup of tea. If a child weighs only 30 pounds, this represents one fifth of 150 pounds, and the child would receive only 1/5 cup (3 tablespoons equals 1/4 cup, so 1/5 cup would be about 2-1/2 tablespoons) of tea. It is important not to overdose. You can make herbal formulas more tasty for children by adding a few drops of maple, rice, or barley malt syrup.

A FEW HERBAL RULES OF THUMB

Herbal formulas for acute conditions such as colds, sore throats, and flu are taken for only a few days (two to three) and modified as symptoms change. If you do not experience improvement in your condition, please consult a licensed health-care professional.

Formulas for chronic conditions will be ingested for longer periods of time. Under ideal conditions, expect to take the formula one month for each year you have experienced the problem. It might take up to a month for you to start feeling the benefits of your herbal therapy. Remember, generally, herbs are gentle foodlike medicines that help give your body a nudge in the right direction. They are addressing the underlying deficiencies or imbalances. It may have taken you many years to arrive at your present state of disharmony, so it's important to be patient and let your body gradually build up its natural defenses. When taking formulas for chronic conditions, herbalists will normally recommend that you consume the herbs only five or six days a week and rest from them for one or two days. You can ingest a formula that treats chronic conditions for three months, then rest from it for two weeks. The formula can be repeated or modified slightly with the change of seasons or a change in your condition. *If you come down with a cold or flu, discontinue all tonifying herbs until you have recovered.* (Tonifying herbs are those that supplement a deficient condition. For example, herbs that Tonify the Blood are those that help build blood, treating such symptoms as anemia, restless fatigue, and general weakness. If you constantly suffer from colds or flu, feel weak and weary, and have a pale, dull complexion, Qi Tonifying herbs could be called for to build your *qi*, or vital energy.)

CREATING YOUR OWN HERBAL FORMULA

A beginning herbalist would probably be wise to start creating herbal formulas by using only four to six herbs. For ease, suggestions regarding common herbal combinations are contained under each of the healing herbs described in Chapter 3. You will choose herbs from four categories of herbal functions:

1. *Major Herbs* are the main herbs you choose to dominate the prescription. These are the herbs that, energetically, best address your main symptoms. At first, pick only one or two herbs that really seem to "hit the nail on the head."

2. *Supporting Herbs* develop the primary effects of the Major Herbs you have chosen. Suggestions for supporting herbs follow the description of each of the herbs listed in the upcoming section.

3. *Assisting Herbs* enhance the effects of the Major Herbs while addressing associated symptoms. For example, if you are suffering from a serious cold, you may want to include kudzu root to relieve neck and shoulder stiffness.

4. *Conducting Herbs* are those that aid assimilation and utilization of the other herbs in your formula. Three commonly used conducting herbs include *ginger, licorice, or jujube dates.* You will almost always put a small amount of at least one of these herbal harmonizers in any formula you create. Read the descriptions of each and decide which one best addresses your individual needs.

Let's look at a classic Chinese herbal formula that comes to us from the Han dynasty. *Ma Huang Tang,* or Ephedra Combination, as it is known in English, is used to treat common colds and associated aching joints, fever, headache, cough, and a feeling of chest distention in persons with strong bodies. It is also used for pneumonia, bronchitis, stuffy nose, rheumatoid arthritis, bronchial asthma, measles, and typhoid fever. See page 50 for the formula, with an explanation of the actions of each of its four herbal ingredients.

Often, herbs that relax the body, known as antispasmodic herbs, such as peony root (white), are added to formulas. By relaxing the muscles, herbs are more easily absorbed and utilized by the body.

In the Orient, sweet herbs such as jujube date or licorice root are often added to formulas to sweeten and protect the digestive organs from excess bitterness. The bitter flavor, when used in excess over a long period of time, can overstimulate the secretion of hydrochloric acid in the stomach, creating

MA HUANG TANG	
Ephedra (6 to 9 grams)	Ephedra is the chief or Major Herb that, in conjunction with Cinnamon Twigs, promotes sweating and improves blood circulation.
Cinnamon Twigs (6 to 9 grams)	Cinnamon is the Supporting Herb that develops the effects of Ephedra by warming and inducing perspiration.
Apricot Seed (6 to 9 grams)	Apricot Seed is the Assisting Herb whose moistening and descending properties soothe the effects of Ephedra and Cinnamon. In combination with Ephedra, it relieves asthmatic coughing.
Licorice Root (3 to 6 grams) or 2 to 4 slices	Licorice Root is the Conducting Herb that coordinates the actions of the other three herbs. It helps prevent unfavorable reactions by protecting the stomach and harmonizing the formula.

chronic digestive weakness. For this reason, you will find most formulas contain a mildly sweet herb to harmonize the actions of the bitter herbs.

BECOMING ACQUAINTED WITH YOUR HERBS

To start, you might want to purchase six to twelve herbs that seem right for you and your family. Break off a small piece of each herb and place it on your tongue. Leave it there for five to ten minutes to truly experience its flavor and unique energies. This takes you back to the ancient roots of herbalism. The flavor of a substance tells you about its unique healing characteristics. Try to distinguish if the primary flavor is sour, bitter, sweet, spicy, or salty. After the herb has been on your tongue awhile, does the flavor change? What is that secondary flavor? (See Chapter 5 for more detail regarding the unique healing characteristics of each of the Five Flavors!)

There's a saying in herbal circles that a good herbalist intimately knows and normally uses only about 75 to 125 herbs. There are truly hundreds, if not thousands, of wonderful healing plants in the world. The best advice, however, is for you to get to know only a few of them in depth and expand your knowledge slowly. Otherwise, it can be completely overwhelming.

UNDERSTANDING THE BASICS
OF ORIENTAL MEDICINE

In Oriental medicine, the fundamental root of all disease is viewed as an imbalance of yin and yang. While you will take a deeper look at this important key to decoding Oriental medicine in Chapters 6 and 7, for now it's important to remember that yang is associated with heat, energy, and conditions tending toward excess dryness, redness, and inflammation such as skin infections, ulcers, acne, and thick yellow discharges. Yin is associated with cold, fatigue, paleness, and disharmonies that involve deficiency, excess moisture, and thin clear or white mucus discharges.

As you start reading descriptions of the herbs in Chapter 3, remember that Traditional Oriental Medical thought views the human body as a "living, dynamic ecological system." Disease is described in terms of climates and weather conditions. A fever might be viewed as a "Heat" imbalance, while chills indicate a "Cold" imbalance. Puffiness or edema is considered a condition related to excess "Damp" while cracking of the skin and lips are a sign of "Dryness."

CREATING SUNNY SKIES IN YOUR HUMAN GARDEN

Oriental Medical Diagnosis	Symptoms	Herbs that Might Help
Wind Relates to Wood Element	Are you sensitive to drafts and changes in the weather? Other symptoms include itching and sneezing; pains that travel or migrate; as well as intermittent pains.	Ginger (fresh) Kudzu Peony Root (white) Schizonepeta
Heat Relates to Fire Element	Do you easily overheat or suffer from sensations of heat in your head and limbs? Other symptoms include agitation and tendencies to overreact.	Gardenia Honeysuckle Forsythia Licorice
Dampness Relates to Earth Element	Do you suffer from water retention and puffiness? Other symptoms include sore joints and muscles, thick, sticky mucus, and swelling in humid weather.	Alisma Astragalus Atractylodes Poria Cocos Stephania

Oriental Medical Diagnosis	Symptoms	Herbs that Might Help
Dryness Relates to Metal Element	Do you suffer from dry skin and lips with painful cracking? Other symptoms include lack of urine and other body secretions, becoming easily warm and flushed, and frequent thirst.	American Ginseng Anemarrhena Ophiopogon Schisandra
Cold Relates to Water Element	Are you easily chilled and suffer from coldness in your limbs and torso? Other symptoms include frequent, clear urination as well as feeling weary and withdrawn.	Cinnamon Bark Ginger (Dried) Fennel Seeds Licorice Root (Honey-Baked)

In working with herbs for nearly 25 years, I have rarely seen reactions—and those were a couple of minor cases of nausea. While most herbs are far safer than many modern pharmaceutical drugs, *all herbs are not safe all of the time for all people.* Please carefully read the contraindications accompanying each herb described in the upcoming section. Herbs that are classified as either "Hot" ☼ or "Cold" ● should be treated with respect and recommended dosages should be carefully followed. "Neutral" � herbs are generally more gentle, or foodlike in nature—often you can add these herbs to some of your favorite soups or stews. "Warm" ▲ and "Cool" ◑ herbs are also coded to help you balance your formula energetically. (For example, if you are suffering from a "Hot" condition with such symptoms as high fever, inflammation, or yellow mucus you will want to use more Cold or Cooling herbs in your formula. On the other hand, Hot or Warming herbs treat "Cold" conditions with such symptoms as chills, clear or white mucus, poor digestion, and diarrhea.) If you experience nausea or vomiting, reduce the dosage or discontinue taking the herb.

Herbal formulas are easily modified to cool them down or warm them up as needed simply by adding a particular herb. For example, if you find an herb that, symptomatically, is perfect for your disharmony, but energetically seems too cold for your constitution, a small amount of ginger or cinnamon (1 to 2 grams) may be added to the herbal prescription to warm it up.

Please remember—the herb that works wonders for you is probably not the right herb for your spouse, neighbor, friend, or dog. The universal laws of Yin and Yang are at work here. Opposites do tend to attract, so chances are your best friend or better half probably needs a completely different healing herb from the one you do. Wonderful pointers for healing energetically versus symptomatically with herbs can be found in Chapters 6 and 7—these are the true secrets of Oriental herbal healing.

Achyranthes Root
An Herbal Aid for Your Poor Aching Back
Botanical Name: *Achyranthes bidentata*

A Brief History of Achyranthes
Mandarin: Niu Xi; **Japanese:** Goshitsu; **Korean:** Usûl

Achyranthes, a weedy perennial of the amaranth family, grows mostly in the tropics and subtropics of Africa, Australia, and Eurasia, but has also been widely naturalized, mostly in the southern states of the United States. The literal translation of its Mandarin name, Niu Xi, means "ox knees." The stem of this plant has enlarged nodes, which make it resemble the knees of an ox. Rich, sandy, slightly acidic soil in Henan Province, China, produces very large roots—some reaching 3 to 4 feet in length. The root is harvested in wintertime once the leaves and stems have withered. When shopping for achyranthes, look for thick, long roots of a pale color, firm flesh, and fine cortex with no speckles or dirt.

While relatively unknown outside the Orient, this wonderful healing herb has been used as food and medicine for thousands of years. Seeds of *A. bidentata* make a good substitute for grains and have been used to make bread in India during times of famine. In Java, the leaves of one species, *A. aspera,* are commonly eaten as a veggie, while burnt leaves yield vegetable salt.

——— 🌍 ———

Healing Qualities of Achyranthes
Bitter, Sour, Neutral Energy
Treats Liver and Kidney Organ Systems
Category: Herb that Invigorates the Blood (see page 350)

In Traditional Oriental Medicine, achyranthes belongs to a category of herbs that increase circulation or "Invigorate the Blood." If not caused by infection or injury, pain is thought to be the result of Congestion or Stagnation of Blood and Qi. Just imagine a clogged irrigation ditch in your garden; debris accumulates and life-giving water and nutrients do not reach the plants. The same is true in our human garden. Due to lack of exercise and many hours driving to work and then sitting at our desks, our blood, lymph, and energy do not flow as they should. Our cells are denied oxygen and food; toxins are not carried away. The result is often localized pain that is deep, sharp, and colicky in nature. This type of pain is most often associated with lower abdominal pain (dysmenorrhea or amenorrhea), low-back and knee pain, chest pain, or lingering pain caused by an old accident.

In the Orient, achyranthes roots are treated in various ways to increase their therapeutic actions. Uncooked root helps remove congestion and reduce swelling while root prepared in wine enhances circulation. Achyranthes root treated with brine strengthens bones and tendons. Roasted, or stir-fried root, supplements Liver and Kidney functions while strengthening bones and tendons.

The bitter and sour properties of achyranthes stimulate our digestive and circulatory systems, liver, and kidneys. Acting primarily on the lower part of the body, this herbal ally can greatly aid in the relief of pain by stimulating circulation.

If you have problems with delayed or painful menstruation, low back or knee pain and weakness, or pain due to kidney stones, you might wish to try one of the following herbal combinations.

Herbal Combinations Using Achyranthes

Achyranthes is often used in conjunction with *eucommia bark* for low-back and knee pain and weakness.

For difficult menstruation, achyranthes is combined with *safflower, dang gui,* and *cinnamon bark.*

Achyranthes, *dang gui* and *scutellaria* are combined to treat painful urinary tract disorders and kidney stones.

Contraindications: Do not use achyranthes if you are weak, have diarrhea, suffer from excessive bleeding during menstruation, or were recently injured. Achyranthes should not be used during pregnancy since research indicates that it dilates the cervix.

Other Herbs that Invigorate the Blood

If the healing properties of achyranthes are not quite right for your condition, but Congestion or Stagnation are a problem, please see other herbs in this category: *Ligusticum, Peony Root (Red), Safflower Flower, Salvia.*

Maximum Daily Dosage: 9 to 15 grams
1/4 ounce to 1/2 ounce

Aconite

Keeps the Home Fires Burning

English Name: Aconite or Monkshoods
Botanical Name: *Aconitum carmichaeli*

A Brief History of Aconite

Mandarin: Fù zi; **Japanese: Bushi;** Korean: Puja

Aconite belongs to a genus consisting of about 100 hardy, tuberous, poisonous perennials. Yes, it is poisonous—extreme caution with this herb is called for. In Greek mythology, Cerebus is the name of a three-headed dog that Hercules had to drag from Hades as his twelfth punishment. According to the legend, poison foam dripped from the dog's mouth and wherever the saliva landed, aconite plants sprouted. Another legend has it that witches combined aconite with deadly nightshade to concoct a wicked brew that enabled them to fly. Monkshood was also once used to make arrow poisons. It gets its English name from the hooded shape of its deep-blue delphinium-like flowers. This hood shape restricts pollination of aconite to only bees. *A. carmichaelii* grows in China while *A. napellus* is found in central and western Europe. The aconite plant prefers growing near water in northern temperate wooded or grassland regions.

Aconite contains a toxic phytochemical called aconitine. *A. ferox* has one of the deadliest and fastest-acting poisons known, followed by *A. napellus*. However, several species are used medicinally in the Orient and have valuable therapeutic properties when used properly. References to the use of *A. carmichaelii* are first found in Chinese medical texts dating around AD200. In Chinese, this herb has two names—the fresh root is called *wu tou,* while fu zi refers to the root that is cooked with sugar and salt. The Chinese first soak the hard tubers in vinegar for a month, then in salt water for a month; they alternate and repeat this process three times to diminish the effects of the poisonous compounds. If one senses a numbing sensation in the mouth when drinking a tea made with aconite, this indicates that the poisons have not been totally neutralized. The tea should be discarded, as well as any remaining dry herb.

Dried aconite root is basically spindle-shaped with a pointed bottom. It comes prepared in a number of forms—blast-fried root is a translucent golden color; whereas roots that are skinned, sundried, and treated with sulfur are white in color; another type is lighter yellow (again translucent), but black on the cut edges. Most medicinal quality aconite comes to us from Sichuan and Shaanxi provinces of China.

Aconite is legally restricted in some countries. It should be prescribed only by qualified, licensed herbal practitioners.

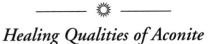

Healing Qualities of Aconite

Spicy, Hot, Toxic Energy
Treats Heart, Kidney and Spleen Organ Systems
Category: Herb that Warms the Interior and Expels Cold (see page 351)

In Traditional Oriental Medicine, Aconite belongs to a category of herbs that Warm the Interior and Expel Cold. It is the "Hottest" or most Yang herb used in the Orient and is the number one herb used to restore Devastated Yang conditions (extreme weakness and fatigue). Aconite can warm those dwindling Kidney Fires that are signaled by impotence, frequent or insufficient urination, and spermatorrhea. It is used to treat vomiting of clear fluid, diarrhea, abdominal pain and cold extremities that are the result of Deficient Spleen and Kidney Yang. Recent research has shown it to be effective in cases of congestive heart failure. Aconite stops pain and has diuretic and antirheumatic effects, as well as being one of the best metabolic stimulants known. It is used as a restorative in cases of severe shock or trauma.

Herbal Combinations Using Aconite

Aconite is combined with *cinnamon bark* for low back/knee pain and weakness, cold hands and feet, impotence, and frequent urination.

For Collapse of Spleen and Kidney Yang (chills and cold extremities and diarrhea with undigested food), aconite is combined with *ginger root* and a large dosage of *licorice root.*

Aconite is combined with *astragalus* to treat spontaneous sweating and chills due to Deficient Yang Energy.

Atractylodes is combined with aconite to stop pain and eliminate coldness from the abdomen. Fluid congests in the Middle Burner (Stomach and Spleen area) due to excess Cold Dampness and Deficient Yang energy; symptoms include vomiting, diarrhea, and edema.

Contraindications: Aconite should be administered by qualified, licensed professionals only. It *should not* be taken by pregnant women or severely weak persons.

Other Herbs that Warm the Interior and Expel Cold

If the healing properties of aconite seem right for you, be sure to consult a licensed professional. As a beginning herbalist, you might find other herbs in this category helpful: *Fennel Seeds, Ginger*
Maximum Daily Dosage: 2 to 5 grams
1/12 ounce to 1/6 ounce
(This is a tiny amount!)

Acorus Rhizome

Stops Sour Belching
English Name: Across or Sweetflag Rhizome
Botanical Name: *Acorus gramineus*

A Brief History of Acorus
Japanese: Shōbu, **Korean:** Ch'angp'o, **Mandarin:** Shí Chāng Pu

Two species of aquatic acorus, or sweetflag, grow wild in northern and eastern Asia, as well as in North America. Cultivated and traded in the Orient for well over 4,000 years, acorus spread into eastern Europe from Mongolia and Siberia sometime during the thirteenth century; gradually making its way into western Europe by the sixteenth century. *A. calamus* was cultivated in large quantities in Norfolk, England, and was gathered annually at the "gladdon harvest." In the eighteenth century, medicinal lozenges for indigestion, coughs, and infection prevention were made by crystallizing slices of calamus root. In order to prevent sickness while traveling, Native American people of the Penobscot tribe living in Maine would chew on a piece of sweetflag rhizome.

Harvested during the autumn and winter months, most medicinal roots of *A. gramineus* come to us from three provinces in China—Jiangsu, Zhejiang, and Sichuan. The rhizome of acorus does not break easily; it should be firm, aromatic, and not very fibrous. Look for roots that are clean, dry, and plump, with a white cross section. Generally, the rhizomes can be purchased precut in longitudinal slices, ready for decocting.

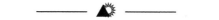

Healing Qualities of Acorus Rhizome
Spicy, Slightly Warm, Aromatic Energy
Treats Heart and Stomach Organ Systems
Category: Aromatic Substance that Opens the Orifices (See page 355)

This warm, spicy herb eliminates Damp and dissipates Wind, according to Traditional Oriental Medicine and is used for Cold, Wind, and Damp Bi-Syndromes. In Western terms, acorus would be considered a tonic, aromatic herb with antibacterial properties. It stimulates digestion, aids depression, and helps clear bronchial congestion and excess mucus. It also possesses mild sedative qualities.

Contraindications: Acorus should not be given to patients who perspire easily and it is contraindicated in cases of Excess Yang due to Yin Deficiency with cough and spitting of blood.

Herbal Combinations Using Acorus

To open the chest, relieve pain, Open the Sensory Portals (our senses of smell, taste, sound, and sight) and warm the Stomach, acorus is stir-fried with *ginger* juice; to strengthen the Spleen and Open the Portals, it is stir-fried with *bran* and *honey.*

Magnolia bark and *tangerine peel* are combined with acorus to relieve chest and upper-digestive-tract discomfort due to Dampness in the Middle Burner (the area of the body roughly below the sternum and above the navel).

Lotus seed, coptis, and *acorus* are used to treat dysentery-like disharmonies that result in poor digestion.

If you suffer from heartburn accompanied by sour belching, chew on a few small pieces of sweetflag root for a few minutes. Swallow the juice and discard the root.

Maximum Daily Dosage: 3 to 6 grams
1/10 to 1/5 ounce

Aduki Beans

Help Overcome Edema

English Name: Aduki Bean
Botanical Name: *Phaseolus calcaratus*

A Brief History of Aduki Beans

Mandarin: Chì Xiao Dòu; **Japanese:** Sekishozu; **Korean:** Chôksodu

A member of the legume family, the aduki bean is a small red bean that can be purchased at most Oriental markets or health-food stores. Always look for beans that are not shriveled but are full, round, and dark-red in color. Adukis are grown for food in Japan and China. Most commercially grown beans come to us from three Chinese provinces—Guangdong, Guangxi, and Jiangxi.

——— 🐦 ———

Healing Qualities of Aduki Beans

Sweet, Sour, Neutral Energy
Treats Heart and Small Intestine Organ Systems
Category: Herb that Drains Dampness (see page 347)

Aduki (sometimes seen written as azuki or adzuki) has the ability to relieve what is known in Traditional Oriental Medicine as "True Dampness," or edema in the lower region of the body. Just think of a flooded river valley—numerous ponds have formed and the soil is completely waterlogged. Now imagine someone digging small trenches down to the river to help drain those fields. The nature of this herb food promotes urination, draining our human bodyscape of Excess Dampness. Excess moisture damages the Earth Element (Stomach and Spleen). Think of the soggy soil of house plants that have been overwatered for a few weeks and how the roots and stem near the soil start to rot. Excess water can also extinguish the Fire Element (Heart and Small Intestine), impairing digestion and assimilation of nutrients. These small beans tone the Heart and Spleen while treating edema and urinary problems, including urinary infections, eczema, and suppurative skin infections. Aduki beans clear Damp-Heat and are helpful in treating sores, carbuncles, and mild cases of jaundice.

These nutrient-packed, naturally high-fiber, low-fat beans are a great addition to almost all diets. Persons with damp constitutions will find aduki beans to be a wonderful herbal ally that can be consumed frequently. However, if you tend to have symptoms relating to dryness, you should eat adukis less frequently and concentrate on moistening, full sweet foods that pertain to the Earth Element. You need to irrigate those dry fields in your human garden.

Traditionally, aduki bean sprouts are eaten to control bleeding during pregnancy and for blood in the stool. Flowers of the aduki plant are used to relieve alcoholism, detoxicate, and relieve headaches due to intoxication. They are also used in cases of malaria, dysentery, and diabetes.

There is some great news regarding these little red jewels. You're familiar with the age-old reputation beans have for creating intestinal gas (known as "Evil Wind" in the Orient). Adukis are usually much easier on your system in this regard. However, remember to soak all beans 18 to 24 hours before cooking, preferably with a piece of kombu seaweed, and be sure to change the rinse water at least two or three times. This not only minimizes their "Evil Wind" potential, but, by actually starting the sprouting process, you increase the protein content up to 70 percent. Do not soak more than 24 hours, however, since once beans sprout, the protein content rapidly drops again.

Herbal Combinations Using Aduki Beans

Aduki, combined with *dang gui,* is applied topically in plaster form to treat toxic swellings, abscesses, and bleeding hemorrhoids from Damp Heat.

It is combined with *ephedra, forsythia fruit,* and *white mulberry* root bark for mild cases of Damp-Heat jaundice.

In the Orient, adukis are cooked with *peanuts* and *red jujube dates* for edema that stems from deficiency or malnutrition.

Other Herbs that Drain Damp

If the healing properties of aduki beans are not quite right for your condition, but edema or water retention is a problem, please see other herbs in this category: *Alisma, Coix, Dioscorea, Poria Cocos, Stephania, Zhu Ling*
Maximum Daily Dosage: 9 to 30 grams
1/4 ounce to 1 ounce

JANET, LIVER CANCER, AND ADUKI BEAN SOUP   In 1989, I received a phone call from a dear friend who had moved to New Mexico. Janet was 63 years old and had retired from teaching the previous year. In 1984, she suffered from colon cancer, which was removed surgically. The cancer had now spread to her liver. After two surgeries and extensive chemotherapy, Janet's doctors sent her home to die, saying it was a hopeless situation—she had two to four weeks to live. During our conversation, Janet told me she was in terrible pain due to fluid retention that had created severe abdominal swelling. We talked a great deal about food and herbs that might help. I gave Janet's husband a recipe for what I call "Aduki Soup" (see Chapter 5 for the recipe), as well as the names of herbal formulas that might help, including Silymarin (an extract from Milk Thistle seeds).

Three weeks later, Janet called to say she was eating aduki bean soup every day and the abdominal swelling was nearly gone. Almost pain free, she had been able to get out of bed for the first time in months to take out the trash. The food and herb therapy did not cure Janet's liver cancer. But she was able to vacation with her husband and enjoy the company of her grandchildren for nearly another five years, living in relative comfort. Janet passed on in 1994. She will always be remembered.

Agastache

Settles the Tummy

English Name: Patchouli or Pogostemon cablin (Blanco)
Botanical Name: *Agastache rugosa*

A Brief History of Agastache

Mandarin: Huò Xiang, **Japanese:** Kakko, **Korean:** Kwakhyang

Agastache rugosa, also known as Korean mint or patchouli, belongs to a genus composed of 30 species of aromatic perennials native to northern Vietnam, Laos, Japan, China, North America, and Mexico. *A. rugosa* grows in eastern Asia and is the variety used in Chinese Medicine. *A. foeniculum* (found in North and Central America) is a long-flowering border plant whose rich nectar attracts bees. In the 1870s, North American beekeepers widely planted this later variety to produce a special honey with a mild flavor of aniseed. Leaves from *A. foeniculum* were collected by Native Americans to make a pleasant, mintlike tea. Some tribes used the tea medicinally to relieve coughs. Agastache has also been used as a flavoring for meat and salad dishes.

Most of the medicinal quality herb comes from Guangdong, China, or the Philippines. The best quality agastache gives off a strong, though pleasant aroma.

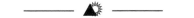

Healing Qualities of Agastache

Spicy, Slightly Warm Energy
Treats Lung, Spleen, Stomach Organ Systems
Category: Aromatic Herb that Transforms Dampness (see page 349)

Aromatic Herbs that Transform Dampness are used medicinally in the Orient to treat abdominal distention and fullness, nausea, diarrhea, vomiting, or the regurgitation of sour fluids. This type of "Dampness" is sometimes caused by food poisoning or other acute digestive disorders. Agastache is also taken internally to relieve headache, fever and chills, malaria, dysentery, bad breath, morning sickness, and Summerheat-Damp colds and flu. If you suspect food poisoning, please consult a qualified health-care practitioner immediately.

Contraindications: Agastache should not be taken if there are Heat signs accompanying Yin Deficiency.

Herbal Combinations Using Agastache

Agastache and *cardamom seed* are effective in relieving morning sickness.

Combined with *pinellia* and *atractylodes,* agastache is used to treat nausea and vomiting, a feeling of epigastric and abdominal distention, or reduced appetite and diarrhea due to "Dampness" blocking the Middle Burner. (The Middle Burner corresponds to the area in the human body just below the sternum that houses the liver, spleen and pancreas, stomach, and small intestines.)

For Damp Warm febrile diseases such as malaria and dysentery, agastache is combined with *scutellaria, forsythia fruit,* and *talcum.* The symptoms include fever, abdominal distention, achy limbs, lethargy, and dark, scanty urine.

Other Herbs that Transform Dampness

If the healing properties of agastache are not quite right for your condition, but dampness is a problem, please see other herbs in this category: *Cardamom Seed, Magnolia Bark*

Note: It is important not to simmer this herb for more than 15 minutes.
Maximum Daily Dosage: 5 to 9 grams
1/6 ounce to 1/4 ounce

Agrimony
Nature's Own Coagulant
Botanical Name: *Agrimonia pilosa*

A Brief History of Agrimony
Mandarin: Xian Hè Cao, **Japanese:** Senkakuso, **Korean:** Sônhakch'o

Agrimony is still an ingredient in a French herbal lotion that was once used as a battlefield remedy on fifteenth-century long-barreled gunshot wounds. Fifteen species of agrimony, a member of the rose family, are found in South American and Northern temperate regions. Agrimony measures about two feet tall and has small yellow flowers that are used as a source of golden-yellow dye. The African Zulu people drink a decoction of agrimony leaves to expel tapeworms. *A. pilosa* has a high vitamin K content, which promotes the clotting of blood, making it an excellent herb to control bleeding.

---------- 🌏 ----------

Healing Qualities of Agrimony
Bitter, Spicy, Neutral
Treats Lung, Liver and Spleen Organ Systems
Category: Herb that Regulates the Blood and Stops Bleeding (see page 350)

In Traditional Oriental Medicine, agrimony belongs to a category of herbs that Regulate the Blood by Controlling Bleeding. It's used extensively to control nosebleed, bleeding gums, blood in the urine, uterine bleeding, and vomiting or coughing blood. Because of its neutral nature, agrimony is easily combined with other herbs to control conditions known in the Orient as Hot, Cold, Deficient, or Excessive Bleeding.

Herbal Combinations Using Agrimony

Rectal suppositories are made from agrimony to treat diarrhea and tapeworm.
    Sophora is combined with agrimony for bloody stool.

Other Herbs that Stop Bleeding

If the healing properties of agrimony are not quite right for your condition please see other herbs in this category: *Mugwort, Pseudoginseng (see "Ginseng"), Sanguisorba, Sophora*
    Contraindications: Taken in excess, agrimony can cause nausea or vomiting.
    Excessive bleeding can be life-threatening. Please consult a licensed medical professional.
    Maximum Daily Dosage: Dry—9 to 15 grams or
                 1/4 ounce to 1/2 ounce
                 Fresh—15 to 30 grams or
                 1/2 ounce to 1 ounce

Alismatis

**Relieves Water Retention and
Lowers Blood Pressure**

English Name: Alismatis or Water Plantain Rhizome
Botanical Name: *Alisma plantago-aquatica*

A Brief History of Alisma

Mandarin: Zé Xiè, **Japanese:** Takusha, **Korean:** T'aeksa

Alisma or water plantain is a marginal aquatic perennial belonging to a genus composed of ten species. *A. plantago-aquatic's* attractive, pale-lilac flowers open in the afternoon and make it a popular garden-pond plant in temperate parts of Eurasia. The plant used medicinally in the Orient has white flowers. At one time, alisma was called "mad-dog weed" because it was thought to be a cure for rabies. This gentle healing herb was first mentioned in Chinese Medical texts around A.D. 200.

Most medicinal-quality alisma comes to us from Jiangxi, Sichuan, Yunnan, and Guizhou provinces in China. The best rhizomes are large, hard, yellow-white in color, and round or oval in shape. Pieces purchased for decocting come in round slices—those treated with brine are a little darker in color.

Healing Energies of Alisma

Sweet, Bland, Cold, Non toxic
Treats Kidney and Bladder Organ Systems
Category: Herb that Drains Dampness (see page 347)

The nature of this herbal ally promotes urination—draining our human bodyscape of Excess Dampness and Heat, while lowering blood pressure, cholesterol, and blood sugar levels. Alisma stir-fried with brine acts on the Kidney and Bladder pathways and is specific for Kidney weakness with such symptoms as dizziness, ringing in the ears, or deafness. Raw alisma strengthens the Spleen while relieving water retention. In Western terms, alisma is used to treat diabetes, kidney inflammation, painful urination, vertigo, lumbago, edema, and acute diarrhea.

Because of alisma's gentle nature, it has less tendency to injure the Yin than do other herbs in this category.

Herbal Combinations Using Alisma

Moutan peony cortex is combined with alisma to treat the sensation of deep, hot pain in the bones, dizziness, and vertigo.

Alisma is combined with *pinellia* to treat abdominal distention with scanty urine due to damp-heat in the Middle Burner (stomach/spleen/pancreas/small intestine area of the body).

Contraindications: In cases of spermatorrhea or leukorrhea due to Damp Cold or Deficient Kidney Yang energy (extreme weakness and exhaustion).

Other Herbs that Drain Dampness

If the healing properties of alisma are not quite right for your condition but you need to Drain Dampness, please see other herbs in this category: *Aduki Bean, Coix, Dioscorea, Poria Cocos, Stephania, Zhu Ling*
Maximum Daily Dosage: 6 to 12 grams
1/5 ounce to 1/3 ounce

Allium sativum see Garlic

Aloe

Is a Gentle Purgative
English Name: Aloe Leaf (dried juice concentrate)
Botanical Name: *Aloe vera* L. or *A. ferox* Mill.

A Brief History of Aloe
Mandarin: Lú Huì, **Japanese:** Rokai, **Korean:** Nohwa

There are 325 species of *Aloe vera* native to Africa, Arabia, and the Cape Verde Islands. The African variety was used to antidote poisons from arrow wounds. An evergreen perennial and member of the lily family, aloe plants vary greatly in size and shape. Some are shrubs, while others are trees or climbers. All of them have thick, pointed foliage and colorful flower spikes. Most *Aloe vera* comes to us from Africa and the West Indies, *Aloe ferox* from southern Africa, and *Aloe vera chinensis* from China.

Ancient Egyptians took *A. vera* to treat excess mucus; it can still be identified in some of their famous wall paintings. It was used for embalming by the Jewish people—the body of Jesus was wrapped in linen soaked with myrrh and aloes. The Greeks and Romans applied aloe gel to wounds, and it was a favored purgative herb during the Middle Ages. Bitter tasting aloe extracts were also applied to children's fingertips to stop nail biting.

Often, aloe gel or liquid is taken for various reasons as a dietary supplement in Western herbalism (to aid digestion and liver function). Its energy and therapeutic value is somewhat different from the bitter, cold, dried aloe-leaf concentrates used in Oriental medicine. *A. ferox* comes in extremely concentrated shiny reddish brown or black coal-like chunks, while *A. vera* resembles a black, nontranslucent mass.

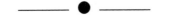

Healing Energies of Aloe

Bitter, Cold Energy
Treats Large Intestine, Liver, and Stomach Organ Systems
Category: Downward-Draining Herb—Purgative (see page 346)

Aloe is an antifungal agent used in treating infections such as ringworm. The anti-inflammatory properties of the gel and liquid promote healing of damaged tissues. In Oriental medicine, dried aloe leaf concentrate is used to treat constipation, eliminate menstrual block, and destroy intestinal parasites or worms. Aloe clears excess heat from the Liver Meridian accompanied by such symptoms as dizziness, headache, ringing in the ears, epigastric discomfort, constipation, and fever. Of the Purgatives, aloe is considered one of the most mild—it can be used for chronic constipation.

Contraindications: Avoid aloe during pregnancy. Vomiting can result from high doses of leaf concentrate. Not to be used by persons suffering from rectal bleeding or persons with digestive weakness—Cold, Deficient Spleen and Stomach disharmonies.

Other Purgative Herbs

If the healing properties of aloe are not quite right for your condition, please see other herbs in this category: *Rhubarb Rhizome*

Maximum Daily Dosage: 0.5 to 1.5 grams

This is a small amount! 1.5 grams is about 1/20th of an ounce

American Ginseng see *Ginseng, American*

Anemarrhena
Treats Infectious Disease
Botanical Name: *Anemarrhenae asphodeloides*

A Brief History of Anemarrhena
Mandarin: Zhi Mu; Japanese: Chimo; Korean: Chimo

There is only one species of this attractive, night-flowering plant that is a member of the lily family. Small, fragrant, yellow-white, six-petaled flowers are borne on three foot spikes. Found in northern China and Japan, anemarrhena has been collected in the wild for medicinal use since A.D. 200. Research is currently being conducted in China regarding the feasibility of cultivating anemarrhena.

The soft anemarrhena rhizome breaks easily. Look for smooth, large, plump rhizomes with a slightly spongy pale-yellow interior.

●

Healing Qualities of Anemarrhena
Bitter, Cold Energy
Treats Lung, Stomach, and Kidney Organ Systems
Category: Herbs that Clear Heat and Drain Fire (see page 345)

Anemarrhena nurtures the Yin and moistens Dry conditions. It is a mucilaginous tonic herb that effectively clears fungal and bacterial infections. This rare lily is taken internally to reduce high fevers accompanying infectious diseases, tuberculosis, urinary problems, and chronic bronchitis. It also reduces blood-sugar levels.

Contraindications: Persons suffering from diarrhea should not take anemarrhena. Taken in excess, anemarrhena may cause a sudden drop in blood pressure.

Herbal Combinations Using Anemarrhena
Anemarrhena is combined with *phellodendron cortex* to relieve Yin Deficiency accompanied by dizziness, night sweats, and vertigo.

Cinnamon bark is combined with anemarrhena to treat Damp Heat in the Lower Burner (the area of the body below the naval that includes the reproductive organs, intestines, and kidney and bladder complex) resulting in retention of urine and afternoon fevers.

Ophiopogon and *trichosanthes* are combined with anemarrhena to treat Dryness in the Lung and Stomach Organ Systems.

Other Herbs that Quell Fire

If the healing properties of anemarrhena are not quite right for your condition, please see other herbs in this category: *Gardenia, Gypsum*
Maximum Daily Dosage: 5 to 10 grams
1/5 ounce to 1/3 ounce

Angelica Sinensis see Dang Gui

Apricot Kernel
Relieves Coughing, Wheezing, Constipation
Botanical Name: *Prunus armeniaca*

A Brief History of Apricot Kernel
Mandarin: Xìng Rén or Ku Xìng Rén; Japanese: Kyonin; Korean: Sa'in

Many of our favorite fruits and nuts come from the rose family, including cherries, apricots, plums, peaches, and almonds. There are more than 430 species of deciduous, occasionally evergreen trees and shrubs that belong to this genus. *P. armeniaca* (wild apricot) and *P. persica* (peach) were cultivated in China for well over 2,500 years. Historical texts indicate they reached Greece around the fourth century B.C. and were grown in Italy during Roman times.

Many species of *Prunus* have been used medicinally throughout history. They are first mentioned in Chinese medical texts around 500 A.D.. The seeds of some species contain a phytochemical known as hydrocyanic acid, which breaks down in water to form cyanide. This compound is exceedingly poisonous, but in small quantities promotes a sense of well-being, improves digestion, and stimulates respiration. Apricot seeds used medicinally in the Orient are steamed or stir-fried to reduce toxicity. Laetrile (used in cancer therapy) is extracted from seeds of *P. armeniaca* (wild apricot). Its oils are used in the cosmetic industry for the manufacture of skin-care products, while the fruits are used to make liqueurs.

─────── ▲ᴹ ───────

Healing Qualities of Apricot Kernel

Bitter, Warm, Slightly Poisonous Energy
Treats Lung and Large Intestine Organ Systems
Category: Herb that Relieves Coughing and Wheezing (see page 348)

Herbs in this category treat the "symptom" by stopping coughing and wheezing. It is important, however, to use them in conjunction with herbs that address the "root" problem. If the cough is due to an external factor (such as a cold or flu), they should be combined with herbs that Release the Exterior such as ginger, ephedra, or magnolia flower; if the cough is due to internal weakness or injury, they are combined with Tonifying herbs; if the cough is Cold (producing clear or white mucus), they are combined with Warming herbs; if the cough is Hot (producing thick, yellow mucus), they are combined with herbs that Clear Heat.

Apricot seed is used broadly to treat many kinds of coughs stemming from Heat or Cold. It is particularly useful for coughs or difficult breathing of a dry nature, since this herb is moistening. It effectively relieves dry constipation by moistening the intestines. Apricot seed also treats bronchitis, asthma, and emphysema.

Contraindications: Do not exceed the maximum daily dosage; over-dosage can cause respiratory failure. Apricot kernel should not be used in cases of diarrhea.

Herbal Combinations Using Apricot Kernel

Apricot seed is often used in conjunction with *ophiopogon* for Dry coughs due to Heat injuring the Lungs.

For asthma, apricot seed is combined with *ephedra*.

Apricot seed and *hemp seed* are combined to treat constipation from Deficient Qi and Dry intestines.

Other Herbs that Relieve Coughing and Wheezing

If the healing properties of apricot kernel are not quite right for your condition, but coughing and wheezing are a problem, please see other herbs in this category: *Coltsfoot, Mulberry Root Bark*

Maximum Daily Dosage: 5 to 10 grams
1/5 ounce to 1/3 ounce

Astragalus

Builds Immunity

English Name: Milk vetch or Yellow vetch root
Botanical Name: Astragalus membranaceus

A Brief History of Astragalus

Mandarin: Huáng Qí; **Japanese:** Ogi; **Korean:** Hwanggi

Astragalus has been used for thousands of years in the Orient as a tonic herb to build resistance to infection. There are more than 2,000 species of annuals, perennials, and shrubs related to the medicinal variety grown in the dry, sandy soils of eastern Asia. Some astragalus species are used as food and fodder crops while others, known as "locoweed," are actually toxic to livestock. Other species of this remarkable plant accumulate minerals and were used by prospectors as indicators of ore-rich deposits. Another 100 species or so are grown as ornamentals for their colorful flower spikes. Astragalus, a slightly sweet-tasting root, is used frequently in Chinese cooking to create delicious, nourishing soups and broths that Tonify the Qi.

You can usually find this yellowish-white root in Oriental markets, sold in a form that resembles irregularly shaped tongue depressors. The outer skin of the root is grayish-brown to black in color. Good quality roots are long, dry, unwrinkled, and do not have a hollow or black core. They are somewhat flexible and should resist snapping when gently bent.

―――――― ▲ ――――――

Healing Qualities of Astragalus

Sweet, Slightly Warm Energy
Treats Spleen and Lung Organ Systems
Category: Herb that Tonifies the Qi (see page 352)

If Your Get Up and Go, Got Up and Went . . .

Astragalus might be right for you. Considered a superior herb in Traditional Oriental Medicine, astragalus is extremely safe and health-enhancing. For well over 5,000 years in the Orient, special herbs known as Qi Tonifiers have been used to "Strengthen the Exterior" or enhance the body's Defensive Qi— astragalus is one of those herbs. Modern studies confirm this herb has many powerful immune-stimulating properties. Research on a compound composed of Astragalus and Codonopsis demonstrated improved action of the thymus gland and spleen (glands responsible for producing immune cells). This compound increased the activity of killer T-cells and reduced the generation of T-suppressor cells, thus enhancing the body's immunity.

Astragalus also lowers blood pressure and blood-sugar levels and is used in treating diabetes, kidney problems, slow-healing skin eruptions, and prolapsed organs. Astragalus promotes urination and relieves edema.

Cook with Your Cure!

If you lack appetite, feel fatigued, suffer from frequent colds and flu, shortness of breath, spontaneous sweating, or diarrhea, during the fall and winter months you might consider adding a slice of astragalus root to broths, soups, stews, or grain dishes that will be simmering for 30 minutes or more. After the food is prepared, remove and discard the root. Although it's next to impossible to "eat" a tough astragalus root, you may want to chew on it for a few minutes. The flavor of astragalus is slightly sweet and will not make any noticeable difference in the flavor of your dish.

Herbal Combinations Using Astragalus

Astragalus is combined with *ginseng* to treat general weakness, lack of appetite, fatigue, and spontaneous sweating due to Qi Deficiency.

Aconite is combined with astragalus to help eliminate spontaneous sweating due to Yang Deficiency.

Dang gui and astragalus are combined to treat Deficient Blood and Qi, fatigue and poor circulation.

Codonopsis is combined with astragalus to treat prolapsing organs and increase immunity.

Cohosh, bupleurum, and astragalus are combined for excessive uterine bleeding and for rectal and uterine prolapse.

Other Herbs that Tonify Qi

If the healing properties of astragalus are not quite right for your condition, but you feel that Tonification of Qi is what you need, please see other herbs in this category: *Atractylodes, Codonopsis, Dioscorea, Ginseng, Jujube Date Fruit, Licorice*

Maximum Daily Dosage: 5 to 10 grams

1/5 ounce to 1/3 ounce

Atractylodes

Strengthens the Digestive System
Botanical Name: Atractylodes macrocephala

A Brief History of Atractylodes

Mandarin: Bái zhú; **Japanese:** Byakujutsu; **Korean:** Paekch'ul

Atractylodes, or Chinese thistle daisy, adorned with purple, thistlelike flowers that are one to two inches in diameter, grows wild in waste and pasture-
lands throughout China, Korea, and Japan. There are actually seven species
of this rhizomatous perennial plant; all are used in Traditional Oriental
Medicine. Because of the great demand for these healing plants, they are now
grown on a large-scale basis.

First mentioned in the Chinese Tang Materia Medica recorded in A.D.
659, atractylodes is a hard rhizome with knobby protuberances located on
the lower extremities. When shopping for atractylodes, look for clean, large,
dry rhizomes with a white interior and light-brown skin.

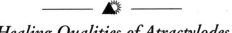

Healing Qualities of Atractylodes

Bitter, Sweet, Warm Energy
Treats Spleen and Stomach Organ Systems
Category: Herb that Tonifies the Qi (see page 352)

Herbs that Tonify the Qi are commonly used in treating weakness of the
Spleen or Lung Organ Systems. Think of it this way: In Oriental Medicine
the Spleen is responsible for extracting Qi (or vital energy) from our food,
while the Lungs are responsible for extracting Qi (another form of vital energy) from the air. If we lack Qi, then one of these systems is probably not
functioning up to par. Symptoms of Deficient Spleen Qi include lack of
appetite, loose stools or diarrhea, a feeling of heaviness in the arms and legs,
and tiredness. Lung Qi Deficiency is signaled by a pale complexion, weak
voice, shallow breathing, shortness of breath, and spontaneous sweating.

Qi Tonifying herbs are usually rich and sweet in nature, so it's important to combine them with small quantities of herbs that Move and Regulate
the Qi such as cyperus or tangerine peel.

Atractylodes is commonly prescribed for cases involving weak or disturbed digestion. It possesses diuretic and antibacterial qualities and lowers
blood-sugar levels.

Herbal Combinations Using Atractylodes

Atractylodes is combined with *codonopsis* and *ginger* to treat abdominal pain, diarrhea, and vomiting due to Cold and digestive weakness.

Poria cocos and *cinnamon twigs* are combined with atractylodes to help eliminate chest distension, congested fluids, and edema due to weak digestion.

Scutellaria and atractylodes are combined to calm a restless fetus due to internal Heat.

Other Herbs that Tonify Qi

If the healing properties of atractylodes are not quite right for your condition, but you feel that Tonification of Qi is what you need, please see other herbs in this category: *Astragalus, Codonopsis, Dioscorea, Ginseng, Jujube Date Fruit, Licorice*

Maximum Daily Dosage: 5 to 10 grams
1/5 ounce to 1/3 ounce

Bamboo Sap and Shavings
Clear Lung Infections
Botanical Name: *Phyllostachys nigra*

A Brief History of Bamboo Sap and Shavings
SAP: **Mandarin:** Zhú Lì; **Japanese:** Chikureki; **Korean:** Chikujo
SHAVINGS: **Mandarin:** Zhú Rú; **Japanese:** Chikujo; **Korean:** Chukchu

You're probably familiar with the graceful foliage of bamboo so beautifully depicted in Oriental artwork. Used medicinally since at least A.D. 500 (as well as for musical instruments, paper, drainpipes, scaffolding, furniture, fishing poles, and human and panda food) bamboo is probably one of the most widely used plants. There are 60 species of medium- to large-sized bamboos growing in China, Burma, and India. Large quantities of tender shoots of a number of species, particularly *P. pubescens,* are canned and exported for a delicious addition to stir-fries and other Oriental dishes. While a number of members of the bamboo family are used medicinally in China, *P. nigra* is most frequently mentioned in Chinese medical texts. It has slender stems that turn from greenish brown to black in the second or third year of their growth. Cultivated in gardens and large containers for hundreds of years, *P. nigra* flourishes in wild, damp areas of central and eastern China.

—— ● ——

Healing Qualities of Bamboo Sap
Sweet, Very Cold Energy
Treats Heart, Lungs, and Stomach Organ Systems
Category: Herb that Cools and Transforms Phlegm Heat (see page 348)

Bamboo sap is a sweet, cold herbal expectorant that is effective against bacterial infections (particularly lung with cough and phlegm). It lowers fevers and controls vomiting and nosebleed.

Herbal Combinations Using Bamboo Sap
Bamboo sap is used in combination with *pinellia* to control cough, wheezing, and a feeling of chest constriction due to Hot, bacterial lung infections.
Contraindications: In cases of loose stool due to digestive weakness or coughs due to Cold.

—— ◖ ——

Healing Qualities of Bamboo Shavings
Sweet, Cool Energy
Treats Lung, Stomach, Gall Bladder Organ Systems
Category: Herb that Cools and Transforms Hot Phlegm (see page 348)

Bamboo shavings Cool the Blood and stop nosebleeds and vomiting of blood. It is used to treat Heat in the Lungs (infections) accompanied by thick phlegm and coughing up of blood. It is given to stop vomiting sour or bitter material, bad breath, nausea, and yellow greasy tongue coating that are indicative of Stomach Heat patterns in Oriental Medicine.
Contraindications: Bamboo shavings should not be given to patients with nausea, vomiting, or food stagnation due to Cold symptoms.

Herbal Combinations Using Bamboo Shavings
Bamboo shavings are combined with *scutellaria* and *trichosanthes* for coughs due to Lung Heat.
Codonopsis and *licorice* are combined with bamboo shavings to treat hiccups due to Deficient Stomach Qi with symptoms of Heat.
Bamboo shavings, *pinellia,* and *green citrus peel* are used to treat insomnia and palpitations caused by Hot Phlegm.
Fresh *ginger root* juice added to tea made with bamboo shavings helps eliminate vomiting.

Other Herbs that Cool and Transform Hot Phlegm

If the healing properties of bamboo are not quite right for your condition, please see other herbs in this category: *Fritillary, Kelp (Seaweed), Trichosanthes*
Maximum Daily Dosage: 5 to 10 grams
1/5 ounce to 1/3 ounce

Black Cohosh see Cohosh, Black

Biota Seed
Relieves Insomnia and Palpitations
English: Thuja or Arborvitae Seed
Botanical Name: *Biota orientalis* or *Thuja orientalis*

A Brief History of Biota Seed
Mandarin: Bai Zi Rén; **Japanese:** Hakushinin; **Korean:** Paekchain

Thuja, a genus consisting of five evergreen coniferous trees, was used by many Native North Americans to make baskets, bows, canoes, cordage, and roofing. *B. orientalis* is a pyramidal-shaped tree or shrub, ranging from 15 to 40 feet in height, with fine, deep-green, scalelike leaves. Its grayish-colored cones reach about three quarters of an inch long.

When shopping for biota, look for full, oily seeds that are yellowish white in color.

———— 🌏 ————

Healing Qualities of Biota Seed
Sweet, Neutral Energy
Treats Heart, Kidney, and Large-Intestine and Spleen Organ Systems
Category: Herb that Nourishes the Heart and Calms the Spirit (see page 355)

Biota seed, a gentle sedative herb, treats irritability, forgetfulness, insomnia and palpitations accompanied by anxiety, night sweats, constipation in the elderly, and debilitation in postpartum women. Biota *leaf* stimulates the uterus and is contraindicated for pregnant women; however, it is prescribed for arthritis pain, as well as for premature balding.

Contraindications: Persons suffering from loose stools or excess mucus should avoid biota seed. According to some traditional sources, biota should not be combined with chrysanthemum flower.

Herbal Combinations Using Biota Seed

Biota, *schisandra* and *oyster shell* treat night sweats due to Yin Deficiency.

Polygala, zizyphus seeds, and biota are combined to eliminate insomnia and palpitations due to anxiety (Heart Blood Deficiency in Oriental terms).

Other Herbs that Nourish the Heart and Calm the Spirit

If the healing properties of biota are not quite right for your condition, please see other herbs in this category: *Polygala, Zizyphus Seed*
Maximum Daily Dosage: 5 to 18 grams
1/5 ounce to 2/3 ounce

Bupleurum Root
A Great Aid for the Liver
English Name: Hare's Ear Root
Botanical Name: *Bupleurum scorzoneraefolium, B. chinensis*

A Brief History of Bupleurum
Mandarin: Chái Hú; **Japanese:** Saiko; **Korean:** Siho

There are approximately 100 species of bupleurum, including annuals, perennials, and evergreen shrubs that grow throughout temperate Asia, North America, and Europe. Bupleurum's woody rootstock gives rise to hollow stems that bear narrow stem leaves. Tiny yellow flowers are borne in umbels from late summer through autumn.

B. scorzoneraefolium, or *B. chinensis,* was first mentioned in classical Chinese medical texts around A.D. 200. Its light, brittle roots are long and contorted. Good quality roots should snap easily to reveal pale-brown and white wood. They should be thick and long and slightly aromatic. Taste a small piece of the bupleurum root—the flavor should be slightly bitter. Medicinal quality root comes to us from a number of provinces in China.

Healing Qualities of Bupleurum

Bitter, Slightly Spicy, Cool Energy
Treats Liver and Gall Bladder Organ Systems
Category: Herb that Releases Exterior Conditions (see page 344)

A bitter herb that has antiviral effects and lowers fevers, bupleurum is also a liver and circulatory tonic. It is taken raw with wine for feverish illnesses and with vinegar to stimulate circulation. Bupleurum is also administered internally for malaria, menstrual disorders, emotional instability, dizziness, vertigo, abdominal bloating, herpes simplex, hemorrhoids, and uterine and rectal prolapse. Herbalists refer to bupleurum as a liver dredge because it effectively treats a sluggish liver (frequently associated with emotional instability).

In Oriental terms, bupleurum treats Lesser Yang Heat patterns with such symptoms as alternating chills and fever, flank pain, irritability, a bitter taste in the mouth, vomiting, and a sense of chest constriction.

Herbal Combinations Using Bupleurum

Bupleurum, a drying herb, is frequently combined with moistening herbs such as *dang gui* or *lycii berries* to help counteract its drying action.

Bupleurum combined with *peony root (white)* treats menstrual irregularity, costal pain, vertigo, and dizziness that is the result of Liver Qi Congestion or Obstruction.

Ligusticum and *dang gui* are combined with bupleurum to Harmonize the Blood.

Bupleurum and *licorice root* treat hepatitis and pain in the liver area.

Mint and bupleurum are useful for emotional instability acompanied by a feeling of chest constriction and irregular menstrual cycle due to obstructed Deficient Liver Blood.

Note: There are a number of classical bupleurum formulas that are excellent for various female complaints, from irregular cycles to menopausal symptoms. See Chapter 4.

Contraindications: Occasionally, bupleurum may cause nausea or vomiting. Simply reduce the dosage. Persons with dry coughs or Liver Fire Rising to the head (symptoms might include severe headaches and red eyes) should not take bupleurum. In this case, check if the healing qualities of cyperus are not more appropriate for your condition.

Other Herbs that Release Exterior Conditions

If the healing properties of bupleurum are not quite right for your condition, please see the other herbs in this category: *Chrysanthemum flower, Cohosh, Peppermint, Pueraria*

Maximum Daily Dosage: 3 to 5 grams
1/10 ounce to 1/5 ounce

Cardamom Seed (White)

Eases Nausea

Botanical Name: Amomum cardamomum

A Brief History of White Cardamom Seed

Mandarin: Bái Dòu Kòu; **Japanese:** Byakuzuku; **Korean:** Paektugu

Several species of cardamom make up this aromatic genus that belongs to the ginger family. They produce orchid-like flowers on dense spikes that attach to short, leafy stalks at the base of the plant. Like many orchids, cardamom plants prefer minimum temperatures of about 64°F. This tender rhizomatous perennial has reedlike stems that can reach up to 10 feet in height. *Elettaria cardamomum,* known as "true cardamom," possesses the most pleasant flavor. However, *Amomum cardamomum* is considered the superior medicinal herb.

Round, brownish-white or tan-colored cardamom fruits easily break into three equal portions to reveal irregular light- to dark-brown seeds. Each of the three portions or compartments holds seven to ten seeds. Look for cardamom fruits that are full, large, and unbroken.

──────── ▲ ────────

Healing Qualities of White Cardamom Seed

Spicy, Warm Aromatic Energy
Treats Lung, Spleen, and Stomach Organ Systems
Category: Aromatic Herb that Transforms Dampness (see page 349)

In Traditional Oriental Medicine, white cardamom seed belongs to a category of herbs that "Transform Dampness." This type of dampness is one that settles into our Middle Burner or Stomach and Spleen area giving rise to such symptoms as a sensation of fullness or congestion—as if the food is just sitting there and not digesting. Cardamom helps break up that Qi Stagnation, causing it to descend. Cardamom is useful to stop vomiting and lack of appetite that results from Deficient Spleen and Stomach Cold conditions.

In Western terms, this spicy, warming herb stimulates appetite, controls nausea and vomiting, and relieves indigestion. Cardamom helps relieve the symptoms of irritable bowel syndrome and morning sickness.

Contraindications: Do not use cardamom in cases of Yin and Blood Deficiency and use it cautiously with persons who do not have Cold Damp symptoms.

Other Herbs that Transform Dampness

If the healing properties of cardamom are not quite right for your condition please see other herbs in this category: *Agastache, Magnolia Bark*

Herbal Combinations Using Cardamom Seed

Cardamom seed is often used in conjunction with *orange peel* for belching, nausea, vomiting, diarrhea, and sensation of abdominal fullness due to Spleen and Stomach Deficiency and Accumulation of Dampness.

For poor appetite and epigastric pain due to Cold Dampness or Food Congestion, cardamom seed is combined with *agastache.*

Cardamom seed and *magnolia bark* are combined to treat Congested Qi or Cold Dampness that has accumulated in the Middle Burner (Spleen and Stomach and Small Intestine area of the body).

Ginger and cardamom seed help relieve morning sickness.

Maximum Daily Dosage: 1.5 to 3 grams
1/20 ounce to 1/10 ounce

Chrysanthemum Flower

Soothes and Brightens the Eyes

Botanical Name: Chrysanthemum morifolium

A Brief History of Chrysanthemum

Mandarin: Jú Hua; **Japanese:** Kikuka; **Korean:** Kukhwa

There are approximately 20 species of aromatic perennials that were once classified as *Chrysanthemum* but are now named *Dendranthema.* The popular florists' variety, *dendranthema x grandiflorum,* as well as the medicinal variety come from a hybrid group that were grown in China prior to 500 B.C.

Florists' chrysanthemums came to the West from China in the eighteenth century. First mentioned in classical Chinese medical texts in the first century A.D., chrysanthemum leaves and flowers have long been a part of Oriental cuisine. Edible leaves are called "chop suey greens."

Medicinal quality chrysanthemum flowers come from China and should be intact and bright-yellow colored.

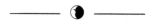

Healing Qualities of Chrysanthemum

Sweet, Slightly Bitter, Slightly Cold Energy
Treats Lung and Liver Organ Systems
Category: Cool, Spicy Herb that Releases Exterior Conditions (see page 344)

Chrysanthemum is taken internally to relieve hypertension, angina, and coronary artery disease (it dilates the coronary artery, thus increasing blood flow to the heart). This herb has antibiotic properties, soothes inflammations, reduces fevers, and is used to treat feverish colds. It is used for liver-related disorders (including headaches). Chrysanthemum relieves red, itchy, irritated eyes due to strain or allergy.

Herbal Combinations Using Chrysanthemum

This herb has recently been used by itself to treat hypertension or as an infusion with *dandelion root* and *honeysuckle flowers*.

Dandelion root, honeysuckle flowers, and chrysanthemum flowers are used to treat furuncles.

Note: Flowers are steamed in China prior to drying to reduce bitterness.

Contraindications: Chrysanthemum is the most gentle of herbs; it is considered nontoxic. However, a few people may find it to be a skin allergen.

Other Cool, Spicy Herbs that Release Exterior Conditions

If the healing properties of chrysanthemum flowers are not quite right for your condition, please see other herbs in this category: *Bupleurum, Cohosh, Peppermint, Pueraria*

Maximum Daily Dosage: 3 to 10 grams
1/10 ounce to 1/3 ounce

Cimicifuga see Cohosh, Black

Cinnamon Bark

Rekindles that Inner Flame

Botanical Name: *Cinnamomum cassia*

A Brief History of Cinnamon Bark

Mandarin: Ròu Guì; **Japanese:** Nikkei; **Korean:** Yukkye

There are more than 250 species of evergreen shrubs and trees belonging to the genus of Cinnamomum that provide two widely used, yet very different commodities—camphor and cinnamon. Camphor is used in the manufacture of medicinal oils that are applied externally to relieve joint and muscle aches and pains. As a balm, it is applied to chapped lips and cold sores, and as an oil, it is rubbed on the chest and back of cold sufferers. Camphor is a major ingredient in the manufacture of mothballs.

C. zeylanicum, the source of our popular cinnamon spice, comes from Sri Lanka and southern India. Cinnamon, without a doubt, is one of the world's oldest spices. The use of cinnamon was first recorded in China in 2700 B.C. and later in Egypt in 1600 B.C. By the fourteenth century, cinnamon bark was being used in Europe, not as a table spice, but to mull wine as well as to produce incense, drugs, and oil. In 1536, the Portuguese invaded Ceylon to monopolize cinnamon production. The Dutch began cultivating cinnamon in 1770 and dominated its world trade from 1796 through 1833.

A native to lowland China, *C. Cassia* is widely used in Oriental medicine. It is considered by the Chinese to be one of the "five spices"—along with anise, star anise, cloves, and fennel seeds. Medicinal-quality cinnamon bark comes to us from three provinces in China—Guangdong, Guangxi, and Yunnan. It is dark reddish brown in color unless the cork has not been stripped off, in which case it is brown. Look for bark with a strong aroma and a full, sweet, spicy taste.

———— ☀ ————

Healing Qualities Cinnamon Bark

Spicy, Sweet, Hot Energy
Treats Heart, Kidney, Liver, and Spleen Organ Systems
Category: Herb that Warms the Interior and Expels Cold (see page 351)

The inner bark of *C. cassia* is very hot, sweet, and spicy—it fortifies Yang energy. Cinnamon bark stimulates circulation, relieves spasms and vomiting, improves digestion, controls chronic diarrhea, and curbs infections. In Oriental medicine, the heating energies of cinnamon bark are used to Tonify the Kidney and Adrenal system in cases of low vitality, cold, weak legs and back, impotence, spermatorrhea, and rheumatism. It is used to treat gynecological symptoms that stem from deep inner Cold conditions, including painful menses.

Cinnamon bark is often used as a supporting herb in chronic cases of Qi and Blood Deficiency.

See Cinnamon Twigs, which follows.

Herbal Combinations Using Cinnamon Bark

Cinnamon bark and *aconite* are used to restore failing Kidney Yang energy.

Ginseng, rehmannia, and cinnamon bark are combined to treat Deficient Heart and Kidney conditions with shortness of breath and palpitations.

Astragalus and cinnamon bark are combined to treat Yin boils, which are chronic sores that ooze clear liquid and are usually concave. This combination also treats Blood and Qi Deficiency.

Cinnamon bark and *dang gui* are used for painful or absent menses due to Cold Deficiency patterns.

Contraindications: Cinnamon bark is a very hot herb and should not be used if there are any Heat symptoms, by persons with Yin Deficiency, or during pregnancy.

Other Herbs that Warm the Interior and Expel Cold

If the healing properties of cinnamon bark are not quite right for your condition, please see other herbs in this category: *Aconite, Fennel Seeds, Ginger*

Maximum Daily Dosage: 1 to 5 grams

1/25 ounce to 1/5 ounce

Cinnamon Twigs

Bring that Cold or Flu to the Surface

Botanical Name: *Cinnamomum cassia*

A Brief History of Cinnamon Twigs

Mandarin: Gùi Zhi; **Japanese:** Keishi; **Korean:** Kyechi

Please see preceding history of Cinnamon Bark.

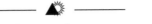

Healing Qualities of Cinnamon Twigs

Spicy, Sweet, Warm
Treats Heart, Lung, and Bladder Organ Systems
Category: Warm, Spicy Herb that Releases Exterior Conditions (see page 344)

Cinnamon twigs (considered less warming than bark), are often used for acute cold and flu symptoms. This is especially true where sweating occurs but there is no improvement in the patient's condition. Cinnamon twigs are used to stimulate circulation and warm cold hands, feet, and joints. Twigs are said to strengthen Heart Yang energy and stop palpitations due to Deficiency. Cinnamon twigs are often used in herbal formulas for gynecological problems such as painful cramping.

Contraindications: Do not take cinnamon twigs in case of high fevers, Heat symptoms accompanying Yin Deficiency, or during pregnancy.

Herbal Combinations Using Cinnamon Twigs

Peony root (white) is often combined with cinnamon twigs to treat cold and flu symptoms with chills and low fevers as well as to warm and Tonify the Middle Burner (Stomach and Spleen and Small Intestine area of the body).

Cinnamon twigs are combined with *aconite* to treat cold, painful hands and feet.

Toasted licorice root and cinnamon twigs treat shortness of breath and palpitations due to Yang Deficiency in the Upper Burner (upper chest region).

Other Warm, Spicy Herbs that Release Exterior Conditions

If the healing properties of cinnamon twigs are not quite right for your condition, please see other herbs in this category: *Ephedra, Ginger (Fresh), Magnolia Flower*

Maximum Daily Dosage: 1.5 to 5 grams
1/20 ounce to 1/5 ounce

Clematis
Helps Say Good-bye to Rheumatism and Gout
English Name: *Chinese Clematis Root*
Botanical Name: *Clematis chinensis*

A Brief History of Clematis
Mandarin: Wei Líng Xian; **Japanese:** Ireisen; **Korean:** Wôjôksum

Most of us are familiar with the beautiful variety of showy flowers produced by ornamental clematis that grow in our gardens. In Greek, the word *klematis* means "climbing plant." There are about 230 species of clematis, mostly found in temperate regions. A few species are used medicinally in homeopathic remedies for skin eruptions and rheumatism including *C. recta* and *C. vitalba,* both found in Europe. *C. vitalba,* was called "beggar's weed" in France because beggars would irritate their skins, simulating sores in order to gain sympathy and a possible hand-out. Clematis contain glycosides, a plant constituent that creates a blistering effect and burning taste. The Australian Aborigines use *C. glycinoides* as a traditional cold and headache remedy. The spicy fragrance of clematis foliage, when inhaled, causes profuse watering of the eyes and nose.

    C. chinensis grows in central and western China and bears panicles of fragrant small white flowers that are produced in fall. This species has been used medicinally in the Orient for well over 1,000 years. Numerous clematis roots are bound together on a root tuber. Good-quality roots are brown, long, and firm—it is best if no woody stem remains attached to the tuber; their fragrance is slightly fetid. Most medicinal quality herb comes to us from China's provinces of Anhui, Jiangsu, and Zhejiang.

Healing Qualities of Clematis
Spicy, Salty, Warm, Poisonous Energy
Treats Urinary Bladder Organ System
Category: Herb that Expels Wind Dampness (see page 347)

Clematis is a spicy, warming herb that has sedative and painkilling qualities. It is frequently taken with wine to dispel Wind-Damp conditions such as arthritis and rheumatism. Clematis lowers fevers, relieves spasms, has diuretic properties, and is used to treat malarial disease, gout, tonsillitis, and pain due to Cold that has settled in the knees and lower back.

Herbal Combinations Using Clematis

Clematis is combined with *achyranthes* to treat joint pain in the lower back and extremities.

Cardamom and clematis relieve epigastric pain.

Caution: Harmful if eaten; also mild irritant to the skin. Clematis should not be taken by persons with Deficient Qi and Blood.

Other Herbs that Expel Wind Dampness

If the healing properties of clematis are not quite right for your condition, please see other herbs in this category: *Cocklebur Fruit, Du Huo*
Maximum Daily Dosage: 3 to 10 grams
1/10 ounce to 1/3 ounce

Cocklebur Fruit

Great for Sinusitis, Rhinitis, and Lumbago!
Botanical Name: *Xanthium sibiricum or X. strumarium*

A Brief History of Cocklebur Fruit

Mandarin: Cang Er Zi; **Japanese:** Sojishi; **Korean:** Ch'angija

There are only two species of Xanthium. *X. strumarium* can be found growing from Europe to eastern Asia. Its spiny burs cling to anything that passes—the furry coats of creatures or human clothing. While cocklebur is subject to statutory weed control in parts of Australia, it has been used as medicine in the Orient for hundreds of years.

Back on our small farm in Kansas, I was often sent out on "cocklebur weed patrol." What a task! I could never understand why there was any room in creation for such a thorny plant. But, yes, Oriental medicine found a good use for what is considered a rather rude, invasive "weed" by most us. First mentioned around A.D. 618-907 in the *Thousand Ducat Prescriptions,* cocklebur is a common ingredient in Chinese Patent medicines.

The seed of the cocklebur is light gray in color and found inside a tough, thorny yellow- to brownish-green-colored outer shell. Most medicinal-quality herb comes to us from Shandong, Jiangxi, Hubei, and Jiangsu, China. Look for full, yellow fruits. Cocklebur is poisonous; it is stir-fried to remove the toxin.

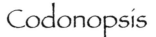

Healing Qualities of Cocklebur
Sweet, Slightly Bitter, Warm, Poisonous Energy
Treats Lung Organ System
Category: Herb that Dispels Wind Dampness (see page 347)

Cocklebur is a rather pleasant-tasting herb that relieves pain and relaxes spasms (particularly in rheumatoid arthritis, rheumatism, and lumbago). It has antifungal and antibacterial properties and is taken internally for relief of sinusitis, allergic rhinitis, toothache, and excess mucus. It is often used as an assisting herb in cold and flu formulas accompanied by splitting headaches that tend to wrap around the head to the back of the neck.

Contraindications: Cocklebur should not be used by persons with Deficient Blood.

Herbal Combinations Using Cocklebur Fruit

Magnolia flower is combined with cocklebur to treat headache and sinusitis or rhinitis.

Cocklebur and *clematis* treat Wind Damp conditions such as lumbago and rheumatism.

Other Herbs that Expel Wind Dampness

If the healing properties of cocklebur are not quite right for your condition, please see other herbs in this category: *Du Huo, Clematis*

Maximum Daily Dosage: 5 to 10 grams

1/5 ounce to 1/3 ounce

Codonopsis
Combats Stress and Fatigue
Botanical Name: Codonopsis pilosula

A Brief History of Codonopsis
Mandarin: Dang Shen; **Japanese:** Tojin; **Korean:** Tangsam

In Greek, *Codonopsis* means "bell-like." Codonopsis is an attractive twining climber with whitish-yellow to olive-green bell-shaped flowers that have purple spots or veins (particularly visible on the inside of the bell). When crushed, its heart-shaped leaves have a strong fragrance. There are approximately 30 species of codonopsis found growing throughout the Himalayas to Japan.

C. tangshen is cultivated extensively in upland fields in China for medicinal use. Considered a superior herb by the Chinese, it is sometimes substituted for *Panax ginseng*. These wrinkled brown roots are light and supple—they snap with difficulty to reveal a lighter tan-colored interior. Look for clean, firm, thick, tight-skinned roots that are sweet-flavored.

——— 🜩 ———

Healing Qualities of Codonopsis
Sweet, Neutral Energy
Treats Spleen and Lung Organ Systems
Category: Herb that Tonifies the Qi (see page 352)

A sweet, soothing herb that is less stimulating and less expensive than ginseng, codonopsis strengthens the immune system, lowers blood pressure, fights fatigue, improves appetite and digestion, and helps alleviate anemia. Codonopsis strengthens the lungs and is used to treat bronchitis. It is a particularly effective herb in combating debility after illness.

In Oriental medicine, ginseng is generally used to combat more serious disorders such as Collapsed Qi and Yang. In contrast, codonopsis is considered a better herbal ally to treat normal, day-to-day kinds of stresses and fatigue.

Contraindications: None noted.

Herbal Combinations Using Codonopsis

Codonopsis is combined with *astragalus* to create a powerful immune-enhancing formula that treats fatigue, poor appetite, shortness of breath, and diarrhea.

Dang gui and codonopsis treat general weakness, fatigue, and dizziness associated with Deficient Qi and Blood.

When it comes to codonopsis, like astragalus, you can cook with your cure. Add a root or two to your favorite chicken- or bean-soup recipe. But don't throw out the tasty codonopsis root once the soup's done. It can be eaten along with the other veggies.

Other Herbs that Tonify Qi

If the healing properties of codonopsis are not quite right for your condition, please see other herbs in this category: *Atractylodes, Ginseng, Astragalus, Dioscorea, Jujube Date Fruit, Licorice*

Maximum Daily Dosage: 5 to 10 grams
1/5 ounce to 1/3 ounce

Cohosh (Black)

Brings Rashes to the Surface

English Name: Bugbane or Black Cohosh Rhizome
Botanical Name: *Cimicifuga foetida, C. dahurica* or *C. heracleifolia*

A Brief History of Black Cohosh

Mandarin: Sheng Má; **Japanese:** Shoma; **Korean:** Sûngma

Cimicifuga, or black cohosh, is also known as "bugbane"; its Latin name, when translated, means *cimex,* "bug," and *fugere,* "to run away." As its name implies, this herb is commonly used to repel insects. Cimicifuga is a hardy perennial belonging to a genus of 15 species found in northern temperate regions. Also known as "squawroot," *C. racemosa* was traditionally used by Native North Americans for female complaints. A number of different species are used interchangeably for similar purposes.

The cohosh rhizome is very irregular in shape, light, hard, and not easily broken. Its surface is brownish-black in color, often with some fine roots attached. Slices of the rhizome reveal porous, yellowish-white wood. Look for clean, large, black rhizomes with the hair removed.

———— ◗ ————

Healing Qualities of Cohosh

Sweet, Spicy, Cool Energy
Treats Large-Intestine, Lung, Spleen and Stomach Organ Systems
Category: Herb that Releases Exterior Conditions (see page 344)

In the Orient, cimicifuga is used in the early stages of measles to encourage the rash to come to the surface. It helps combat Stomach Heat symptoms, which include canker sores, sore or painful teeth and gums, ulcerated gums or lips, or swollen throat. It is also used to raise the Yang Qi and counteract prolapse of internal organs such as the bladder and uterus.

Black cohosh is effective in treating menstrual and menopausal problems; it also relieves labor and postpartum pains and arthritic, rheumatic, and sciatica pains. More specifically, *C. dauhurica* and *C. foetida* lower fevers and relieve pain and are taken internally for colds, coughs, headaches, feverish infections (measles), and gum disease. *C. racemosa* controls coughs, lowers fevers, soothes aches and pains, and stimulates uterine muscles.

Note: This herb is legally restricted in some countries.

Contraindications: Not to be taken by persons with fully erupted measles or who have difficulty breathing. To be avoided by persons with Heat conditions that are due to Yin Deficiency. Taken in excess, this herb can cause nausea and vomiting.

Herbal Combinations Using Black Cohosh

Bupleurum and black cohosh, in combination, treat rectal and uterine prolapse due to Yang Qi Deficiency. They are also effective in combating chronic dysentery-like illnesses.

Other Herbs that Release Exterior Conditions

If the healing properties of black cohosh are not quite right for your condition, please see other herbs in this category: *Bupleurum, Chrysanthemum Flower, Peppermint, Pueraria*

Maximum Daily Dosage: 3 to 5 grams

1/10 ounce to 1/5 ounce

Coíx

Eases Joint Pain

English Name: Seeds of Job's Tears
Botanical Name: *Coix lachryma-jobi*

A Brief History of Coix

Mandarin: Yì Yi Rén; **Japanese:** Yokuinin; **Korean:** Uiiin

Since antiquity, Job's tears, or coix, has been grown as an ornamental. An upright robust annual or perennial grass, six species make up this tropical Asian swamp-loving genus. Green tear-shaped female flowers are enclosed in a hard husk that later turns to gray or grayish-mauve in the fall. Male flowers appear in clusters at the end of a flower spike. In the Orient, coix seeds are often used as beads to make jewelry. Coix was eaten as a dietary staple in ages past, in much the same way rice is eaten today and is still consumed in Southeast Asian countries.

Most Coix comes from the Fujian, Hebei, and Liaoning provinces of China. The seeds are white to yellowish-white in color. They are smooth, with the exception of a broad, deep, rough, light-brown groove that runs lengthwise; at the base is a dark-brown spot. Look for big, unbroken, plump white seeds.

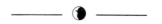

Healing Qualities of Coix

Sweet, Bland, Cool Energy
Treats Spleen, Lung, and Kidney Organ Systems
Category: Herb that Drain Dampness (see page 347)

In Oriental herbal medicine, the properties of coix are considered to be sweet, bland, and cooling. It is taken in raw, powdered form to reduce edema, increase joint mobility, stop muscle spasms in chronic conditions, and clear Damp Heat. It is often stir-fried for use in the treatment of digestive problems.

One herbal prescription, known as Coix Combination, comes to us from the Tang dynasty, 652 A.D.; it has been used for more than thirteen centuries in the treatment of rheumatoid arthritis (see Chapter 4 for this formula). Coix reduces inflammation, lowers fevers, and controls bacterial and fungal infections. It is considered a spleen tonic and has sedative effects. Blood-sugar levels are reduced with large doses of Coix.

Contraindications: Coix should be used with caution during pregnancy.

Herbal Combinations Using Coix

Coix is combined with *Poria cocos* and *Atractylodis macrocephalae* to treat diarrhea resulting from Spleen Defiency.

Ephedra, apricot kernel, and *licorice root* are combined with coix to treat generalized body pain.

In Chaper 5, you will find my favorite Spring Green Lentil and Barley Soup recipe that calls for coix.

Other Herbs that Drain Dampness

If the healing properties of coix are not quite right for your condition, please see other herbs in this category: *Aduki bean, Alisma, Dioscorea, Poria Cocos, Stephania, Zhu Ling*

Maximum Daily Dosage: 10 to 30 grams
1/3 ounce to 1 ounce

Coltsfoot

Stops Coughing and Wheezing

Botanical Name: Tussilago farfara

A Brief History of Coltsfoot

Mandarin: Kuan Dong Hua; **Japanese:** Kantoka; **Korean:** Kwandonghwa

Coltsfoot was smoked as a cough remedy by Native Americans, while the smoke of coltsfoot leaves and roots, burned over cypress charcoal, was swallowed rather than inhaled by ancient Romans. There are 15 species of coltsfoot found growing in northern temperate regions in Europe, and in northern Africa and Asia. *T. farfara* is a very robust creeping perennial with yellow dandelion-like flowers that appear in the early spring on wool-ly, scaly stalks before the large heart-shaped to rounded, toothed leaves appear.

The leaves of coltsfoot can be eaten raw in salads or added to stir-fries or soups; the flowers can be used to make wine. Coltsfoot leaves are used in curing pipe tobaccos as well as an ingredient in herbal tobaccos. In traditional Oriental herbalism, only the coltsfoot flowers are used. When dry, the buds resemble a rough-looking club, being full at the tip and tapering toward the stalk. Look for large mauve-colored buds without stalks.

———— ▲☀ ————

Healing Qualities of Coltsfoot

Spicy, Warm Energy
Treats Lung Organ System
Category: Herb that Transforms Phlegm and Stops Coughing (see page 348)

Coltsfoot has a bittersweet, licorice-like flavor and is used in Oriental herbalism to direct Qi downwards. It soothes irritated tissues, reduces inflammation, and relaxes spasms while stimulating the immune system.

Coltsfoot is taken internally to treat coughs, asthma, bronchitis, whooping cough, and excess phlegm.

Contraindications: This herb should not be used in cases of Lung Heat with Yin Deficiency. It should be used cautiously in treating any coughs accompanied by Heat symptoms. In some countries, this herb is subject to legal restrictions. While coltsfoot contains pyrrolizidine alkaloids, tests have shown it to be nontoxic at low dosages.

Herbal Combinations Using Coltsfoot

Apricot kernel and coltsfoot are combined to treat coughing and wheezing due to excess mucus.

Coltsfoot is combined with *lily bulb* to treat dry (Yin Deficient) coughs with bloody sputum.

Other Herbs that Relieve Coughing and Wheezing

If the healing properties of coltsfoot are not quite right for your condition, please see other herbs in this category: *Almond Kernel, Mulberry Root Bark*
Maximum Daily Dosage: 5 to 10 grams
1/5 ounce to 1/3 ounce

Coptis

Controls Bacterial and Viral Infections

English Name: Coptis Rhizome or Golden Thread
Botanical Name: *Coptis chinensis, C. deltoidea, C. omeiensis,* or *C. teetoides*

A Brief History of Coptis

Mandarin: Húang Lían; **Japanese:** Oren; **Korean:** Hwangnyôn

Sometimes grown in rock gardens for its anemone-like flowers, coptis is a moisture-loving, low-growing perennial found distributed throughout the northern temperate regions. Fine yellow roots grow near the surface of the ground, giving coptis its common English name of "goldthread." Coptis roots contain bright yellow pigments used in dyeing. There are a total of ten species of coptis; at least five of these have been used medicinally.

C. trifolia (Indian goldthread) was used by many Native North American tribes to treat inflammations of the eyes and mouth. *C. Chinensis* is found mentioned in ancient Chinese medical texts dating back to A.D. 200. Native to damp coniferous wood and bogs in China, *C. chinensis* bears three to four small yellow-white flowers.

Irregularly shaped coptis rhizomes are brownish-yellow in color and often resemble the closed foot of a chicken. Thin slices of the rhizome are quite porous, and the inner wood is bright yellow in color. Look for clean, long, heavily noded rhizomes without hair. Most medicinal-quality coptis comes from the Sichuan, Hubei, and Shaanxi provinces of China.

——— ● ———

Healing Qualities of Coptis
Bitter, Cold Energy
Treats Heart, Liver, Stomach, and Large Intestine Organ Systems
Category: Herb that Clears Heat and Dries Dampness (see page 345)

Coptis is a very bitter, cold herb that Clears Fire and Dries Dampness. It is used to control viral and bacterial infections. Coptis stimulates circulation, lowers fevers, and relaxes spasms. Coptis is a specific herbal aid for "Hot" conditions and is taken internally for high fevers, enteritis, dysentery-like disorders, conjunctivitis, middle-ear infections, and inflammation of the mouth or tongue. Externally it is applied to inflamed mucous membranes in the mouth and eyes. To prepare an excellent gargle or mouthwash to help clear minor sore throats, mouth irritations, or canker sores, simmer 2 ounces of coptis in a quart of water for 30 to 40 minutes; strain the liquid and add 1 teaspoon of glycerin or honey if desired. Refrigerate the liquid for up to three days and warm as needed.

Contraindications: Prolonged use of coptis can injure the Spleen and Stomach. It should not be used in Yin-Deficient patterns or given to patients with Cold-Deficient Spleen and Stomach or Kidney Organ Systems.

Herbal Combinations Using Coptis

Coptis is combined with *rehmannia* to treat insomnia and delirium due to excess Heat conditions.

Saussurea root is combined with coptis to treat Hot dysentery-like disorders.

Other Herbs that Clear Heat and Dry Dampness

If the healing properties of coptis are not quite right for your condition, please see other herbs in this category: *Gentian, Phellodendron, Scutellaria, Sophora Maximum Daily Dosage:* 1 to 3 grams
1/30 ounce to 1/10 ounce

Cornus
Stops Night Sweats
English Name: Asiatic Cornelian Cherry Fruit
Botanical Name: *Cornus officinalis*

A Brief History of Cornus

Mandarin: Shan Yú Ròu or Shan Zhu Yú; **Japanese:** Sanyuniku; **Korean:** Sansuyôk

Grown mostly as ornamentals, cornus shrubs or trees produce tiny yellow flowers along bare branches in late winter. These flowers later turn into bright-red cornelian cherries. *C. officinalis* was first described in Chinese medical texts around A.D. 200. Other species that have been used therapeutically include *C. sericea*, American red osier, which is traditionally used to treat diarrhea, vomiting, and indigestion. The fruit of *C. florida*, flowering dogwood, relieves tension headaches and serves as a tonic for nervous exhaustion.

The dried cornus fruit is wrinkled and purplish red to black in color with a glossy, translucent skin. The flesh should be sticky and soft. Look for plump, shiny, dark-red fruit with a good strong sour flavor that makes you pucker.

Healing Qualities of Cornus
Sour, Slightly Warm Energy
Treats Liver and Kidney Organ Systems
Category: Astringent Herb that Stabilizes and Binds (see page 354)

Cornelian cherry fruits have sour, astringent, and slightly warming qualities. This herb acts mainly on the Liver and Kidneys as an energy tonic aiding urinary dysfunction and impotence, excessive menstruation, and nocturnal sweats (especially in cases of extreme Yang and Qi Deficiency). It relieves the pain associated with a weak lower back and knees, dizziness, ringing in the ears, and loss of hearing. Cornus also lowers blood pressure, controls bacterial and fungal infections, and helps stop bleeding. It is used in cases of Deficiency with excessive or prolonged menstruation.

Contraindications: Not to be used by persons with difficult or painful urination. Cornus should be used cautiously by persons with Kidney Yang Deficiency.

Herbal Combinations Using Cornus

Rehmannia, dioscorea, and cornus are combined to treat frequent urination, dizziness, lower-back pain, and ringing in the ears.

Cornus and *schisandra* treat palpitations, shortness of breath, and abnormal sweating due to Liver and Kidney Yin and Yang Deficiency.

Other Astringent Herbs that Stabilize and Bind

If the healing properties of cornus are not quite right for your condition, please see other herbs in this category: *Ginkgo, Pomegranate Husk, Schisandra*
Maximum Daily Dosage: 5 to 10 grams
1/5 ounce to 1/3 ounce

Cuscuta

Treats Impotence and Helps Prevent Miscarriage

English Name: Dodder Seeds
Botanical Name: *Cuscuta chinensis* or *C. japonica*

A Brief History of Cuscuta

Mandarin: Tû Si Zi; **Japanese:** Toshishi; **Korean:** T'osacha

Cuscuta is an unusual parasitic plant that has no roots or green parts—it penetrates its host plant with a threadlike stem used to siphon off nutrients. Cuscuta leaves resemble scales, and the pale yellow stems are striped or red-spotted. Cuscuta prefers temperate and warm regions and is found growing at low altitudes in eastern Asia. *C. japonica* produces numerous pale-yellow, bell-shaped flowers on short spikes in the late summer. Descriptions of *C. japonica* appear in first century A.D. Chinese medical literature based on texts from 1500 B.C. Common dodder *(C. epithymum)* was once a popular cure used by European herbalists to treat "melancholy diseases" and disorders of the liver, spleen, and kidneys.

Tiny, uncooked cuscuta seeds are a light tan color while those that have been steamed are light brown to brownish-red in color. Cuscuta seeds are quite hard, making them difficult to break. Look for clean, plump seeds.

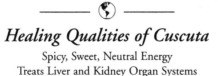

Healing Qualities of Cuscuta

Spicy, Sweet, Neutral Energy
Treats Liver and Kidney Organ Systems
Category: Herb that Tonifies the Yang (see page 353)

Cuscuta seeds act mainly as a stimulant to the Kidneys and Liver; they are used specifically to treat Deficient Kidney Yang and increase the Yin with symptoms such as nocturnal emission, premature ejaculation, vaginal discharge, ringing in the ears, frequent urination, or a painful lower back. Cuscuta is taken internally to aid poor eyesight (blurred vision and spots before the eyes) due to energy weakness of Liver and Kidneys. This gentle herb helps stop diarrhea due to Spleen and Kidney Deficiency. Cuscuta is also an important herbal ally to help prevent miscarriage.

Contraindications: Cuscuta is considered a neutral herb but has the tendency to Tonify the Yang more than the Yin. It should not be used by persons with scanty, dark urine or by those persons with Heat symptoms due to Yin Deficiency.

Herbal Combinations Using Cuscuta

Astragalus, lycii berries, and cuscuta treat blurred vision, ringing in the ears, and dizziness.

Cuscuta, *dioscorea,* and *codonopsis* are combined for lack of appetite and diarrhea due to Deficient Kidney and Spleen energy.

Rehmannia, cornus, psoralea, and cuscuta treat Deficient Kidney Yin with lower back pain, premature ejaculation, or spermatorrhea. Deer Antler is added to increase Kidney Yang energy.

Other Herbs that Tonify the Yang

If the healing properties of cuscuta are not quite right for your condition, please see other herbs in this category: *Epimedium, Eucommia, Fenugreek Seed*

> *Maximum Daily Dosage:* 9 to 15 grams
> 1/4 ounce to 1/2 ounce

Cyperus
Relieves Painful, Irregular Menstrual Cycles
English Name: Nut-grass Rhizome or Sedge
Botanical Name: *Cyperus rotundus*

A Brief History of Cyperus
Mandarin: Xiang Fù; **Japanese:** Kobushi; **Korean:** Hyangbu

Cyperus is found growing worldwide—there are more than 600 species of grasslike annuals and perennials in this genus. *C. rotundus* loves damp places and is probably one of the world's most invasive "weeds"; however, it has long been important in both traditional Chinese medicine and in Ayurvedic (East Indian) medicine. Its oval-shaped tubers contain fragrant essential oils. They can be burnt like incense and used as an insect repellent. Other members of the cyperus family include *C. papyrus,* from Egypt, which is used to make Egyptian papyrus paper. The volatile oils in *C. longus* are used in the perfumery industry. *C. articulatus* has an aroma similar to lavender and is used to treat nausea and dyspepsia.

The exterior surface of the cyperus rhizome is purplish black in color and is covered by a number of flat-lying hairs. It is very hard and breaks with great difficulty to reveal a dark brownish-red interior. Look for cyperus slices that are firm, large, reddish in color, and possessing a strong aroma.

—— 🌍 ——

Healing Qualities of Cyperus
Spicy, Slightly Bitter, Sweet, Neutral
Treats Liver and Triple Warmer Organ Systems
Category: Herb that Regulates the Qi (see page 349)

Cyperus is taken internally for digestive complaints that are related to Blocked Liver Energy. Cyperus also treats menstrual irregularities and pain that are, once again, due to blocked or Congested Liver Qi. It relieves pain below the ribs and abdominal distension.

Contraindications: Not to be used by persons with Yin Defiency or Heat in the Blood. Cyperus should not be used by persons with Deficient Qi without Congestion.

Herbal Combinations Using Cyperus
Cyperus and *bupleurum* treat distension and pain in the chest and flanks.

Dang gui and cyperus treat irregular menstruation and pain due to congested Blood and Qi.

Saussurea and cyperus are used to eliminate abdominal pain, indigestion, vomiting, and diarrhea due to Liver and Spleen Organ System Qi Obstructions.

Other Herbs that Regulate Qi
If the healing properties of cyperus are not quite right for your condition, please see other herbs in this category: *Persimmon Calyx, Tangerine Peel*
Maximum Daily Dosage: 5 to 10 grams
1/5 ounce to 1/3 ounce

Dandelion

Eases Joint Pain and Clears Sores and Abscesses

Botanical Name: *Taraxacum mongolicum*

A Brief History of Dandelion

Mandarin: Pú Gong Ying; **Japanese:** Hokoei; **Korean:** P'ogongyông

Dandelion (that poor, humble, life-giving plant we so persecute with pesticides) is grown as a vegetable in many European countries, especially France. In springtime, the Greeks harvest wild dandelion greens to be steamed and served with olive oil and lemon. There are approximately 60 species of Taraxacum growing in northern temperate regions and parts of South America.

Throughout history, many cultures have found multiple uses for dandelion. Its roots are roasted and ground for the manufacture of a caffeine-free coffee substitute. Dandelion roots and leaves are utilized as flavoring for soft drinks and herbal beers. Dandelion flower petals flavor wines, and the steamed greens are consumed in many countries. This healing plant was first mentioned in Chinese medical texts around A.D. 650. Prescribed and praised by Arab physicians in the eleventh century, dandelion became a popular European herb in the late 1400s. *T. officinale* contains large quantities of potassium salts, making it a potent diuretic. The bitter flavor of dandelion makes it one of the best natural digestive aids known. Its healing properties stimulate liver function and help reduce swelling and inflammation. Dandelion's anti-rheumatic effects ease joint pain. So don't kill your cure—steam the greens in spring and harvest the roots in autumn!

————— ● —————

Healing Qualities of Dandelion

Bitter, Sweet, Cold Energy
Treats Liver and Stomach Organ Systems
Category: Herb that Clears Heat and Toxicity (see page 346)

In Traditional Oriental Medicine, dandelion is used to Clear Heat and Detoxify. This group of herbs is often used to treat hot, toxic swellings such as mastitis, appendicitis, pulmonary and breast abscesses, furuncles, and boils, as well as urinary-tract infections and certain viral infections such as mumps. You know that a swelling is "Hot" if it is painful. These herbs have antimicrobial and antiviral effects, reduce inflammation, and also have diuretic qualities.

Dandelion is especially effective in treating red, swollen eyes, mumps, and painful, swollen throats. Dandelion is taken internally for liver and gallbladder complaints, including jaundice, cirrhosis, and gallstones. Because of its high potassium content, dandelion is used to treat edema accompanying high blood pressure and heart weakness. It is also quite effective in treating eczema, acne, constipation, and chronic joint pain due to Excess Heat conditions such as gout.

Contraindications: Do not use dandelion if your symptoms are related to Deficiency Cold patterns.

Herbal Combinations Using Dandelion

Dandelion, *honeysuckle flowers, forsythia fruit,* and *chrysanthemum* flowers treat Hot, painful, deep-rooted sores like boils.

Chrysanthemum, scutellaria, and dandelion treat red, swollen eyes.

Dandelion, *trichosanthes, fritillaria* and *myrrh* are effective in treating carbuncles, furuncles, and breast abscess.

Other Herbs that Clear Heat and Toxicity

If the healing properties of dandelion are not quite right for your condition, please see other herbs in this category: *Forsythia Fruit, Honeysuckle Flower*
Maximum Daily Dosage: 9 to 30 grams
1/4 ounce to 1 ounce

Dang Guí
Is the Queen of Women's Herbs
English Name: Tangkuei Root
Botanical Name: *Angelica sinensis*

A Brief History of Dang Gui
Mandarin: Dang Gui; **Japanese:** Toki; **Korean:** Tanggwi

The use of *Angelica sinensis* as an important tonic herb dates back to about A.D. 200 in China. One of its cousins, *A. archangelica,* was so widely used in Europe during the 15th century that it became known as the most important of all herbs. As one story goes, the "angelic" healing properties of angelica were revealed to a monk in a dream by an angel. Reputed to cure every conceivable disease, including the plague, angelica also warded off evil spirits and witchcraft. It is still eaten as a veggie in the Scandinavian countries and Greenland. Candied, tender young stalks are used for decorating cakes and desserts. Liqueurs are flavored with angelica roots and seeds, and its oils are used in perfumery.

There are approximately 50 biennial and perennial plants belonging to this genus—all natives to temperate regions of the northern hemisphere. Robust, hollow-stemmed angelica plants bear umbels of greenish-white flowers in the springtime. The penetrating fragrance of angelica is reminiscent of that of its close cousin—the celery plant. When shopping for dang gui roots, look for those with a strong smell, pale-yellowish flesh, and large, plump main root. Slices of large roots are usually preferred for herbal prescriptions while small whole knobs are used for making soup. Since a number of varieties of angelica are used medicinally, be sure to specify that you want Angelica *sinensis.*

Healing Qualities of Dang Gui

Sweet, Spicy, Bitter, Warm Energy
Treats Heart, Liver, and Spleen Organ Systems
Category: Herb that Tonifies the Blood (see page 352)

Dang gui is known as the queen of women's herbs because of its ability to tonify and invigorate the entire female system. It nourishes the blood, eliminating anemia and constipation due to anemia; it regulates menses and is used for almost all gynecological problems, including irregular menstruation, dysmenorrhea, and amenorrhea. Dang gui is also used to treat palpitations, ringing in the ears (tinnitus), blurred vision, abdominal pain, dry skin, and skin eruptions. Dang gui increases circulation, treating rheumatic pains and pain from traumatic injury in both men and women.

Contraindications: Avoid the use of dang gui in the presence of diarrhea or Deficient Heat symptoms. Persons suffering from chronic water retention, poor digestion, chronic infection, night sweats, or skin rashes should use this herb with caution.

Herbal Combinations Using Dang Gui

Dang gui and *astragalus* treat weakness, pallor, and/or low-grade fever associated with excessive loss of blood.

Cinnamon twigs, gentian, and dang gui treat absent or painful menses due to Cold.

Salvia and dang gui are combined to treat faulty circulation in the hands and feet.

Honeysuckle, peony root (red), and dang gui eliminate the pain and swelling of sores and abscesses.

Peony root (white), rehmannia (cooked), ligusticum, and dang gui are prescribed for painful and/or irregular menstrual cycles due to anemia or congested blood.

Astragalus, fresh ginger, and dang gui are combined to treat postpartum abdominal pain as well as exhaustion and weakness.

Cook with your cure. If you are anemic, tired, and weak, throw a couple of slices of dang gui into your favorite chicken soup or stew recipe, along with a piece of *codonopsis* and *astragalus.*

Other Herbs that Tonify the Blood

If the healing properties of dang gui are not quite right for your condition, but you need to tonify blood, please see other herbs in this category: *Longan Berries, Lycii Fruit, Peony Root (White), Polygonum, Rehmannia (Cooked)*
Maximum Daily Dosage: 3 to 15 grams
1/10 ounce to 1/2 ounce

Dendrobium

Eases Low Back Pain and Strengthens Vision
Botanical Name: Dendrobium nobile

A Brief History of Dendrobium
Mandarin: Shí Hú; **Japanese:** Sekkoku; **Korean:** Sôkkok

Tree-dwellers by nature, there are more than 1,000 species of lovely dendrobium orchids. *D. nobile* is an alpine perennial native to China, Laos, Thailand, and northeastern India. This lovely plant is cultivated worldwide for its beautiful flowers that smell like fresh grass in the morning, honey at noon, and have the delicate fragrance of primrose at dusk.

Use of dendrobium in the Orient has been traced back to at least 2000 B.C. It was frequently used in Taoist longevity herbal formulations and has the reputation of being an aphrodisiac.

Look for pliable, soft, shiny golden-yellow stems with brown nodes revealing a fibrous interior when snapped. Most medicinal quality herb comes from the Taiwan and Hubei and Sichuan provinces, China.

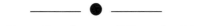

Healing Qualities of Dendrobium
Sweet, Slightly Salty, Bland, Cold Energy
Treats Kidney and Stomach Organ Systems
Category: Herb that Tonifies the Yin (see page 353)

Dendrobium is specifically used to treat Yin-Deficiency conditions. It nourishes the body's fluids, eliminating a parched mouth and severe thirst. It increases salivation. Dendrobium treats Stomach Yin Deficiency with such symptoms as dry heaves, stomach pain, and a shiny tongue with little coating. This herb also treats low back pain, muscular aches and pains, and blurred vision accompanying the later stages of a febrile disease.

Contraindications: This herb should not be used in patients experiencing conditions related to Excess Dampness. Dendrobium is a cold herb and should not be prescribed to weak persons who do not have Heat symptoms.

Herbal Combinations Using Dendrobium

Rehmannia, glehnia, scrophularia, and dendrobium treat conditions associated with the later stages of a febrile disease, which include such symptoms as low-grade fever, blurred vision, thirst, and aching muscles due to lack of body fluids.

Dendrobium, *ophiopogon,* and *trichosanthes* treat dry heaves, abdominal pain, and shiny tongue accompanying Stomach Yin Deficiency.

Achyranthes, lycii berries, and dendrobium are prescribed for a weak, sore lower back due to Kidney Yin Deficiency.

Other Herbs that Tonify the Yin

If the healing properties of dendrobium are not quite right for your condition, please see other herbs in this category: *American Ginseng (see "Ginseng"), Glehnia, Lily Bulb, Ophiopogon*
Maximum Daily Dosage: 5 to 10 grams
1/5 ounce to 1/3 ounce

Dioscorea
Helps Overcome Weakness and Fatigue
English Name: Chinese Yam Root
Botanical Name: *Dioscorea opposita*

A Brief History of Dioscorea

Mandarin: Shan Yào; **Japanese:** Sanyaku; **Korean:** Sanyak

Dioscorea gets it botanical name from Dioscorides, a famous Greek naturalist and physician who lived during the first or second century A.D. However, its common name, "yam," comes to us from the West African dialect and means "eat." During the mid-1800s, when Europe was threatened by the potato blight, this Oriental yam became the subject of experimentation as a possible potato substitute. The Dioscorea genus is composed of about 600 species of tropical and subtropical twining climbers. *D. opposita* is probably the hardiest of the commercially cultivated yams that thrive in northern parts of Japan, Korea, and China. Some dioscorea are grown exclusively as ornamentals, while many are cultivated for food in warm regions. One species, *D. alata* (white yam) produces large edible tubers that can reach up to 50 kilos, or 110 pounds.

Many species of dioscorea yam are used by the pharmaceutical industry in the preparation of steroids. One species of Mexican yam *(D. macrostachya)* was the only source of diosgenin, used in the manufacture of contraceptive pills, until 1970, when the hormone was synthesized. *D. villosa* (wild Mexican yam) contains substances that are very similar to the human progesterone hormone. Phytochemicals from other yam species are used in the manufacture of hydrocortisone-based creams used for inflammations of the skin such as eczema. A number of species of yam have been used in Traditional Oriental Medicine as well as East Indian Ayurvedic medicine for hundreds of years.

Good-quality dioscorea is heavy, hard, and chalky in appearance. Look for oval-shaped slices that are straight, firm, and pure white in color.

———— ✹ ————

Healing Qualities of Dioscorea
Sweet, Neutral Energy
Treats Kidney, Lung, and Spleen Organ Systems
Category: Herb that Tonifies the Qi (see page 352)

Chinese yam is a sweet, soothing herb that Tonifies the Kidney and Adrenals, Spleen, and Lung Organ Systems. It is used to treat Spleen Qi Deficiency with such symptoms as lack of appetite, vomiting, chronic diarrhea, and fatigue. Dioscorea is taken internally to relieve frequent urination, asthma, dry coughs, diabetes, and emotional instability associated with Qi Deficiency. It stops spontaneous sweating due to Deficient Qi.

Contraindications: This herb should not be used in treating Damp-Heat conditions or Excess patterns.

Herbal Combinations Using Dioscorea

Poria cocos and dioscorea are combined to treat loose, watery stools that are the result of Spleen Deficiency.

Trichosanthes and dioscorea are used to reduce thirst and irritability caused by depletion of fluids due to Warm-febrile illnesses.

Dioscorea and *codonopsis* treat poor appetite, watery stools, fatigue, and weakness related to Kidney and Spleen Deficiency.

Cornus, rehmannia, and dioscorea treat night sweats and spermatorrhea due to Deficient Kidney energy.

Other Herbs that Tonify the Qi

If the healing properties of dioscorea are not quite right for your condition, please see other herbs in this category: *Astragalus, Atractylodes, Codonopsis, Ginseng, Jujube Date Fruit, Licorice*
Maximum Daily Dosage: 9 to 30 grams
1/4 ounce to 1 ounce

Dodder Seeds see *Cuscuta*

Dragon Bone
Calms the Spirit
English Name: Fossilized Vertebral and Extremity Bones (Usually of Mammals)
Pharmaceutical Name: Os Draconis

A Brief History of Dragon Bone
Mandarin: Lóng Gu; **Japanese:** Ryukotsu; **Korean:** Yonggol

Dragon bone is not an herb but the fossilized remains of elephants, rhinoceroses, and sometimes camels, antelopes, or cattle. In Traditional Oriental Medicine, substances such as minerals and shells are used to anchor or calm the spirit. Naturally high in mineral salts, dragon bone contains calcium carbonate, calcium phosphate, potassium, iron, and sulfates.

Look for hard, white fossilized material that readily absorbs moisture. You can test this by touching your tongue to the rocklike substance—your tongue will readily stick to the surface because the moisture is so quickly absorbed.

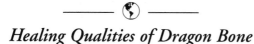

Healing Qualities of Dragon Bone
Sweet, Astringent, Neutral Energy
Treats Heart, Liver, and Kidney Organ Systems
Category: Substance that Settles and Calms the Spirit (see page 355)

Dragon bone treats insomnia, relieves palpitations, dizziness, anxiety, hysteria, nervousness, irritability, night sweats, blurred vision, uterine bleeding, leukorrhea, and nocturnal emissions. Dragon bone powder is applied topically to chronic ulcers and sores to promote healing.

Oyster shell and dragon bone are often combined. Fossilized teeth are also used. The teeth have basically the same qualities as dragon bone, but are more effective in treating insomnia, anxiety, and frequent dreaming. From a Western standpoint, these substances have a tranquilizing, sedative effect.

Contraindications: Persons suffering from conditions involving Damp-Heat should not be given dragon bone.

Herbal Combinations Using Dragon Bone

Note: Dragon bone or teeth should be crushed prior to making decoctions. These substances should be simmered for at least 30 minutes prior to adding herbs.

Cinnamon twigs, peony root (white), and dragon bone are combined to treat diarrhea, excessive uterine bleeding, and vaginal discharge due to Yang Deficiency as well as dizziness, fatigue, and painful lower back, legs, and feet.

Ginseng, aconite, and dragon bone treat profuse perspiration due to extreme weakness and fatigue (Collapsed Qi and Devastated Yang energy).

Polygala, zizyphus seed, and dragon bone are helpful for insomnia, palpitations, loss of memory, and excessive dreaming.

Astragalus, white peony root, and dragon bone treat spontaneous sweating.

Cornus, oyster shell, and dragon bone help in reducing night sweats due to Yin Deficiency.

Other Substances that Calm the Spirit

If the healing properties of dragon bone are not quite right for your condition, please see other herbs in this category: *Oyster Shell, Pearl*
Maximum Daily Dosage: 10 to 15 grams
1/3 ounce to 1/2 ounce

Du Huo

Puts the Spring Back in Your Step

Botanical Name: *Angelica pubescens*

A Brief History of Du Huo

Mandarin: Dú Húo; **Japanese:** Dokkatsu; **Korean:** Tokhwal

Du Huo, also known as *Angelica pubescens*, is a close relative of dang gui *(Angelica sinensis)*. This genus is composed of approximately 50 biennial and perennial plants that grow in northern-hemisphere temperate zones. Angelica's name comes from medieval Latin *herba angelica,* meaning "angelic herb." It was believed that these plants had the capability of protecting against evil and curing all ailments. One of du huo's cousins, *A. archangelica,* was widely used in Europe during the fifteenth century and is still eaten as a veggie in the Scandinavian countries and Greenland. Candied tender young angelica stalks are used for decorating cakes and desserts, while liqueurs are flavored with its roots and seeds.

Good-quality du huo (also spelled "tu huo") roots are yellowish brown in color with irregular wrinkles. The hard, solid root will snap easily to reveal a light-yellow to brown-colored interior. Look for thick, clean roots with a strong fragrance.

------------ ▲ ------------

Healing Qualities of Du Huo

Bitter, Spicy, Warm Energy
Treats Kidney and Bladder Organ Systems
Category: Herb that Dispels Wind Dampness (see page 347)

Du huo is a bitter, spicy warming herb that treats acute and chronic pain in the lower back and legs (rheumatic arthritis and lumbago) called Wind-Cold-Damp Obstruction in Oriental herbal medicine. Du huo is also used to treat headaches and toothache.

Contraindications: Du huo should not be used by persons with Heat signs due to Yin Deficiency.

Herbal Combinations Using Du Huo

Du huo and *ephedra* treat colds and flus accompanied by body aches and pains, but without perspiration.

Gentian, asarum (Chinese wild ginger), and du huo treat numbness, pain, and aching in the neck, back, legs, and feet.

Other Herbs that Expel Wind Dampness

If the healing properties of du huo are not quite right for your condition, please see other herbs in this category: *Clematis, Cocklebur*

Maximum Daily Dosage: 3 to 9 grams

1/10 ounce to 1/4 ounce

Ephedra Stem

Relieves Asthma and Allergies

English Name: Ephedra or Joint Fir

Botanical Name: *Ephedra sinica* or *E. equistestina*

A Brief History of Ephedra

Mandarin: Má Húang; **Japanese:** Mao; **Korean:** Mahwang

Ephedra is considered to be an evolutionary link between flowering plants and conifers. The tiny leaves appear at the nodes and look like scales. There are about 40 species of shrubs and climbers that grow in Asia, subtropical America, southern Europe, and northern Africa. The male plants produce conelike flowers and must be present to pollinate the female plants for red fleshy fruits to appear. Some ephedra species have a high alkaloid content (particularly ephedrine) that is used in many patent medicines to reduce excess mucus and ease asthma, coughs, and hay fever. These species include *E. equisetina, E. intermedia, E. gerardiana* (from East India), and *E. sinica.*

E. trifuca, an American species also known as Mormon Tea, has diuretic properties rather than antiasthmatic effects. Another species, *Catha edulis,* found in southwest Middle East and Ethiopia, contains a stimulant used in geriatric medicine. It is similar to ephedrine and is known as norpseudoephedrine or cathine.

Má Húang, *E. sinica*, has been used in the Orient as an asthma treatment for well over 5,000 years. Ephedra stems or stalks are long, slender, light greenish-yellow in color, and break easily. Look for dry stems with a solid core and bitter, astringent flavor.

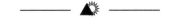

Healing Qualities of Ephedra

Spicy, Slightly Bitter, Warm Energy
Treats Lung and Bladder Organ Systems
Category: Herb that Releases Exterior Conditions (see page 344)

Honey-roasted ephedra stem is given for asthma while the raw herb is prescribed for colds and flu.

This warming, bitter, spicy herb dilates bronchial vessels, promotes perspiration, stimulates the heart and central nervous system, and has diuretic properties. Ephedra is taken internally for relief of asthma, hay fever, and allergic complaints.

Contraindications: Ephedra should not be given to persons taking monoamine oxidase (MAO) inhibitors or suffering from glaucoma, high blood pressure, or hyperthyroidism. Persons who are generally weak, have difficulty breathing, or have night sweats should avoid ephedra.

Note: Ephedra species are legally restricted in some countries.

Herbal Combinations Using Ephedra

Ephedra is combined with *cinnamon* for relief of cold and flu symptoms.

Honey-roasted ephedra, *apricot kernel,* and *licorice root* are combined to treat asthma.

Other Herbs that Release Exterior Conditions

If the healing properties of ephedra are not quite right for your condition, please see other herbs in this category: *Cinnamon Twigs, Ginger, Magnolia Flower, Schizonepeta, Siler*

Maximum Daily Dosage: 1.5 to 6 grams
1/20 ounce to 1/5 ounce

Epimedium

Adds Spice to Your Love Life
Botanical Name: *Epimedium grandiflorum*

A Brief History of Epimedium

Mandarin: Yín Yáng Huò or Xian Líng Pí; **Japanese:** Inyokaku; **Korean:** Umyanggwak

This genus is composed of about 25 species of evergreen or semi-evergreen perennials that grow in eastern and western Asia as well as in Mediterranean regions. *E. sagittatum* can be found in the moist woodlands of central China and has been naturalized in Japan. In the springtime, Epimedium bears tiny white flowers. It is sometimes grown as ground cover in shady borders. The first references to this species being used as a medicinal herb are found in the Chinese *Shen Nong Canon of Herbs* written between A.D. 25 and 220.

The leaves of epimedium are oval shaped with pointed tips and a finely serrated edge. Look for unbroken leaves that are shiny, light olive-green on the surface and grayish-green on the undersurface.

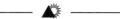

Healing Qualities of Epimedium
Spicy, Sweet, Warm Energy
Treats Kidney and Liver Organ Systems
Category: Herb that Tonifies the Yang (see page 353)

Epimedium acts as an aphrodisiac, but its other properties include Liver and Kidney tonification, dilation of blood vessels, and lowering of blood pressure. This herb is taken internally for asthma, bronchitis, arthritis and lumbago, cold or numb extremities, menstrual irregularity, impotence, involuntary and premature ejaculation, high blood pressure, and absent-mindedness due to Deficient Kidney and Liver Yang.

Herbal Combinations Using Epimedium

Astragalus, lycii berries, schisandra, and epimedium are prescribed for Deficient Kidney energy resulting in impotence and infertility.

Contraindications: Epimedium should not be taken over prolonged periods of time. Taken in excess, this herb can cause vomiting, dizziness, nosebleed, and thirst. Persons with Heat signs due to Yin Deficiency should not take epimedium.

Other Herbs that Tonify the Yang

If the healing properties of epimedium are not quite right for your condition, please see other herbs in this category: *Cuscuta, Eucommia, Fenugreek Seed*
Maximum Daily Dosage: 3 to 10 grams
1/10 ounce to 1/3 ounce

Eucommia Bark

Treats Backache and Hypertension
Botanical Name: *Eucommia ulmoides*

A Brief History of Eucommia

Mandarin: Dù Zhòng; **Japanese:** Tochu; **Korean:** Tuch'ung

The deciduous eucommia tree, a native of central China, gets its name from *eu* and *kommi,* Greek words that mean "good or true gum." The leaves of eucommia are elliptical and elmlike, and its wood contains a high rubber content that is used medicinally. Eucommia bark is harvested in the spring and early summer months, folded with the inside out and tied with rice straws. Once the inner surface has blackened, the bark is untied and left in the sun to dry. Eucommia bark is sliced into very thin strips that remain attached to one another due to white threads of natural latex that hold them together.

The inner surface of eucommia bark is smooth and dark brown in color, while the outer pale grayish-brown cork is wrinkled in appearance. Look for dry, hard bark that is held together by tough rubbery threads.

———— ▲ ————

Healing Qualities of Eucommia

Sweet, Slightly Spicy, Warm Energy
Treats Liver and Kidney Organ Systems
Category: Herb that Tonifies the Yang (see page 353)

This gentle, Yang Tonifying herb treats threatened miscarriage due to Cold Deficient Kidney patterns as well as impotence and early stages of hypertension. Eucommia promotes circulation and is used to treat a weak, sore lower back and knees, fatigue, and frequent urination.

Contraindications: Eucommia should not be combined with *scrophularia,* according to some traditional sources. It should not be given to persons with Heat symptoms resulting from Yin Deficiency.

Herbal Combinations Using Eucommia

Cinnamon twigs, *du huo, gentian,* and eucommia are combined to treat Damp-Cold back pain with a cold, sore, swollen sensation that becomes worse when exposed to cold. The patient's tongue coating would be white and greasy in appearance.

Cuscuta, cornus, and eucommia treat impotence and frequent urination due to Cold Deficient Kidneys.

Eucommia is combined with *dioscorea* and *dipsacus* (Radix Dipsaci Asperi) for habitual miscarriage.

Other Herbs that Tonify the Yang

If the healing properties of eucommia are not quite right for your condition, please see other herbs in this category: *Cuscuta, Epimedium, Fenugreek Seed*
Maximum Daily Dosage: 6 to 10 grams
1/5 ounce to 1/3 ounce

Fennel Seed

Stops Stomach Pain
Botanical Name: *Foeniculum vulgare*

A Brief History of Fennel Fruit

Mandarin: Xiao Hul Xiang; **Japanese:** Shouikyo; **Korean:** Sohoehyang

Since Classical times, fennel has been grown and eaten as a vegetable. Cultivated on imperial farms, *F. vulgare* spread into the central and northern parts of Europe during Charlemagne's time (from A.D. 742 to 814). There is only one species of this anise-flavored biennial or perennial plant that grows on dry, sunny wasteland, with a preference for coastal areas. Some varieties of fennel can reach up to 6 feet in height, producing umbels of tiny yellow flowers followed by the gray-brown fennel fruit or seed. The delicate, thread-like foliage of fennel, as well as its bulbus stalk base are eaten raw in salads or cooked as a vegetable. Italian salami gets it characteristic flavor from fennel seeds, as does the French liqueur, *fenouillette*. Fennel seeds are crushed to make a tasty digestive tea.

Look for fragrant dry, yellowish-green seeds. Most medicinal-quality fennel fruit comes from China, India, Japan, and Southern Europe.

─────── ▲ ───────

Healing Qualities of Fennel Fruit
Spicy, Warm Energy
Treats Liver, Kidney, Spleen, and Stomach Organ Systems
Category: Herb that Warms the Interior and Expels Cold (see page 351)

In the Orient, fennel seed is used to eliminate Cold from the lower abdominal region (Lower Burner). It treats indigestion, colic, and gas (Evil Wind). Fennel regulates and harmonizes Stomach Qi, treating such symptoms as vomiting, poor appetite, and abdominal pain. It can reduce lower back pain due to Cold by warming the Kidneys.

Contraindications: Fennel fruit should be used with caution if Heat signs accompanying Yin Deficiency are present.

Herbal Combinations Using Fennel Fruit

Fennel is used in conjunction with *ginger* and *magnolia bark* for vomiting and for poor appetite due to Stomach Cold.

Other Herbs that Warm the Interior and Expel Cold

If the healing properties of fennel fruit are not quite right for your condition, please see other herbs in this category: *Aconite, Ginger (Dried)*
Maximum Daily Dosage: 3 to 10 grams
1/10 ounce to 1/3 ounce

Fenugreek
Treats Impotence and Aids Digestion
Botanical Name: *Trigonella foenum-graecum*

A Brief History of Fenugreek Seed
Mandarin: Hú Lú Ba; **Japanese:** Koroha; **Korean:** Horop'a

Fenugreek, one of the world's oldest medicinal herbs, was favored by Hippocrates, Father of Western medicine. Fenugreek gets its botanical name, *Trigonella,* from its "triangular" shaped single or paired yellow-white flowers, tinged with violet at the base, which produce yellow-brown seeds in beaked pods. A total of 80 species of annuals are found growing from the

Mediterranean region to southern Africa and Australia. Fenugreek was used in ancient Egypt to ease labor pains and increase milk flow; Egyptian women still use it to soothe menstrual pain. Grown as a fodder crop in Greece and in southern and central Europe, trigonella is used as a spice in most Mediterranean countries, Russia, the Balkans, the Middle East, western Asia, and China.

Fresh trigonella leaves are cooked as a vegetable curry in India; dried leaves flavor root veggies in Middle Eastern and Indian cooking. Slightly roasted to reduce the bitterness, fenugreek seeds are ground to become an important ingredient of curry powder, pickles, and Ethiopian spice mixes. In Egypt these aromatic seeds flavor bread, stew, and fried foods. In northern Yemen, boiled seeds are pureed and served with fried onions and meat. Sprouted seeds are eaten as a salad vegetable. Extracts of fenugreek seeds are utilized by the food industry in the manufacture of synthetic maple syrup, and vanilla, caramel, maple, and butterscotch flavors.

Most fenugreek seed comes to us from India, North Africa, Southern Europe, and China. Look for smooth, clean, plump, red- to yellowish-brown seeds.

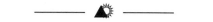

Healing Qualities of Fenugreek Seed
Bitter, Warm Energy
Treats Kidney and Liver Organ Systems
Category: Herb that Tonifies the Yang (see page 353)

Used traditionally as an aphrodisiac, this bitter, spicy, warming herb treats impotence, increases milk flow, stimulates the uterus, reduces blood sugar, improves digestion, soothes irritated tissues, and lowers fevers. The healing properties of fenugreek include diuretic, antiparasitic, antitumor, laxative, and expectorant effects.

In Traditional Oriental Medicine fenugreek is used mainly for Kidney-related imbalances such as low back pain, impotence, premature ejaculation, edema of the legs, and hernia. Medicinally, fenugreek seed is prescribed for insufficient lactation, painful menstruation, labor pains, digestive disorders, gastric inflammation, and late-onset diabetes. It is applied externally for skin inflammations and cellulitis. In Ayurvedic medicine fenugreek is regarded as a rejuvenative and aphrodisiac and is used to treat general debility, poor appetite, digestive and bronchial complaints, allergies, gout, and arthritis.

Contraindications: Fenugreek should be used cautiously by persons with Damp-Heat or Heat signs due to Yin Deficiency.

Herbal Combinations Using Fenugreek Seed

Relieve gas and stomach distress by sprinkling fenugreek powder over foods. A tea of fenugreek seeds can be prepared by bringing a cup of water to a boil; remove from heat and add seeds; cover and let steep 15 to 20 minutes. Drink one cup prior to each meal to aid digestion and relieve minor peptic ulcers.

Herbal Combinations Using Fenugreek

Aconite, psoralea, and fenugreek are combined to treat pain and sensations of coldness in the lower back, lower abdomen, legs, and feet.

Other Herbs that Tonify the Yang

If the healing properties of fenugreek seed are not quite right for your condition, please see other herbs in this category: *Cuscuta, Epimedium, Eucommia*
Maximum Daily Dosage: 3 to 5 grams
1/10 ounce to 1/5 ounce

Forsythia Fruit
Clears Bacterial Infections
Botanical Name: *Forsythia suspensa*

A Brief History of Forsythia Fruit
Mandarin: Lían Qíao; **Japanese:** Rengyó; **Korean:** Yôn'gyo

Forsythia gets it name from William Forsyth (1737–1804), horticulturist and gardener at Kensington Palace in London. A total of seven species of deciduous shrubs belong to this genus. Six of these grow mainly in eastern Asia with only one species coming from Southeastern Europe. A profusion of bright yellow flowers grace the slender, hollow branches of forsythia shrubs long before the leaves appear. Dried, aromatic, woody fruits (mostly without seeds) are the part of the plant used medicinally in the Orient. The use of *F. suspensa* can be traced back in some of the earliest traditional Chinese medical texts to approximately 2000 B.C.

Forsythia fruits that have just begun to ripen are bluish-green in color and are called "green"; though difficult to obtain, these are generally considered the best. "Old" fruits should be golden tan in color with thick shells. Usually, medicinal-quality forsythia fruits come from China.

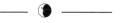

Healing Qualities of Forsythia Fruit
Bitter, Slightly Spicy, Cool Energy
Treats Heart, Liver, and Gall Bladder Organ Systems
Category: Herb that Clears Heat and Relieves Toxicity (see page 346)

Most often, the "old," or dried fruit of the forsythia plant is used in Oriental medicine. Forsythia fruit, an excellent herbal antibiotic, lowers fevers and is taken internally to clear all "Hot" sores including carbuncles, abscesses, and neck lumps. It is used to treat acute bacterial infections, tonsillitis, allergic rashes, and colds and flu accompanied by fever, slight chills, a headache, and sore throat. This diuretic herb stimulates the heart, gall bladder, and nervous system. Forsythia fruit contains vitamin P, which strengthens capillaries.

Contraindications: Not to be used for Cold, Yin ulcers, or in cases of Spleen/Stomach Deficiency accompanied by diarrhea.

Herbal Combinations Using Forsythia Fruit
Forsythia fruit is combined with *chrysanthemum flower* for the first stages of a warm-febrile disease.

Coptis and forsythia fruit treat acute infections such as dysentery.

Ephedra, peony root (red), licorice, and forsythia fruit are combined for allergic rashes.

Other Herbs that Clear Heat and Relieve Toxicity
If the healing properties of forsythia fruit are not quite right for your condition, please see other herbs in this category: *Dandelion, Honeysuckle Flower*
Maximum Daily Dosage: 5 to 10 grams
1/5 ounce to 1/3 ounce

Fritillary
An Herbal Aid for that Coughy, Feverish Feeling
Botanical Name: *Fritillaria cirrhosa*

A Brief History of Fritillary
Mandarin: Chuan Bèi Mu; **Japanese:** Senbaimo; **Korean:** Ch'ônp'aemo

A member of the lily family, fritillary grows in central Asian and western Siberian woodlands and meadows. There are approximately 100 species of fritillary, a hardy and frost-hardy, bulbous perennial that bears cream-colored bell-shaped flowers in the springtime. The plant lies dormant during summer months. Several species are either cultivated or gathered in the wild for medicinal use in China, most commonly *F. pallidiflora* and *F. cirrhosa*.

Most medicinal-quality herb comes from China. Look for plump, dry, heavy bulbs that are pure white.

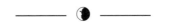

Healing Qualities of Fritillary

Bitter, Sweet, Slightly Cold Energy
Treats Lung and Heart Organ Systems
Category: Herb that Cools and Transforms Phlegm-Heat (see page 348)

Fritillary clears Heat, reducing sores, swellings, and nodules. This herb is used for many types of coughs, particularly those with Heat signs due to Yin Deficiency. Dried bulbs are cooked in decoctions or taken as powders to relieve coughs, bronchitis, pneumonia, feverish illnesses, breast or lung tumors, or abscesses. This is an expectorant herb that relaxes bronchial spasms and lowers fevers and blood pressure.

Contraindications: Fritillary should be administered by qualified practitioners only. The *unprocessed or raw herb is toxic* and is not for internal consumption. In excess, this herb can cause breathing difficulties and heart failure.

Herbal Combinations Using Fritillary

Fritillary, *polygala, poria cocos,* and *trichosanthes* are combined to treat painful obstruction of the chest (a stifling feeling in the chest and upper abdomen) with insomnia and palpitations.

Note: Fritillary is incompatible with *aconite* and counteracts the effects of *gentian* according to some traditional sources.

Other Herbs that Cool and Transform Phlegm-Heat

If the healing properties of fritillary are not quite right for your condition, please see other herbs in this category: *Bamboo Sap and Shavings, Kelp (Seaweed), Trichosanthes*

Maximum Daily Dosage: 3 to 10 grams
1/10 ounce to 1/3 ounce

Gambir

Stops Muscle Spasms

Botanical Name: *Uncaria rhynchophylla* or *U. sinensis*

A Brief History of Gambir

Mandarin: Gou Téng; **Japanese:** Chotoko; **Korean:** Kudûing

Gambir gets its botanical name *Uncaria* from the Latin word *uncus,* which means "hook." The stems of these climbing shrubs bear rather large, downward-curving hooks or thorns that resemble anchors. Native to Japan and China, the gambir vine produces large ball-shaped heads of tiny white flowers.

Look for smooth, unbroken thorns (shaped like fish hooks) with a shiny reddish-brown surface.

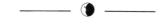

Healing Qualities of Gambir

Sweet, Cool Energy
Treats Heart and Liver Organ Systems
Category: Herb that Extinguishes Wind and Stops Tremors (see page 356)

This wonderful herb stops muscle spasms, extinguishing what is known as Liver Wind in Oriental medicine. Symptoms include seizures, tremors, and eclampsia. It soothes Liver Fire Rising with such symptoms as red eyes, irritability, headache, and hypertension. It is also used for fevers, headaches, and red eyes due to colds/flu.

Contraindications: None noted.

Important Note: Gambir should not be simmered for more than 10 minutes. Decoct the other herbs in your formula first and add in the gambir toward the end of the cooking time.

Herbal Combinations Using Gambir

Scutellaria, prunella, and gambir treat Liver Heat (red eyes, irritability, headaches).

Other Herbs that Extinguish Wind and Stop Tremors

If the healing properties of gambir are not quite right for your condition, please see the other herb in this category: *Gastrodia*

Maximum Daily Dosage: 5 to 10 grams

1/5 ounce to 1/3 ounce

Gardenia Fruit
The Oriental "Herb of Happiness"
Botanical Name: *Gardenia jasminoides*

A Brief History of Gardenia Fruit
Mandarin: Zhi Zi; **Japanese:** Sanshishi; **Korean:** Ch'icha

Everyone is familiar with the lovely fragrance and beautiful blossoms of gardenia, but too few are aware of this flower's wonderful ability to give the gift of gladness. The fruit of the gardenia flower has the ability to eliminate feelings of irritability and frustration, bringing peace of mind. There are more than 200 species of evergreen trees and shrubs in this genus, all natives to tropical and warm regions of Africa and Eurasia. Gardenia flowers yield an essential oil that is used in perfumery. The Chinese flavor tea with a delightful scent of gardenia. It was first mentioned in traditional Chinese medical texts around A.D. 25–220, during the Han dynasty.

The outer surface of the gardenia fruit is glossy and yellowish to reddish-brown in color. A number of oval, reddish-brown seeds are packed together inside the fruit in a solid mass. Look for clean, small, plump, dry fruits that are unbroken and contain red seeds.

Healing Qualities of Gardenia
Bitter, Cold Energy
Treats Heart, Liver, Lung, Stomach, and Triple Warmer Organ Systems
Category: Herb that Clears Heat and Drains Fire (see page 345)

According to Oriental thought, gardenia fruit drains Damp-Heat and Cools the Blood. Besides tranquilizing the mind through its actions of improving liver function and thus releasing blocked emotions, the fruit of the gardenia flower is taken internally for hepatitis, jaundice, feverish illness, and hemorrhage. It lowers fevers and blood pressure, stimulates bile flow, checks bleeding, and promotes healing. Gardenia is applied externally to skin inflammations, sprains, wounds, and toothaches.

Contraindications: Gardenia should not be given to persons with diarrhea due to Cold from Deficiency.

Herbal Combinations Using Gardenia Fruit

Moutan peony cortex and gardenia relieve painful menses, dull headache, dry, itchy eyes, and intercostal pain due to Liver Blood Deficiency.

Rhubarb root, artemisia, and gardenia treat jaundice resulting from Damp-Heat in the Gallbladder/Liver Organ Systems.

For swelling and bruises due to trauma, powdered gardenia fruit can be mixed with vinegar or egg white and applied topically.

Other Herbs that Clear Heat and Quell Fire

If the healing properties of gardenia fruit are not quite right for your condition, please see the other herbs in this category: *Anemarrhena, Gypsum*
Maximum Daily Dosage: 3 to 10 grams
1/10 ounce to 1/3 ounce

Garlic

Nature's Antibiotic

Botanical Name: *Allium sativum*

A Brief History of Garlic

Mandarin: Dà Suàn; **Japanese:** Taisan; **Korean:** Taesan

Everyone is familiar with the fragrance of the lowly garlic bulb. Books can be and have been written about the healing powers of this wonderful gift from nature. Onions, chives, leeks, and shallots all belong to the Allium genus of plants, which contains about 700 species of odoriferous cousins—biennials and perennials native to the northern hemisphere, Mexico, Ethiopia, and southern Africa.

Garlic figures as one of humankind's most ancient herbs. According to one Muslim legend, as Satan left the Garden of Eden after tempting Adam and Eve, wherever his left foot stepped, garlic grew—onions sprang up from his right footprint. More than 5,000 years ago garlic was consumed by the Babylonians; 3,000 years ago it was used by the Egyptians as a cure for tumors, heart problems, headache, and worms; it was even placed in Tutankhamun's tomb. Garlic was eaten in large quantities by ancient Greeks and Romans—a custom that continues to this day. In fact, athletes competing in the first Olympic games consumed garlic for an energy boost. During

A.D. the first century, Dioscorides, chief physician to the Roman army, pre-scribed garlic for the troops to expel intestinal worms. Garlic juice was used by French, British, and Russian army doctors to treat infected battle wounds during World War I.

Garlic gets its characteristic fragrance from the presence of sulfur com-pounds—nature's own antibiotic that stimulates our immune system. It has therapeutic effects on our respiratory, circulatory, and digestive systems.

Garlic with purple skin is most effective in treating toxicity and against parasites. Look for clean, plump, firm bulbs.

Healing Qualities of Garlic

Spicy, Warm Energy
Treats Large Intestine, Lung, Spleen, and Stomach Organ Systems
Category: Herb that Expels Parasites (see page 356)

Garlic kills hookworms, pinworms, yeast and fungal infections, and is used to treat ringworm of the scalp. In Oriental medicine it is utilized to prevent colds and flus and to relieve toxicity. Garlic relieves sudden coughing, diar-rhea, dysentery, bronchitis, consumption, and other lung disorders.

Contraindications: Garlic should not be used in the presence of Deficient Heat symptoms.

Herbal Combinations Using Garlic

Garlic is effective used alone. For a sore throat, steep 4 to 6 cloves of minced garlic in 1/2 cup of water for 8 to 12 hours (do not cook). Gargle the tea for a sore throat and swallow it if you have a cold or flu.

Garlic is applied topically in a sesame- or olive-oil base to toxic swellings. To prepare garlic oil, soak 10 to 12 cloves of minced garlic in 1/2 cup oil for two weeks. Strain the garlic from the oil, cover tightly, and keep in a cool, dark location. A few drops of warm garlic oil does wonders to soothe an earache.

Garlic is also a great insect repellent. Add it to your favorite dishes or consume a few cloves daily. When you perspire, a slight odor is given off that sends insects scurrying.

Garlic and rice gruel is used to treat consumption.

However, don't go overboard! Eating garlic paste by the jar can burn sensitive stomach and esophagus linings, and too much raw garlic can upset the stomach.

Other Herbs that Expel Parasites

If the healing properties of garlic are not quite right for your condition, please see the other herb in this category: *Pumpkin Seeds and Husks*
Maximum Daily Dosage: 3 to 5 cloves of garlic

Gastrodia

Alleviates Muscle Spasms and Migraines

Botanical Name: *Gastrodia elata*

A Brief History of Gastrodia

Mandarin: Tian Má; **Japanese:** Tenma; **Korean:** Ch'onma

A member of the orchid family, gastrodia thrives on organic fungal foods and is native to Siberia, Tibet, China, Korea, and Japan. Though very difficult to cultivate, the Chinese have now devised a means to grow gastrodia due to its increasing scarcity in the wild. This leafless saprophyte reaches 2 to 3 feet in height; its brown stem has a scalelike appearance. The underground rhizomes are preferably harvested in the winter.

The medicinal use of gastrodia is first described in Chinese texts dating back to A.D. 470. The hard, horny gastrodia rhizome is not easily broken. Its pale-brown exterior has irregular wrinkles and the interior is glossy dark brown in color. When shopping for gastrodia, look for thin, translucent slices without a hole in the middle.

——— ✹ ———

Healing Qualities of Gastrodia

Sweet, Neutral Energy
Treats Liver Organ System
Category: Herb that Extinguishes Wind and Stops Tremors (see page 356)

Gastrodia calms the Liver, extinguishing Wind with such symptoms as spasms, tremors, pediatric convulsions, epilepsy, hemiphlegia, numbness of the lower back and extremities, and headaches, including migraines.

Contraindications: In large doses, this herb could be toxic. Do not exceed the recommended dosage.

Herbal Combinations Using Gastrodia

Gambir, scutellaria, achyranthes, and gastrodia treat dizziness and headache due to Liver Yang Rising.

Other Herbs that Extinguish Wind and Stop Tremors

If the healing properties of gastrodia are not quite right for your condition, please see the other herb in this category: *Gambir*
    Maximum Daily Dosage: 3 to 5 grams
                    1/10 ounce to 1/5 ounce

Gentian

Treats Urinary Infections and Conjunctivitis

English Name: Chinese Gentian Root
Botanical Name: *Gentiana scabra;* in Manchuria *G. triflora* is used instead

A Brief History of Gentian

Mandarin: Lóng Dan Cao; **Japanese:** Ryutan; **Korean:** Yongdanch'o

Gentian is named after King Gentius of Illyria (c. 500 B.C.) who was said to have discovered the medicinal properties of *G. lutea.* Roughly, the kingdom of Illyria covered the region that corresponds to the country of Yugoslavia today. Gentian became an important ingredient in *theriac,* a secret medieval alchemical brew reputed to cure all ailments. There are more than 400 species of annuals, biennials, and perennials that compose this genus. Many gentians are grown for their funnel-shaped blue, purple, yellow, or white flowers. *G. macrophylla* and *G. scabra* grow in northern and eastern Asia while *G. lutea* graces alpine pastures and woodlands in Europe.

Bitter-tasting herbs have been used for ages by herbalists all around the world to aid digestion by stimulating gastric secretions. Some of the world's most bitter compounds are found in gentian. *G. lutea* is so bitter that the taste is still evident even when diluted to 1 in 12,000 parts. For this reason, gentian is used in many commercial bitter tonics, aperitifs, and Enzian schnapps.

Gentiana scabra root is actually composed of many long yellow to brownish-yellow roots that are attached to a rhizome. Look for long, thick, flexible roots that are unbroken.

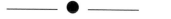

Healing Qualities of Gentian

Bitter, Cold Energy
Treats Liver, Gall Bladder, and Bladder Organ Systems
Category: Herb that Clears Heat and Dries Dampness (see page 345)

G. scabra, a cold and bitter anti-inflammatory herb, is used in Oriental medicine to drain Damp-Heat from the Liver and Gallbladder Organ Systems.
Gentian is an excellent remedy for acute urinary-tract infections, vaginal
infections, genital itch, conjunctivitis, liver disorders, and eye complaints
related to liver disharmony. Gentian increases blood-sugar levels. It also
enhances the analgesic and sedative effects of other herbs. Gentian is used to
treat hypertension accompanied by dizziness or ringing in the ears.

Contraindications: Gentian is a cold herb and should not be given in
case of digestive (Spleen/Stomach) weakness with diarrhea.

Herbal Combinations Using Gentian

Scutellaria, bupleurum, and gentian form an excellent combination to combat Liver Fire or Damp-Heat accompanied by a number of symptoms
including conjunctivitis, testicular swelling and pain, painful urination, a bitter taste in the mouth, and pain in the chest.

Other Herbs that Clear Heat and Dry Dampness

If the healing properties of gentian are not quite right for your condition,
please see other herbs in this category: *Coptis, Phellodendron, Scutellaria*
Maximum Daily Dosage: 3 to 5 grams
1/10 ounce to 1/5 ounce

Ginger (Dried)

Reignites the Digestive Flame
Botanical Name: *Zingiber officinale*

A Brief History of Ginger

Mandarin: Gan Jiang; **Japanese:** Kankyo; **Korean:** Kôngang

Used as a spice in Asia since antiquity, ginger's botanical name, *zingiber,* comes
from the ancient East Indian Sanskrit language. Ginger's East Indian Ayurvedic

name *vishwabhesaj* means "universal medicine." Ginger is an important herb in about half of all Chinese and Ayurvedic herbal prescriptions. It reduces the toxicity and irritant effects of some herbs in the formulas.

This herb has truly made its way around the world. The Romans listed ginger as a taxable commodity in A.D. 200; and the Spaniards introduced it into the Americas. There are approximately 100 species of ginger that produce thick, hard, light-golden-tan aromatic rhizomes (or underground stems). Ginger, a deciduous perennial plant with upright stems that die down in the winter months, yields yellow-green flowers with a deep-purple and yellow-marked lip. Various species of ginger are commercially grown in warm, tropical regions—some of the best come from Jamaica.

Ginger finds it way into many culinary delights including curries, chutneys, cakes, cookies, meat and fish dishes, soups, pickles, candy, soft drinks—you name it. Ginger oil is used in perfumery as well as for food flavoring. First mentioned in Chinese medical texts during the Han dynasty (A.D. 25-200), ginger, in a number of different forms including *fresh, dried,* and *wild,* treats a plethora of complaints. Dried ginger, energetically, is much hotter than the fresh. Look for clean, dry, light cream-colored slices with a strong flavor.

———— ☼ ————

Healing Qualities of Dried Ginger
Spicy, Hot Energy
Treats Heart, Lung, Spleen, and Stomach Organ Systems
Category: Herb that Warms the Interior and Expels Cold (see page 351)

In Traditional Oriental Medicine dried ginger is used to warm the center or Middle Burner consisting of the Spleen/Stomach Organ System. Ginger rescues devastated, weak Yang energy and expels Cold. It warms the Lung and reduces thin, watery, or white phlegm. Ginger stops hemorrhage due to cold, particularly uterine bleeding. In Western terms, dried ginger improves digestion and liver function; it stops nausea and vomiting. Ginger stimulates circulation, reducing muscle spasms and easing pain of rheumatism, lumbago, and menstrual cramps.

If you do not have Heat symptoms but tend to suffer from chronic Cold complaints, you will probably want to add 2 to 4 thin slices of dried ginger root to most of your herbal formulas.

Contraindications: Do not use dried ginger in case of Heat symptoms such as high fever, inflammatory skin eruptions, or in cases of Yin Deficiency with Heat signs. Dried ginger should be used with caution during pregnancy.

Herbal Combinations Using Dried Ginger

Dried ginger and *licorice root* treat Cold Deficiency of the Stomach/Spleen with such symptoms as epigastric pain, nausea, and vomiting.

    Coptis and dried ginger are used for vague stomach pain with a feeling of gnawing hunger accompanied by belching and nausea. This combination treats dysenteric disorders.

    Schisandra, wild ginger, and dried ginger treat coughing and wheezing with watery phlegm that stops the downward flow of Lung Qi.

Other Herbs that Warm the Interior and Expel Cold

If the healing properties of dried ginger are not quite right for your condition, please see other herbs in this category: *Aconite, Fennel Seeds*
    Maximum Daily Dosage: 3 to 10 grams
               1/10 ounce to 1/3 ounce

Ginger (Fresh)

Great for Colds, Coughs, Colic, and Morning Sickness

Botanical Name: *Zingiber officinale*

A Brief History of Ginger

Mandarin: Sheng Jiang; **Japanese:** Shokyo; **Korean:** Saenggang

Please see preceding history of ginger under "Dried Ginger." Note that the Mandarin, Japanese, and Korean names for fresh ginger are different from those for dried ginger. The healing qualities of fresh ginger, which follow, though similar, are distinct. Use dried ginger for severe, chronic problems relating to internal coldness.

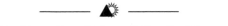

Healing Qualities of Fresh Ginger

Spicy, Warm Energy
Treats Lung, Spleen, and Stomach Organ Systems
Category: Herb that Releases the Exterior (see page 344)

In Traditional Oriental Medicine fresh ginger is used to promote sweating and as an expectorant for coughs due to colds and flus accompanied by chills. Fresh ginger, like dried ginger, is an excellent digestive aid and can be added to herbal formulas to harmonize the effects of the herbs, especially if your tendency is to be on the "Cold" side of the Yin/Yang equation. Fresh ginger is particularly effective in detoxifying *aconite* and *pinellia.*

Contraindications: Do not use fresh ginger in case of Lung or Stomach Heat symptoms such as coughing up of mucus streaked with blood (Lung Heat) or painful peptic ulcers, canker sores in the mouth or on the tongue, or vomiting blood (Stomach Heat).

Herbal Combinations Using Fresh Ginger

If you are suffering from the first stages of a cold or flu with chills, add a teaspoon or so of freshly grated and strained ginger juice to your herbal concoction to harmonize the formula and encourage sweating.

To relieve morning sickness, simmer 2 to 4 slices of fresh ginger in two cups of water for 15 minutes. A touch of *cardamom* can be added to further strengthen the formula. Slowly sip the warm tea.

Jujube dates and fresh ginger strengthen and protect Spleen/Stomach Qi and eliminate epigastric pain, nausea, and vomiting.

Pinellia and fresh ginger treat productive coughs due to Phlegm-Dampness.

Other Warm, Spicy Herbs that Release the Exterior

If the healing properties of fresh ginger are not quite right for your condition, please see other herbs in this category: *Cinnamon Twigs, Ephedra, Magnolia Flower, Schizonepeta, Siler*

Maximum Daily Dosage: 3 to 10 grams
1/10 ounce to 1/3 ounce

Ginkgo Nut
The Herb that Aids Memory
English Name: Ginkgo Nut, Maidenhair Tree
Botanical Name: *Ginkgo biloba*

A Brief History of Ginkgo Nut
Mandarin: Bái Guo; **Japanese:** Ginkyo; **Korean:** Unhaeng

Grown as a sacred tree in Japan and China, the rare *G. biloba* can occasionally be found growing in the wild in central China, Zhejiang, and Guizhou

Provinces. Only one species makes up this genus, and it has no known close relatives. Male and female trees must grow nearby for fruiting to occur; the yellowish-colored oval fruits smell like rancid butter once they have ripened. Ginkgo leaves are quite beautiful—a delicate fan shape approximately 5 inches across, which graces a long, slender stalk. Since ancient times in Japan, ginkgo leaves have been placed between pages of books to discourage the nibbling of insects. The outer coat that protects the ginkgo seed is used as an insecticide.

Ginkgo seeds from Japan and China were sent to Europe around 1727, and soon they were in cultivation. Maidenhair trees growing today are almost identical to those that were discovered in fossil form. For this reason, Ginkgo is often called a "living fossil." One of the main constituents found in maidenhair trees are ginkgolides—a phytochemical (phyto = plant) that has not been found in any other plants. Ginkogolides have a blocker (called PAF, or platelet activating factor) that inhibits allergic reactions. The flavonoids present in ginkgo improve circulation, especially circulation to the brain.

Ginkgo nuts or seeds are considered a delicacy and are eaten roasted in Southeast Asian countries, China and Japan. They are slightly toxic, however, with symptoms of overdose including irritability, difficulty breathing, headache, fever, and tremors. This reaction can be antidoted by simmering 60 grams of raw licorice root in 2 cups of water for 20 to 25 minutes and drinking the liquid; or by simmering 30 grams of ginkgo-seed shells and following the preceding directions. A reaction to herbal formulas containing ginkgo nuts can be avoided by including some of the hard shells and thin linings of the seeds in the prescription.

The ginkgo seed-coat is white; look for plump, full, round seeds of a yellow color.

———— 🜨 ————

Healing Qualities of Ginkgo Nut
Sweet, Bitter, Astringent, Neutral, Slightly Poisonous Energy
Treats Lung and Kidney Organ Systems
Category: Astringent Herb that Stabilizes and Binds (see page 354)

Ginkgo has antibacterial and antifungal qualities; it stimulates circulation, controls allergic responses, and dilates bronchial tubes and blood vessels.

In Oriental thought, it supplements Kidney Yang energy, stabilizing the Lower Burner (or Kidney/Adrenal/Bladder and Reproductive Organs). Ginkgo is taken internally for circulatory complaints such as Raynaud's disease and varicose veins, loss of memory or cerebral insufficiency in the elderly, asthma, and urinary incontinence. Ginkgo expels phlegm and stops coughing and wheezing.

Contraindications: Ginkgo should not be used in Excess. Because of its slightly toxic nature, this herb should not be ingested in large quantities or over a prolonged period of time. Taken in excess, this herb may cause headaches, diarrhea, vomiting, and dermatitis.

Herbal Combinations Using Ginkgo Nut

Gingko is combined with *ephedra, apricot seed,* and *white mulberry root cortex* for asthma and coughs.

Make your favorite chicken soup with *lotus seeds,* plenty of *black pepper,* and gingko nuts to treat a thin, watery vaginal discharge due to Deficiency in the Lower Burner.

Other Astringent Herbs that Stabilize and Bind

If the healing properties of ginkgo nut are not quite right for your condition, please see other herbs in this category: *Cornus, Pomegranate Husk, Schisandra*

Maximum Daily Dosage: 3 to 5 grams
1/10 ounce to 1/5 ounce

Meet the Ginseng Family
American Ginseng
Eleuthero (Siberian) Ginseng
Panax Ginseng
Pseudoginseng

Ginseng figures prominently as one of the most, if not *the* most famous herbs used by humankind. Its botanical name, *Panax ginseng,* comes from *Panakes,* a Greek word meaning "panacea," or "all healing." In Oriental herbalism ginseng is considered a "superior" medicine because it restores our vital energy while balancing organ-system functions, thus enabling the body to heal itself. Used in China for thousands of years, ginseng remains a main ingredient in hundreds of herbal formulas prescribed today.

There are a number of legends regarding the origins of ginseng's medicinal use. One story maintains that fairies gave this healing herb to humankind; for this reason, you will often find fairies decorating advertisements or ginseng boxes (particularly Korean products). Another ancient Chinese legend holds that Confucius was the first person to give a discourse on the medicinal use of ginseng some 2,500 years ago. Still another story credits Lao Tzu, the great Chinese philosopher, with the discovery of ginseng's healing qualities. Yet another myth says that during the Sui dynasty, a man's wailing was heard nightly until villagers finally traced the source of the crying sound. They dug in the soil and uncovered a root that resembled the figure of a man.

The older, the larger, and the more semblance ginseng roots bear to a human form, the more expensive they are. The best ginseng is truly worth its weight in gold. The top grade, known as "heaven grade," is affordable only to the elite in China. Lesser-quality roots are known as "earth grade" and "man grade."

The three types of ginseng most commonly cultivated and marketed today are Chinese or Korean ginseng *(Panax ginseng);* American ginseng *(Panax quinquefolium)* and Russian or Siberian ginseng *(Eleutherococcus senticosus)*. Each of these healing herbs, plus Pseudoginseng are covered individually in the upcoming sections.

In the West, ginseng's popularity has rapidly increased over the past 30 years. There are a number of wonderful adaptogenic herbs with ginseng-like qualities, however, that are more appropriate for different body types, ages, and disease conformations. Before jumping on the ginseng bandwagon, please consider the possible use of other healing medicinal roots such as *codonopsis, astragalus, glehnia* (known as white ginseng, see page 137), *scrophularia* (black ginseng, see page 199), *polygonum* (purple ginseng, see page 179), or *salvia* (called "red ginseng," see page 193). Don't confuse salvia with steamed *Panax ginseng,* which is also known as red ginseng. Each of these herbs possesses unique healing energies that might be more appropriate for your particular constitution and condition.

Ginseng (American)

Is Best Suited for Most Americans

English Name: American Ginseng Root
Botanical Name: *Panax quinquefolium*

A Brief History of American Ginseng Root

Mandarin: Xi Yáng Shen, **Japanese:** Seiyojin, **Korean:** Sôyangsam

Panax quinquefolium, or American ginseng, a member of the aralia family, is native to hardwood forests of Eastern North America. Preferring cool northern slopes, it grows alongside oaks and sugar-maple trees. Native North Americans used American ginseng to reduce fevers and to relieve various ailments such as headache, colic, convulsions, and dysentery.

Like its cousin *Panax ginseng*, there are many stories regarding the discovery of American ginseng in North America and its introduction into China. According to one version, Pére Jartoux, a French Jesuit priest living in China, traveled through Manchuria sometime in the early 1700s. Having used ginseng, it seems Jartoux was impressed by its medicinal effects and wrote an article about it. He said that if ginseng could be found anywhere else in the world, it would probably be Canada, where the landscape was similar to that of Manchuria. Another Jesuit missionary living in Canada, Pére Joseph Francois Lafitau, read Jartoux's article sometime around 1715. Lafitau had been working with the Caughnawage band of Mohawks near Montreal. After reading the article on ginseng, Lafitau began to search systemically for it in the woods where he lived. As luck would have it, one day the missionary stumbled upon a plant growing near his cabin. Samples of the new American ginseng were sent to China, and by 1718 vigorous herbal trade started that involved Native Americans, French fur traders, and frontiersmen such as Daniel Boone.

Unfortunately, overharvested, the once vast stands of wild American ginseng have now been severely depleted, and its price keeps going up. At this time, authentic root can be priced as high as $400 to $600 per pound. Currently, American ginseng is on the threatened- or endangered-species lists in Virginia, Tennessee, Kentucky, and Illinois. Ginseng roots should be harvested only once the red fruits are ripe and can be replanted to ensure its continued growth.

Because of the exorbitant price of wild Ginseng root, woods-grown is probably the best option for most consumers. Cultivated ginseng is also available, but is less effective than wild or woods-grown. Good wild ginseng root is sweet flavored at first, then the taste changes to a pleasant bitter flavor. Commercial or cultivated root is generally sweetly bland in taste. Don't forget that the therapeutic value of an herb is assessed by its flavor, which tells everything about its chemical constituents and inherent healing energy. To be of healing value, the sweet flavor of wild ginseng root must be followed by that bitter aftertaste.

The outside of American ginseng root is an earthy-brown color with transverse wrinkles; the root will snap smoothly to reveal white flesh with reddish-brown resin ducts. Look for roots that are light, hard, and moist on the inside.

---- ☽ ----

Healing Qualities of American Ginseng
Sweet, Slightly Bitter, Cool, Nontoxic Energy
Treats Heart, Kidney, and Lung Organ Systems
Category: Herb that Tonifies the Yin (see page 353)

Of the *Panax ginsengs*, American ginseng is considered to be the most balanced. It serves as both a yin and yang tonic. Because of its cooling nature, American ginseng is especially suited for North Americans who tend to suffer from Heat conditions.

American ginseng counteracts weakness, irritability, fatigue, and thirst associated with chronic, low-grade fevers, as well as wheezing, expectoration of blood, and loss of voice. It aids in recovery from infectious diseases such as chronic bronchitis or tuberculosis.

Contraindications: This cooling herb should not be used by persons with diarrhea and poor digestion due to Cold.

Herbal Combinations Using American Ginseng

American ginseng, *anemarrhena,* and *gypsum* treat high fever, thirst, and diarrhea from infectious diseases.

Other Herbs that Tonify Yin

If the healing properties of American ginseng are not quite right for your condition, please see other herbs in this category: *Dendrobium, Glehnia, Lily Bulb, Ophiopogon*
Maximum Daily Dosage: 3 to 5 grams
1/10 ounce to 1/5 ounce

Ginseng (Eleuthero)
Combats Stress and Builds Immunity
English Name: Eleuthero Ginseng or Siberian Ginseng
Botanical Name: *Eleutherococcus senticosus*

A Brief History of Eleuthero Ginseng
Chinese: Ciwujia

While not a member of the Panax genus, Eleuthero ginseng belongs to the larger Aralia family of the ginsengs. Eleuthero comes to us from the Eastern

Russian forests and for this reason is also known as Siberian Ginseng. It was discovered in the 1950s by a Russian medical doctor, I. I. Brekhman, who was searching for a source of Panax ginseng. After conducting some 20 years of extensive research on eleuthero, Brekhman concluded that this amazing herb helps the human body adapt to stress and normalizes all its functions— a true adaptogenic herb in every sense of the word. Eleuthero is used by athletes to enhance endurance and performance. It enables them to recover more rapidly after strenuous exercise.

Eleuthero is considered to be a more neutral herb that is less stimulating than the Panax ginsengs. Siberian ginseng can be ingested over a longer period of time than can Panax without concern about its estrogenic and testosterone-inducing effects.

———— ▲ ————

Healing Qualities of Eleuthero Ginseng

Spicy, Warm Energy
Treats Kidney, Lung, and Spleen Organ Systems
Category: Herb that Tonifies the Qi (see page 352)

When the healing qualities of Eleuthero ginseng are compared to those of Panax ginseng, eleuthero is preferable if you are under stress. However, if your energy is extremely low and you are recovering from a chronic illness, Panax ginseng is best suited for you. Eleuthero is a true adaptogen in every sense of the word. If blood sugar is too low it brings it up; if it's too high, eleuthero lowers it. Eleuthero possesses the ability to help us adapt to time-zone changes (jet lag) or to higher elevations. Research also indicates this remarkable herb helps protect us from environmental pollutants while supporting the kidney adrenal complex and enhancing immunity.

Eleuthero can be taken for a much longer period of time than can Panax ginseng; one source indicates it may be ingested from two to eight months at a time.

Contraindications: None noted.

Note: Because of eleuthero's relatively recent discovery in Siberia, I am unaware of any classical Oriental herbal formulas containing this herb. However, the root cortex of one of its close cousins, *Acanthopanax gracilistylus,* has been used for hundreds of years by the Chinese as an herb to dispel Wind-Dampness conditions from the body (lumbago, rheumatism, and so forth).

Other Herbs that Tonify the Qi

If the healing qualities of eleuthero ginseng are not quite right for your condition, please see other herbs in this category: *Astragalus, Atractylodes, Codonopsis, Dioscorea, Ginseng, Jujube Date Fruit, Licorice*
Maximum Daily Dosage: 5 to 15 grams
1/5 ounce to 1/2 ounce

Ginseng (Panax)

Is Best Reserved for the "Over-40 Crowd"

English Name: Ginseng Root
Botanical Name: *Panax ginseng*

A Brief History of Ginseng

Mandarin: Rén Shen; **Japanese:** Ninjin; **Korean:** Insam

Panax ginseng, probably one of the most familiar of all Oriental herbs to Westerners, has been used in Oriental medicine for well over 4,000 years as a Qi Tonic. Ginseng actually made its way into Europe several times after the ninth century but gained importance in Western medicine only after the 1950s when Soviet research confirmed its therapeutic value as an "adaptogenic" herb.

There is a dispute regarding the actual number of species of *Panax*—some persons would argue that there are three, others say six. This depends on whether or not *P. pseudo-ginseng* is considered a single species with variants, or whether there are actually four separate species. *P. ginseng* grows wild in wooded, mountainous regions in northeastern China. This perennial plant has a carrotlike aromatic root whose value increases dramatically with age and appearance of the root. Many ginseng roots actually take on the appearance of humanlike figures with a torso, head, arms, and legs. According to one renowned botanical scholar, Dr. Shiu Ying Hu (formerly of Boston's Arnold Arboretum), ginseng represents earth's vital energy concentrated in a root shaped like a human being. Conventional Chinese belief holds that ginseng is, indeed, earth's crystallized essence in the form of humankind. Popular Oriental names for ginseng include "divine herb," "root of life," "long-life root," and "promise of immortality."

However, ginseng is not a great herb for everyone all of the time. *P. ginseng* is reserved in Oriental medicine to be taken for chronic illness, or for debility associated with old age. One common saying in China goes something like this: "If you take ginseng when you're young, what herb are you going to use when you grow old?" The widespread use of ginseng in the United States as a simple energy booster for all ages is off target. In the Orient, ginseng is usually not prescribed for patients under 40 years of age unless they are recovering from chronic illness. And then, use is usually restricted to three weeks or so. Panax ginseng is also not prescribed when symptoms include anxiety, depression, or acute inflammatory disease. Taken in excess, ginseng can cause restlessness, headaches, and high blood pressure. Indeed, this herb should not be taken by persons suffering from high blood pressure unless they are being monitored by a licensed health practitioner. Used appropriately, ginseng is a wonderful life-promoting herb, but it is not a cure-all and certainly is not indicated for all cases of fatigue. Considered more yin than *P. ginseng, P. quinquefolius* (see American Ginseng) is often more appropriate for children and people up to 40 years of age.

Panax ginseng roots are all white in color when peeled. Since most of ginseng's valuable healing constituents are found in the dark, exterior skin, however, the untouched whole root or root pieces are your best buy. Depending upon the processing method, ginseng roots are either white or red in color.

White roots refer to those that are under six years of age; usually considered of second quality, they are often bleached with sulfur gas and dried in the sun. However, fresh-dried Chinese white ginseng roots, the mildest form of the Asian ginsengs, can often be the most beneficial type for persons under 40 years of age. This is because the healing properties of Chinese white ginseng are similar to those of American ginseng. Look for very pale yellow roots.

Red roots must be at least four years of age but are usually more than six. Steam-processing creates chemical changes in the ginseng root, which make it take on its characteristic red color. Red Korean ginseng is the most stimulating of all ginsengs, followed by Chinese Red and then Chinese White.

Although the best ginseng roots are between 50 and 100 years of age, good roots are between 6 and 12 years old. It is easy to accurately determine the age of a ginseng root, but to do so, the neck must be attached. Count the number of scars on the neck of the ginseng root—each scar represents a year of growth. Always look for ginseng roots with the neck attached; a good harvester wants to show you the age of the roots since roots under three years of age are not considered worth the time or effort. It is between the fourth and sixth years that a ginseng root doubles its weight. During this time, the root's content of a healing phytochemical called ginsenoside peaks.

——— ▲ ———

Healing Qualities of Panax Ginseng
Sweet, Slightly Bitter, Slightly Warm Energy
Treats Spleen and Lung Organ Systems
Category: Herb that Tonifies the Qi (see page 352)

In the Orient, red ginseng is almost always found blended with other healing herbs in balanced traditional formulas. It is used in reviving dying patients—for shock and cardiac failure. Ginseng is given to cancer patients to improve appetite and enhance the immune response. It is particularly effective for elderly persons to increase appetite and improve digestion and to aid in assimilation of nutrients. Ginseng is ideal for weak, chronically ill persons suffering from exhaustion and anxiety. For overstimulated persons with strong constitutions, however, ginseng can bring on feelings of anxiety, heart palpitations, and/or insomnia.

Contraindications: Ginseng should not be ingested with alcohol, caffeine, tea, turnips, or bitter or spicy foods. It is best reserved for persons over 40 years of age and should not be taken by those suffering from high blood pressure. Ginseng should not be taken for more than a few weeks at a time. Excessive use of ginseng can lead to imbalances even in elderly persons.

Herbal Combinations Using Ginseng

A few slices of good Ginseng root is sometimes cooked in tonic soups to boost yang energy just prior to the winter season. If you are convalescing from a chronic illness or would like an immune boost prior to cold winter months, throw 3 to 4 slices of ginseng root into your favorite homemade chicken soup and let it bubble away for a couple of hours over low heat. You might want to add a piece of codonopsis, astragalus, dioscorea, and a few jujube dates.

Ginseng, *ophiopogon,* and *schisandra* are combined to treat spontaneous sweating and shortness of breath related to Qi and Yin Deficiency.

Ginseng and *aconite* treat ice-cold extremities, profuse perspiration, and shortness of breath associated with Devastated Yang and Collapsed Qi conditions.

Other Herbs that Tonify the Qi

If the healing properties of Panax ginseng are not quite right for your condition, please see other herbs in this category: *American, Eleuthero or Pseudoginseng, Astragalus, Atractylodes, Codonopsis, Dioscorea, Jujube Date Fruit, Licorice*
Maximum Daily Dosage: 1 gram to 10 grams
1/30 ounce to 1/3 ounce

Pseudoginseng
Treats Traumatic Injuries
English Name: Pseudoginseng Root
Botanical Name: *Panax pseudoginseng* var. *notoginseng*

A Brief History of Pseudoginseng
Mandarin: San Qi; **Japanese:** Sanshichi; **Korean:** Samch'il

Pseudoginseng (also known as Tien Qi ginseng) is a hardy perennial with car-rotlike roots that grows to a height of about three feet in Bhutan and north-eastern India. Small flowers produce round red berries. A member of the Panax genus, this herb is botanically related to ginseng. Unlike Panax ginseng, however, it is not used as an energy tonic. Because of this herb's ability to relieve pain and move blood, it is the herb of choice in China to treat traumatic injuries. During the Vietnam War this herb was used extensively by the Vietcong to improve recovery from gunshot wounds.

P. zingiberensis (used as a substitute for *P. notoginseng*) is on the endangered-species list, and *P. pseudoginseng* is nearly extinct in the wild. There is confusion in medical literature regarding whether or not there are notable differences in the plant constituents between *P. pseudoginseng* and *P. notoginseng.*

For a more detailed history on other members of the Panax genus, please see "Ginseng."

Good-quality pseudoginseng has a thin cortex and dark color; the root is large, solid, and heavy.

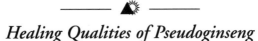

Healing Qualities of Pseudoginseng
Sweet, Slightly Bitter, Slightly Warm Energy
Treats Liver, Stomach, and Large-Intestine Organ Systems
Category: Herb that Regulates the Blood and Stops Bleeding (see page 350)

Pseudoginseng controls bleeding (specifically for hemorrhage from the lungs, digestive tract, or uterus, or from injuries). It has antibacterial properties, relieves pain, improves circulation, and reduces inflammation. The roots are taken internally for heart disease and angina. The flowers are used for vertigo and dizziness.

Contraindications: This herb should not be taken by pregnant women or by persons suffering from Blood or Yin Deficiency.

Other Herbs that Regulate the Blood

If the healing qualities of pseudoginseng are not quite right for your condition, please see other herbs in this category: *Agrimony, Mugwort Leaf, Sanguisorba, Sophora*

Maximum Daily Dosage: 1 to 3 grams taken directly in powder form or 1/30 ounce to 1/10 ounce

Glehnia Root

Strengthens the Lungs
English Name: Root of Beech Silver-top
Botanical Name: *Adenophora tetraphylla* or *Glehnia littoralis*

A Brief History of Glehnia Root

Mandarin: Sha Shen; **Japanese:** Shajin; **Korean:** Sasam

A member of the parsley family, glehnia is native to eastern and southeastern China, Korea, Taiwan, and Japan. Glehnia root is described as one of the five "shens," or medicinal roots, in the *Ben cao gag mu*. Written by Li Shi-Zhen in 1590, this book represents the greatest compilation of Chinese healing plants ever written. While Panax ginseng strengthens our organs of digestion and assimilation (the Spleen Organ System in Oriental thought), glehnia, or "white ginseng," strengthens the Lung Organ System. Botanically, glehnia is not related to ginseng.

Unlike ginseng, which is a Yang Tonic, glehnia is a Yin Tonic. Ginseng is warm and stimulating, while the cooling energy of glehnia actually lowers temperature in animal studies.

Good-quality glehnia roots are long, solid, and yellowish-white in color.

——— ☽ ———

Healing Qualities of Glehnia Root

Sweet, Bitter, Bland, Cool Energy
Treats Lung and Stomach Organ Systems
Category: Herb that Tonifies the Yin (see page 353)

Glehnia is often prescribed after illness marked by fever, when a person feels parched, dry, and dehydrated. It moistens the lungs and relieves dry, hacking coughs. It helps eliminate constipation accompanying these conditions. Glehnia is often used in formulas treating rashes, acne, headaches, or arthritis.

Contraindications: Persons who feel chilled and run-down or who suffer from weak digestion due to Cold from Deficiency should not take glehnia.

Herbal Combinations Using Glehnia

Fritillary, anemarrhena, and glehnia treat dry coughs with phlegm that is difficult to expectorate due to Lung Yin Deficiency.

Raw rhemannia, dendrobium, and glehnia are combined to treat dry mouth and throat, constipation and/or low-grade fevers due to warm-febrile diseases or Stomach Yin Deficiency.

Other Herbs that Tonify the Yin

If the healing properties of glehnia are not quite right for your condition, please see other herbs in this category: *American Ginseng Root (see "Ginseng"), Dendrobium, Lily Bulb, Ophiopogon*
Maximum Daily Dosage: 9 to 15 grams
1/4 to 1/2 ounce

Gypsum
Relieves High Fevers
Chemical Name: *Calcium Sulfate*

A Brief History of Gypsum
Mandarin: Shí Gao; **Japanese:** Sekko; **Korean:** Sôkko

Gypsum, a chemical known as calcium sulfate, has been used since ancient times in the Orient to reduce high fevers resulting from infections. It is also applied externally to rashes, boils, and skin abscesses that have not burst to promote healing. In the Orient, gypsum is commonly used in the culinary sphere as well. Traditionally, it is used as the coagulating agent for bean-curd, made from soybeans. Oriental housewives make a dessert from gypsum called *dao fu fa,* which is similar to bean curd in preparation, taste, and texture.

When shopping for gypsum, look for clean, large lumps that are white and highly fibrous.

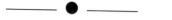

Healing Qualities of Gypsum

Sweet, Spicy, Very Cold Nontoxic Energy
Treats Lung and Stomach Organ Systems
Category: Herb that Clears Heat and Drains Fire (see page 345)

Gypsum relieves high fevers without chills, toothaches, swollen and painful gums, intense thirst, irritability, restlessness, headaches, profuse perspiration, coughing, and expectoration of thick phlegm.

Contraindications: Persons suffering from weak digestion or Cold symptoms should avoid taking gypsum.

Herbal Combinations Using Gypsum

For burns, eczema, and ulcerated sores, gypsum is calcined, mixed with other healing herbs (such as *phellodendron*), and applied topically in powdered form.

Anemarrhena and gypsum treat high fever, irritability, and extreme thirst accompanying febrile diseases.

Gypsum and *wild ginger* treat sore, painful swollen gums and toothache due to Stomach Heat.

Other Herbs that Clear Heat and Drain Fire

If the healing properties of gypsum are not quite right for your condition, please see other herbs in this category: *Anemarrhena, Gardenia*
Maximum Daily Dosage: 10 to 30 grams
1/3 ounce to 1 ounce

Hawthorn Fruit

Aids Digestion and Helps Heal the Heart

Botanical Name: *Crataegus pinnatifida* or *C. cuneata*

A Brief History of Hawthorn Fruit

Mandarin: Shan Zha; Japanese: Sanzashi; Korean: Sanza

Crataegus gets its botanical name from the Greek word *kratos,* meaning "strength"; hawthorn wood is very "strong" or hard. Approximately 280 species of hawthorn, or *Crataegus,* thrive in northern temperate regions. Originally, some 1,000 different species were named, but many of them were probably hybrids. Hawthorn is a small deciduous tree or shrub, densely branched and usually thorny. Fragrant white flowers appear in springtime, followed by egg-shaped, dark-red fruits with one or two stony seeds.

Many rituals have been associated with the hawthorn, including the custom of choosing a May queen. In pagan times, before the Christian era, the King and Queen of May were sacrificed at the end of the growing season. Oddly, to this day, the hawthorn tree still symbolizes hope, as well as an omen of death.

Traditionally, in the countryside, tasty young leaves of the hawthorn were added to sandwiches, like lettuce, which gave it the common name, "bread-and-cheese." Since the Middle Ages, hawthorn fruit has been used in Europe as a remedy for the heart. *C. pinnatifida,* native to northern China, is used medicinally in Oriental herbalism. Practitioners of Traditional Oriental Medicine use this sour, but pleasant-tasting herb as a digestive aid.

Look for large, dry, thick-fleshed fruit with a deep red skin. If the hawthorn fruit is sliced, you will see yellow seeds surrounded by yellowish-brown fruit flesh.

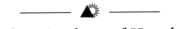

Healing Qualities of Hawthorn
Sour, Sweet, Slightly Warm Energy
Treats Spleen, Stomach, and Liver Organ Systems
Category: Herb that Relieves Food Stagnation (see page 349)

In Oriental medicine, "Food Stagnation" is a term used to cover a number of digestive-tract disturbances from irritable-bowel syndrome to gall-bladder weakness. Often, something as simple as an emotional disturbance can cause Qi and Blood to congest in the Middle Burner or Stomach/Spleen region of the body, giving rise to poor digestion. That's why it is often best not to eat if you are unduly upset. *C. pinnatifida* has antibacterial properties and is a circulatory, uterine, and digestive stimulant. Hawthorn fruits are ingested raw for circulatory disorders, and baked fruit is eaten to aid digestive disturbances. Hawthorn reduces hypertension associated with coronary-artery disease and is utilized to reduce postpartum pain, hernial pain, or in cases of absent menstruation.

Contraindications: Many medicinal plants that act on the heart can be toxic—hawthorn is relatively nontoxic. However, it is always important to consult with qualified medical practitioners before using hawthorn for serious conditions. Use this herb with caution in case of Spleen/Stomach Deficiency (digestive weakness) or if there is acid regurgitation.

Herbal Combinations Using Hawthorn Fruit

Dang gui, ligusticum, and hawthorn relieve menstrual and postpartum pain due to blood stasis.

Fennel seed and hawthorn are used for testicular pain and swelling from prolapse associated with hernias.

Hawthorn and *salvia* relieve chest pain due to blood stasis in the Heart Acupuncture Meridian.

Other Herbs that Relieve Food Stagnation

If the healing properties of hawthorn are not quite right for your condition, please see the other herb in this category: *Radish Seeds*
Maximum Daily Dosage: 5 to 10 grams
1/5 ounce to 1/3 ounce

Honeysuckle Flower
A Superior Herbal Antibiotic
Botanical Name: *Lonicera japonica, L. hypoglauca, L. confusa,*
and *L. similis* are used instead in different parts of China

A Brief History of Honeysuckle Flower
Mandarin: Jin Yín Hua; **Japanese:** Kinginka; **Korean:** Kûmûnhwa

The honeysuckle plant was once an object of worship in ancient Greece; later, its juice was used by European herbalists to treat snake bites. *Lonicera's* botanical name comes from that of a German naturalist and physician—Adam Lonicer (1528-1586)—while its popular name comes from the erroneous belief that bees make "honey" from the pollen of its fragrant flowers. The white flowers produced by *Lonicera japonica* turn yellow the second day and are followed by poisonous black berries. There are over 180 species of honeysuckle shrubs and climbers growing throughout the northern hemisphere. Native to eastern Asia, *L. japonica* has been naturalized in the United States and Australia. This popular, sweet-smelling ornamental plant is now considered a serious weed in some parts of the United States.

Honeysuckle was first mentioned in the Chinese *Tang Materia Medica* written around A.D. 659. For medicinal use, honeysuckle flowers are collected in the early morning before they open and are dried. Stems, harvested in the fall and winter months, are dried for use in poultices, decoctions, powders, tinctures, and pills. Look for large, yellowish-white, unopened buds.

●

Healing Qualities of Honeysuckle Flowers
Sweet, Cold Energy
Treats Large Intestine, Lung, and Stomach Organ Systems
Category: Herb that Clears Heat and Relieves Toxicity (see page 346)

Honeysuckle flowers have a sweet, cooling energy that reduces fevers and inflammation. Often compared to echinacea, this herbal ally has antibacterial and diuretic properties. Honeysuckle also reduces blood pressure, increases perspiration, and relaxes spasms.

Honeysuckle flowers are taken internally for acute rheumatoid arthritis, upper respiratory tract infections (including pneumonia), conjunctivitis, sore throats, high fevers, childhood infections (for example, measles, chickenpox), gastroenteritis, food poisoning, urinary-tract infections, mastitis, and breast cancer. Honeysuckle stems are used for hepatitis, while its stems and flowers treat dysentery. The flowers are also utilized for external applications to treat infectious rashes, skin inflammations, and sores.

Contraindications: Honeysuckle flowers should not be given to persons experiencing diarrhea from Spleen and Stomach Deficiency due to Cold. The flowers should not be used in treating Yin sores or ulcers due to Qi Deficiency (these are concave ulcerations that exude a clear liquid).

Herbal Combinations Using Honeysuckle Flower
Honeysuckle and *forsythia fruit* are often combined with the following herbs:
Add *scutellaria* and *coptis* for high fever.
Add *dandelion, chrysanthemum flower*, and *viola root* for sores and furuncles.
Add *scutellaria* for boils that have not ulcerated and are not discharging pus.

Other Herbs that Clear Heat and Relieve Toxicity
If the healing properties of honeysuckle flowers are not quite right for your condition, please see the other herbs in this category: *Dandelion, Forsythia Fruit*
Maximum Daily Dosage: 10 to 15 grams
1/3 ounce to 1/2 ounce

Job's Tears see *Coix*

Jujube Date Fruit

Helps Keep the Doctor Away
Botanical Name: *Ziziphus jujuba* var. *inermis*

A Brief History of Jujube Date Fruit
Mandarin: Dá Zao or Hóng Zao; **Japanese:** Taiso; **Korean:** Taecho

Jujube is considered a fruit in the Orient and consumed in much the same way that Americans eat apples. However, persons in China did not want to keep their doctors away. Prevention is the key word in Oriental medicine. Oriental health practitioners were paid to keep their patients healthy and did not charge for services if the patient became ill.

Jujube fruit, or Chinese date, is native to temperate Asia and is rarely encountered outside botanic gardens today. These plants were introduced to western Asia, from China, about 3,000 years ago. There are approximately 85 species of this deciduous tree or large shrub growing in tropical and subtropical regions with spiny twigs that reach up to 45 feet in height. Small yellow flowers develop into one-inch-long oval-shaped fruits. A dark reddish-brown to black skin covers the sweet, whitish pulp. Jujube has been cultivated in China for ages and was first mentioned in Chinese medical literature during the Han dynasty (A.D. 25-220). The ancient Romans and Greeks also grew jujubes; they introduced the plant to Spain, where it became naturalized.

Jujubes are eaten fresh or cooked once they become spongy and wrinkled. This increases their sweetness. Usually, red jujube dates are utilized medicinally while the black ones are used in cooking. Look for thick, plump fruits with sweet flesh and small seeds.

———— 🌳 ————

Healing Qualities of Jujube Dates
Sweet, Neutral Energy
Treats Spleen and Stomach Organ Systems
Category: Herb that Tonifies the Qi (see page 352)

Jujube dates find their way into many herbal formulations to moderate the actions of the other herbs and minimize side effects. They have a sedative or calming action and help prevent the formation of ulcers due to stress. Jujubes Tonify the Stomach and Spleen, increasing Qi. They control allergic responses, protect the liver, soothe damaged or irritated tissues, and relieve coughing.

Jujube fruits are ingested for nervous exhaustion, hysteria, chronic fatigue, loss of appetite, and diarrhea. Jujube date seeds (see Zizyphus Seeds) are effective in preventing night sweats, insomnia, palpitations, and excessive perspiration.

Often added to herbal formulas to harmonize, sweeten, and flavor, the long-term usage of jujube is said to improve the complexion.

Contraindications: Since jujube dates increase moisture in the body, they should not be consumed by persons with symptoms pertaining to Dampness, Food Stagnation, or intestinal parasites.

Herbal Combinations Using Jujube Dates

Jujube is often used in Tonifying formulas, especially with *Panax ginseng* and *dang gui*.

Cook with your cure! Please see Chapter 5 for some delicious recipes containing jujube dates.

Other Herbs that Tonify the Qi

If the healing properties of jujube dates are not quite right for your condition, please see the other herbs in this category: *Astragalus, Atractylodes, Codonopsis, Dioscorea, Ginseng, Licorice*

Maximum Daily Dosage: 10 to 15 grams or 2 to 8 pieces

Kelp see Seaweed

Kudzu Root

Relieves Neck and Shoulder Tension

Botanical Name: *Pueraria lobota, P. omeiensis,* or *P. thomsanii*

A Brief History of Kudzu Root

Mandarin: Gé Gen; **Japanese:** Kakkon; **Korean:** Kalgûn

A member of the legume family, pueraria was named after a professor of botany in Copenhagen, Marc Puerari (1766-1845). Also known as kudzu (sometimes spelled kuzu), or Japanese arrowroot, pueraria is native to thickets and sparse woodlands in Japan and southeast Asia. In the 1870s, it was introduced into the southern United States, where it is now considered an unwelcome, invasive intruder. In contrast, pueraria is cultivated in both Japan and China, where its fibers are utilized in the manufacture of textiles. In a single season, this climber can grow up to 60 feet in length while producing fragrant purple flowers that are followed by flat, hairy fruits. Pueraria produces one of the world's largest vegetable roots that can reach 7 feet in length and average 200 pounds in weight. Used as a thickener for Oriental dishes (much like cornstarch in the United States), kudzu root was first mentioned as a medicinal herb in the *Shen Nong Canon of Herbs* written during the Han dynasty in China (206 B.C.–23 A.D.).

The flowers and roots of kudzu have phytochemicals (daidzin and daidzein) that are reputed to suppress the desire to drink alcohol. Oriental medicine has long used kudzu to effectively treat alcohol abuse. Harvard medical researcher Wing-Ming Keung compiled more than three hundred case studies during a recent visit to China in which kudzu root, along with other herbs, proved to be effective in suppressing cravings for alcohol while improving vital organ function. No toxic side effects were reported.

Dried, unprocessed pueraria root is cream colored on the exterior while the interior wood is white and highly fibrous. Look for mealy- or starchy-textured roots that are not too stringy.

——— ◗ ———

Healing Qualities of Kudzu

Sweet, Spicy, Cool Energy
Treats Spleen and Stomach Organ Systems
Category: Herb that Releases Exterior Conditions (see page 344)

Kudzu is considered a sweet, cooling herb that relaxes muscle spasms (particularly in the neck and shoulders), relieves pain, lowers blood pressure, increases perspiration, and soothes the digestive system. It is also taken internally to relieve colds, flu, fevers, headaches, dizziness, chronic diarrhea, measles and other skin eruptions, thirst, dehydration, and stiff neck. The flowers are used for abdominal bloating, gastritis, nausea and vomiting, as well as for drug and alcohol poisoning.

Herbal Combinations Using Kudzu Root

Do you carry tension in your neck and shoulders? Kudzu root is a veritable miracle cure for relieving upper-body muscular tension. Use this wonderful healing herb in your cooking. The first thing you need to do is to go to your cupboard and throw out the cornstarch. Next, buy a couple of packages of lumpy white kudzu-root powder at your health-food store. Now, whenever you need a thickener for sauces, gravies, stir-fries, puddings, pies—you name it—pull out the kudzu-root powder. It takes approximately 1 level tablespoon of kudzu powder to thicken 1 cup of liquid. Always dissolve the powder in about 1/4 cup cold water before stirring it into the dish you are preparing. At first, kudzu is cloudy when added to the liquid in a soup or sauce, but it becomes clear as it cooks and thickens.

Pueraria (kudzu) is combined with *trichosanthes* and *ophiopogon* to treat dehydration and thirst.

Dioscorea and pueraria treat diarrhea due to digestive weakness, or in Oriental terms, Deficient Spleen and Stomach Qi.

Coptis, scutellaria, and pueraria are used to clear dysentery-like disorders (Damp Heat with Hot diarrhea).

Kudzu root plus *kudzu flower* or *chrysanthemum flower* treats hangovers and relieves drunkenness.

Ephedra, cinnamon twigs, peony root (white), and pueraria relieve neck and shoulder stiffness due to colds and flus (of the "Cold" type with low fever, chills, and body aches).

Pueraria and *bupleurum* are combined to treat Wind Heat or flu symptoms accompanied by high fever.

Contraindications: None noted.

Other Cool, Spicy Herbs that Release the Exterior

If the healing properties of kudzu are not quite right for your condition, please see the other herbs in this category: *Bupleurum, Chrysanthemum, Cohosh, Peppermint*

CASE HISTORY: Over the years, I have seen many cases in which pueraria has been the ultimate answer for relief of pain from whiplash and neck and shoulder tension. However, one case stands out in my mind. Betty was 37 years of age when she came to the clinic in October of 1992, complaining of severe neck and shoulder pain due to whiplash. Betty had been injured in a car accident when she was only 8 years old and had never fully recovered. Over nearly three decades she tried virtually every form of conventional and nonconventional therapy known, and as she put it, "was at her wit's end." She did not want to continue taking pain medication for the rest of her life, but the neck and shoulder pain was intolerable. Betty received one acupuncture treatment and, of course, a lesson on cooking with kudzu. Six months later a wonderful note came in the mail. Betty said she couldn't believe that she had been pain free for six months—one acupuncture treatment and a humble herb (considered a "noxious weed" in southern parts of the United States) had changed her life.

Maximum Daily Dosage: 3 to 12 grams
1/10 to 1/3 ounce

Licorice Root

Is the Herbal Harmonizer that Heals Peptic Ulcers

Botanical Name: *Glycyrrhiza uralensis*

A Brief History of Licorice Root

Mandarin: Gan Cao; **Japanese:** Kanzo; **Korean:** Kamch'o

There are 20 species of licorice, a perennial with sticky leaflets and light-blue-to violet-colored flowers that grow in the Americas, Eurasia, and Australia. *G. uralensis,* a key herbal tonifier and detoxifier, known as the "grandfather of herbs" in Oriental medicine, is native to Asia, Japan, and China. Another species, *G. glabra,* was an important herb for the ancient Egyptians, Chinese, and Assyrians; it eventually reached Europe by the fifteenth century.

Since at least 500 B.C., licorice has been used in folk medicine around the world. Dominican friars from Pontefract, Yorkshire, made lozenges (known as pomfrets) from licorice. An American variety of licorice, *G. lepidota,* was used by early settlers and native North Americans as an herbal aid for childbirth and menstrual-cycle problems. African people make a tea of licorice stems and roots to treat eye diseases, appendicitis, and pulmonary tuberculosis. People in Vietnam take powdered licorice root to induce sweating and as a diuretic and purgative. The East Indians treat sore throats, asthma, hoarseness, and intestinal and urinary-tract inflammations with licorice. Extracts from boiled roots are used to make licorice candy as well as flavorings for soft drinks, beer, tobacco, commercial laxatives, and other pharmaceutical products. The foaming agent in beers and fire extinguishers is produced from licorice extracts.

Glycyrrhiza, the botanical name for licorice, comes from the Greek and means "sweet root." *G. glabra* contains a substance known as glycyrrhizin, which has cortisone-like effects. Glycyrrhiza is 50 times sweeter than sugar and is now becoming widely recognized as an incredibly effective aid to heal ulcers.

Licorice, an important herbal harmonizer, has long been used to antidote poisons. Utilized in ancient China to remedy henbane poisoning, licorice was combined with soya beans in the eighteenth century to counter-act poisons in general.

Licorice roots are long and cylindrical. Look for sweet slices, with an earth-brown exterior and light-yellow interior. Root slices that have been stir-fried with honey are quite sticky and reddish-brown in color.

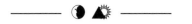

Healing Qualities of Licorice Root

Sweet, Neutral Energy (Raw); Sweet, Warm (Toasted)
Treats all 12 Primary Channels (principally Spleen and Lung)
Category: Herb that Tonifies the Qi (see page 352)

A slice or two of licorice root is added to the majority of Chinese herbal for-mulas to harmonize and direct the effects of the other herbs. It is a sweet tonic herb that reduces pain and inflammation, controls coughing, relaxes muscle spasms (particularly of the legs and abdomen), neutralizes toxins, bal-ances blood-sugar levels, and stimulates adrenocorticol hormones.

Licorice root is taken internally for peptic ulcers, Addison's disease, and asthma. For external use, it can be combined with honeysuckle flowers for application to acne and boils.

Contraindications: The use of licorice is contraindicated during preg-nancy or with hypertension, kidney disease, or for patients taking digoxin-based medications. Taken in excess, licorice can raise blood pressure and cause water retention—it should not be taken by persons with edema. According to traditional sources, licorice should not be combined with poly-gala, euphorbia, daphnes, or seaweed.

Herbal Combinations Using Licorice Root

Dried licorice can be chewed like candy, and many children love its flavor. In China, parents give it to their children to promote the growth of muscle tissue.

Licorice is often combined with *Panax ginseng* as an energy tonic.

Codonopsis and licorice treat fatigue, loose stools, and lack of appetite.

Dandelion and licorice can be taken internally and applied externally for boils, abscesses, and other "Hot" swellings.

Licorice and *peony root (white)* stop muscle cramps and are taken to relieve intestinal and abdominal pain, as well as muscle spasms.

Apricot seed, fritillary, and licorice relieve dry coughs due to Heat.

Other Herbs that Tonify Qi

If the healing properties of licorice are not quite right for your condition, please see the other herbs in this category: *Astragalus, Atractylodes, Codonopsis, Dioscorea, Ginseng, Jujube Date Fruit*
Maximum Daily Dosage: 2 to 10 grams
1/12 ounce to 1/3 ounce

Ligusticum

Increases Circulation and Relieves Pain

English Name: Cnidium or Szechuan Lovage Root
Botanical Name: *Ligusticum chuanxiong,* also known as *L. wallichii*

A Brief History of Ligusticum

Mandarin: Chuan Xiong; **Japanese:** Senkyu; **Korean:** Ch'onkung

Ligusticum is a celery-like plant with small white flowers that is often used as a pot herb. There are a total of 25 species that grow in northern temperate regions, several of which are used medicinally. The Flathead people of North America use *L. canbyi* for colds. The leaves and stems of *L. scoticum* are freshly cut in spring for use as a veggie.

Many Western, Chinese, and Ayurvedic herbalists feel *L. porteri* (also known as *osha,* Colorado cough root, or Porter's lovage) is superior to *L. sinense. L. sinense* is native to Nei Mongol, as well as to the southern Yellow River basin in China. Please note that *L. sinense* is used as a Warm, Spicy herb to Release the Exterior (specifically for Wind Cold symptoms). However, the ligusticum being covered in this section is *L. chuanxiong*—this species has properties different from the former. It is used to Invigorate the Blood. Be sure to ask for *L. chuanxiong* or *L. wallichii* when purchasing this dark-brown, irregularly fist-shaped rhizome covered with many nodes. The interior is light yellow. Look for plump, heavy rhizomes with a strong aroma.

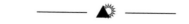

Healing Qualities of Ligusticum

Spicy, Warm Energy
Treats Liver, Gall Bladder, and Pericardium Organ Systems
Category: Herb that Invigorates the Blood (see page 350)

The roots of Szechuan lovage are aromatic, spicy, and warm in energy. They stimulate circulation, lower blood pressure, and have antibacterial and sedative properties. Ligusticum relieves pain and causes uterine contractions; it is used to treat menstrual disorders such as dysmenorrhea, amenorrhea, and endometriosis. Ligusticum is taken internally for aches and pains caused by cold, poor circulation, coronary heart disease, and postpartum bleeding.

Contraindications: Do not use ligusticum in cases of excessive menstrual bleeding, weakness, fatigue, or in case of Deficient Heat symptoms. Overdosage of this herb can result in dizziness and nausea. Ligusticum should not be combined with astragalus, coptis, or cornus according to traditional sources.

Herbal Combinations Using Ligusticum

Ligusticum, *bupleurum,* and *peony root (red)* are combined to treat headache and/or chest pain due to Congested Liver Qi and Blood.

Dang gui and ligusticum treat menstrual disorders as well as Wind-Dampness and Stagnation blocking the channels resulting in moving pains, numbness, and paralysis.

Other Herbs that Invigorate the Blood

If the healing properties of ligusticum are not quite right for your condition, please see the other herbs in this category: *Achyranthes, Peony Root (Red), Safflower Flower, Salvia, Turmeric*

Maximum Daily Dosage: 3 to 6 grams

1/10 ounce to 1/5 ounce

Lily Bulb
Eases Dry Coughs
Botanical Name: *Lilium brownii* var. *colchesteri, L. pumilum,* or *L. longiflorum*

A Brief History of Lily Bulb
Mandarin: Bai Hé; **Japanese:** Byakugo; **Korean:** Paekhap

Few flowers are quite as lovely as a lily in its elegant simplicity, and very few people in the Americas realize that some of the 100 species are actually edible. Lilies serve as an important vegetable for the Japanese, Chinese, and some North American natives who cultivate them as a food source. One variety, *L. candidum,* was recorded by Pliny as being a cure for skin problems and foot complaints. While *L. candidum* has a long record of medicinal use, it is rarely used today because of its scarcity.

The flowers of *L. brownii* are rose-purple on the exterior and pure white on the inside. In the Orient, lily bulbs are valued as one of the few herbs that nourishes Kidney Yin. Lily is more food than medicine, however, and regularly appears in soups year-round. Fresh bulbs are consumed raw or lightly cooked.

Dried lily-bulb slices are yellowish-white in color, semitranslucent, hard, and break cleanly. Look for heavy, white bulbs with a bitter flavor.

Healing Qualities of Lily Bulb
Sweet, Slightly Bitter, Slightly Cold Energy
Treats Lung and Heart Organ Systems
Category: Herb that Tonifies the Yin (see page 353)

Lily bulb nourishes the Yin and Moistens Dryness in our human garden, treating restlessness, irritability, palpitations, insomnia, dry coughing, thirst, sore throats, and lingering low-grade fevers.

Contraindications: If you're Cold and Damp, this herb is not ideal for you. However, if you want to throw a few slices of lily bulb into your aduki-bean soup, along with a slice of ginger to warm it up, it would be quite all right. Therapeutic dosages of this herb should be avoided in case of diarrhea or coughing accompanied by clear or white phlegm.

Herbal Combinations Using Lily Bulb
Again, with this wonderful healing herb food, please feel free to cook with your cure. Persons suffering from Yin Deficiency and Dryness can consume the larger portion of lily bulb that is added to any soup or stew being prepared for the whole family.

Lily bulb is combined with *coix* to treat dry cough, thick mucus, and Lung abscess.

Codonopsis and lily bulb treat Yin and Qi Deficiency as well as relieve chest pain due to congestion.

Other Herbs that Tonify the Yin
If the healing properties of lily bulb are not quite right for your condition, please see the other herbs in this category: *American Ginseng Root (see "Ginseng"), Dendrobium, Glehnia, Ophiopogon*
Maximum Daily Dosage: 5 to 15 grams
1/5 ounce to 1/2 ounce

Longan Berries
Fight Fatigue, Forgetfulness, and Insomnia
Botanical Name: Euphoria longan

A Brief History of Longan Berries
Mandarin: Lóng Yan Ròu; **Japanese:** Ryuganniku; **Korean:** Yonganyuk

Longan fruit, native to India, is now widely cultivated in southern China and the Malay Archipelago. *Euphoria longan,* an evergreen tree, produces small, yellowish-white flowers that later bear round, grayish-yellow fruits. The outer protective skin of the longan berry is very thin, brittle, and easily broken to reveal white, juicy flesh surrounding a shiny, dark-brown seed. As the fruit dries, the interior flesh changes from white to dark brown and shrinks to become a sticky, semitranslucent mass.

When shopping for longan fruit, look for large, soft brown berries with a strong, sweet flavor. In the Orient, longan berries are frequently added to confections, desserts, soups, and drinks.

———— ▲ ————

Healing Qualities of Longan Berries
Sweet, Warm Energy
Treats Heart and Spleen Organ Systems
Category: Herb that Tonifies the Blood (see page 352)

This delicious Blood-Tonifying and Yin-enriching fruit treats anemia, anxiety, restlessness, insomnia, palpitations, dizziness, ringing in the ears, and forgetfulness often due to fatigue, stress, and overwork. Longan is also reputed to halt the premature graying of hair.

Contraindications: Not to be consumed by persons with diarrhea due to Spleen Deficiency (or digestive weakness).

Herbal Combinations Using Longan Berries
You can make delicious desserts with the naturally sweet longan fruit—simply add a few berries to cookies, pies, cakes, or other desserts.

Rehmannia root and longan berries treat dizziness, insomnia, and blurred vision due to Yin and Blood Deficiency.

Ophiopogon, trichosanthes, and longan relieve dryness of the throat and mouth. This combination also treats irritability and anxiety stemming from dehydration and Blood Deficiency.

Other Herbs that Tonify the Blood

If the healing properties of longan fruit are not quite right for your condition, please see the other herbs in this category: *Dang Gui, Lycii Fruit, Peony Root (White), Polygonum, Rehmannia (Cooked)*
Maximum Daily Dosage: 5 to 15 grams
1/5 ounce to 1/2 ounce

Lonicera see Honeysuckle Flower

Lycii Fruit
Aids Vision and Relieves Anemia
English Name: Wolfberry or Fruit of the Matrimony Vine
Botanical Name: *Lycium chinense,* in other parts of China, *L. barbarum* is used

A Brief History of Lycii Fruit
Mandarin: Gou Qi Zi; **Japanese:** Kukoshi; **Korean:** Kugicha

In European folklore, lycii fruit, or wolfberry, was never planted near a home because it was reputed to cause disharmony between husband and wife. To this day, lycii is known as "matrimony vine." It seems, however, that folks in the Orient had a different spin on the properties of this herb. An ancient Chinese adage warns men not to eat lycii berries far from home, alluding to the herb's reputation of being an aphrodisiac.

Native to Japan and China, there are approximately 100 species of deciduous and evergreen lycium shrubs that now grow in most temperate and subtropical regions. Small purple flowers are followed by small, orange- to reddish-colored fruit. Both *L. chinense* and *L. barbarum* are used in Oriental medicine. References to the use of lycium can be found in Chinese medical texts dating back to 206 B.C.

Most medicinal-quality lycii comes to us from China. Look for soft, moist, plump fruits of a bright-red color. Sweet fruits with few seeds are the best.

------ 🜨 ------

Healing Qualities of Lycii

Sweet, Neutral Energy
Treats Liver, Lung, and Kidney Organ Systems
Category: Herb that Tonifies the Blood (see page 352)

Lycii berries can be added to soups and desserts. Try making a batch of your favorite oatmeal cookies and adding lycii berries instead of raisins. You can also add 1 to 2 tablespoons of this blood-building herb to soups and stews.

Sweet, tonic lycii fruit Tonifies the Blood, treating anemia, dizziness, and palpitations. It lowers blood pressure and cholesterol. Lycii fruit is pre-scribed for poor eyesight, dry eyes, blurred vision, photosensitivity, night blindness, vertigo, lumbago, impotence, diabetes, and menopausal complaints.

Herbal Combinations Using Lycii Fruit

Lycii is combined with *rehmannia (raw), cuscuta,* and *eucommia* for Blood and Yin Deficiency and such symptoms as impotence, dizziness, ringing in the ears, and weakness.

Chrysanthemum flowers and lycii treat poor vision, photosensitivity, headaches, and ringing in the ears due to Liver and Kidney Deficiency.

Lycii, *ophiopogon, anemarrhena,* and *fritillary* treat consumptive coughs.

For a delicious breakfast treat, throw a teaspoon or two or lycii berries into your oatmeal. Lycii berries can also be used sparingly in oatmeal cookies, puddings, fruit cakes, as well as in soups, stews, and casseroles.

Contraindications: While you might not want to plant this herb near your home, lycii berries are a delicious and healthful fruit that truly heals as it nourishes. It should not be eaten by persons with colds or flu accompanied by Heat signs (high fevers) or in cases of digestive weakness with loose stools.

Other Herbs that Tonify the Blood

If the healing properties of lycii fruit are not quite right for your condition, please see the other herbs in this category: *Dang Gui, Longan Fruit, Peony Root (White), Polygonum, Rehmannia (Cooked)*

Maximum Daily Dosage: 5 to 10 grams

1/5 ounce to 1/3 ounce

Lycii Root Cortex

Stops Night Sweats Due to Weakness

English Name: Cortex of Matrimony Vine or Wolfberry Root
Botanical Name: *Lycium chinense*

A Brief History of Lycii-Root Cortex

Mandarin: Dì Gu Pí; **Japanese:** Jikoppi; **Korean:** Chigolp'i

Please see the preceding history of lycii fruit.

Look for large, thick, dry, hard pieces of cortex without any wood or other impurities.

———— ● ————

Healing Qualities of Lycii Root Cortex

Sweet, Cold Energy
Treats Lung, Liver, and Kidney Organ Systems
Category: Herb that Cools the Blood (see page 345)

In Oriental herbal medicine, herbs that Cool the Blood are used for the most serious stage of an infectious disease, which should always be treated by a qualified health-care professional. At this stage, internal organs become inflamed and congested; common symptoms include nosebleed and spitting up blood. Herbs in this healing category reduce fevers and promote coagulation of blood.

Herbs that Cool the Blood are also used for treating Heat symptoms that come as a result of deficiency; symptoms can include chronic low-grade fevers in the afternoon or evening, night sweats, thirst, irritability, reddish or purple tongue, and dry throat.

Lycii-root bark is ideal for draining Heat associated with Yin Deficiency described in the preceding paragraph. Lycii-root cortex is antibacterial, and it not only lowers fevers, but cholesterol and blood pressure as well. It treats coughs, asthma, tuberculosis, nosebleed, and childhood eczema. Lycii-root cortex is applied externally to soothe genital itching.

Contraindications: Lycii-root cortex should not be used for symptoms associated with acute colds or flus or in case of loose stools due to Stomach/Spleen Deficiency Cold conditions.

Herbal Combinations Using Lycii Root Cortex

Lycii root cortex and *moutan peony-root cortex* treat nosebleeds and menstrual irregularities due to Blood Deficiency.

Other Herbs that Cool the Blood

If the healing properties of lycii-root cortex are not quite right for your condition, please see the other herbs in this category: *Moutan Peony Cortex, Scrophularia*
Maximum Daily Dosage: 5 to 10 grams
1/5 ounce to 1/3 ounce

Magnolia Bark

Relieves Chronic Digestive Problems
Botanical Name: *Magnolia officinalis* or *M. officinalis* var. *biloba*

A Brief History of Magnolia Bark
Mandarin: Hòu Pò; **Japanese:** Koboku; **Korean:** Mubak

Magnolia gets its name after a botanist from Montpelier, France—Pierre Magnol (1638-1715). In all, there are about 125 species of deciduous and evergreen shrubs and trees in this genus found growing in North America to Venezuela, in the Himalayas to eastern and southeastern Asia. The fragrant, lotus-like blossoms of magnolia range in color from white, yellow, and pink to deep purple. *M. liliflora* grows throughout most of China, while *M. officinalis* is native only to western and central China.

Magnolias have been used medicinally by Native North Americans for hundreds of years. Early pioneers took bitter, alcoholic extracts of magnolia bark to prevent malaria. The use of magnolia bark and flowers dates back more than 2,000 years in traditional Chinese herbal medicine.

The outer layer of good-quality magnolia bark is thicker than the inner layer. Look for bark with a sweet, spicy flavor and strong fragrance, indicating a high oil content.

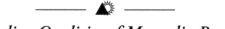

Healing Qualities of Magnolia Bark
Bitter, Spicy, Warm, Aromatic Energy
Treats Spleen, Stomach, Lung, and Large-Intestine Organ Systems
Category: Herb that Transforms Dampness (see page 349)

Magnolia bark used medicinally in Oriental medicine comes from *M. officinalis*. The bark from this species is a warming, relaxant herb with antibacterial and antifungal properties that lowers blood pressure and improves digestion.

This fragrant herb treats chronic digestive disturbances with such symptoms as colic, bloating, gas, acid stomach, loss of appetite, diarrhea, abdominal fullness, stomach pain, and vomiting. Magnolia bark is also used to treat coughs with excess mucus, lumps in the throat, and asthma.

Contraindications: Magnolia bark should not be combined with alisma according to traditional sources. It should not be used during pregnancy.

Herbal Combinations Using Magnolia Bark

Apricot seed, ephedra, and magnolia bark treat coughing and wheezing with excess mucus.

Ginseng, licorice root, and magnolia bark are combined to relieve abdominal distension and dullness from Cold due to Deficiency.

Rhubarb, immature (green) orange peel, and magnolia bark treat constipation due to accumulation and congestion.

Other Aromatic Herbs that Transform Dampness

If the healing properties of magnolia bark are not quite right for your condition, please see the other herbs in this category: *Agastache, Cardamom Seed (White)*

Maximum Daily Dosage: 3 to 9 grams
1/10 ounce to 1/3 ounce

Magnolia Flower
Clears that Stuffy Nose
Botanical Name: *Magnolia liliflora*

A Brief History of Magnolia Flower
Mandarin: Xin Yí Hua; **Japanese:** Shini; **Korean:** Sinihwa

Please see the preceding history of magnolia under magnolia bark.

Look for dried, oval-shaped buds covered with velvety, long, whitish-beige hairs. The dry, unopened buds have a slightly green hue. Buds with no stalks attached are best.

─────── ▲ ───────

Healing Qualities of Magnolia Flower
Spicy, Slightly Warm Energy
Treats Lung and Stomach Organ Systems
Category: Herb that Releases Exterior Conditions (see page 344)

This herb unblocks stuffed nasal passages. Flowers and flower buds of *M. liliiflora* are ingested to treat sinusitis, allergic rhinitis, colds with excess mucus, or runny nose. The main action of this warming, sedative herb is to constrict blood vessels in nasal passages. It also relieves pain, lowers blood pressure, and has antifungal properties.

Contraindications: Taken in excess, magnolia flower may cause dizziness or redness of the eyes. Magnolia flower should not be combined with astragalus.

Herbal Combinations Using Magnolia Flower
Magnolia flower buds and *cocklebur* are combined to relieve sinus headache and nasal congestion due to Wind-Cold (colds and flu with low fevers and chills).

Other Herbs that Release Exterior Conditions
If the healing properties of magnolia flower are not quite right for your condition, please see the other herbs in this category: *Cinnamon Twigs, Ephedra, Ginger (Fresh), Schizonepeta*
Maximum Daily Dosage: 3 to 5 grams
1/10 ounce to 1/5 ounce

Moutan Cortex
Eases Menstrual Discomforts
English Name: Cortex of the Tree Peony Root
Botanical Name: *Paeonia suffruticosa*

A Brief History of Moutan Cortex
Mandarin: Mu Dan Pí; **Japanese:** Botanpi; **Korean:** Moktanp'i

It is interesting to note that even the Greek gods required a physician. His name was Paeon, and that's where the paeonia flower got its name. According to legend, Paeon was the first person in our Western world to use peony root medicinally. According to ancient Greek mythology, the lovely peony plant was of divine origin. Since it came from the moon, peony reputedly had the unique ability to shine at night.

Necklaces made from peony were worn by children in England during the Victorian period to aid in teething and prevent convulsions. Necklaces made with seeds of the peony plant kept witches at bay for children born during the Elizabethan Age. Peonies planted near houses warded off evil spirits, while seeds ingested morning and night served as nightmare prevention. Rinses made from peony root were used to cleanse the womb after childbirth.

Tree peony or *P. suffruticosa,* native to the region from Bhutan to China and Tibet, was the flower favored by Chinese emperors for well over 1,000 years. Peony has been used medicinally in the Orient since the twelfth century. The first reference to its use is found in a Chinese medical text entitled *Pouch of Pearls.*

Look for tree-peony root bark that is round, straight, and evenly sized with a thin skin and thick flesh. The roots should be clean with no fine roots or wood attached.

——— ◑ ———

Healing Qualities of Moutan Cortex
Spicy, Bitter and Cool Energy
Treats Heart, Liver, and Kidney Organ Systems
Category: Herb that Cools the Blood (see page 345)

Tree-peony root bark is a spicy, bitter herb that cools the blood, tranquilizes the spirit, and lowers blood pressure. Moutan is taken internally to reduce fevers, to clear gastrointestinal infections, ulcers, nosebleeds, boils, menstrual complaints, and irritability. Moutan helps to reduce lumps and bruises resulting from traumatic injury. This herb also has antibacterial and antiallergenic properties.

Contraindications: Do not ingest moutan cortex if your condition is due to Cold, during pregnancy, in case of profuse menstruation, or if excessive perspiration is one of your symptoms.

Herbal Combinations Using Moutan Cortex

Moutan cortex is combined with *peony root (red)* to treat irregular menstrual cycles due to Heat and Congestion from Blood Deficiency.

Cinnamon twigs and moutan cortex treat abdominal and chest pain due to blood stasis.

Moutan cortex, *honeysuckle,* and *forsythia* treat carbuncles.
Chrysanthemum and moutan cortex are combined to relieve dizziness
and red, swollen eyes (in Oriental medicine, we call this "Liver Fire Rising").

Other Herbs that Cool the Blood

If the healing properties of moutan cortex are not quite right for your condition, please see the other herbs in this category: *Lycii Root Cortex,
Rehmannia (Raw), Scrophularia*
    Maximum Daily Dosage: 5 to 10 grams
             1/5 ounce to 1/3 ounce

Mugwort
Helps Prevent Miscarriage
Botanical Name: *Artemisia argyi, A. vulgaris* or *A. vulgaris,* var. *indica*

A Brief History of Mugwort
Mandarin: Aì Yè; **Japanese:** Gaiyo; **Korean:** Aeyôp

There are about 300 species of Artemisia, many of which have been used
medicinally; a few others, such as tarragon, are used as flavorings in cooking.
Many Artemisias are grown ornamentally for their interesting aromas and
delicate, sometimes silky, silver foliage. Members of the Artemisia genus are
often referred to as sage brush or wormwood. Southern wormwood, *A.
abrotanum,* has been cultivated for ages to ward off infection and repel
insects. Wormwood has an intensely bitter taste and gets its name from the
medicinal capability to aid in expelling intestinal worms.
    Artemisia is frequently mentioned in Greek and Roman writings dating
back to A.D. the first-century. The plant had a reputation for soothing sore
feet. Various sources indicate it was planted along roadsides by the Romans for
soldiers to use in their sandals on long marches. Known as the "Mother of
Herbs," *A. vulgaris* was one of nine herbs used in Druidic and Anglo-Saxon
times to ward off evil and poisons. This species is still used as a cooking spice
in Spain, Germany, and the United Kingdom. It's added to dishes of carp and
eel, as well as to stuffings for duck, goose, pork, and wild game.
    References to mugwort first appear in Chinese medical texts dating back
to around 500. A.D. *A. anomala* is applied externally for the relief of burns and
skin inflammations in China, while *A. vulgaris* is taken internally. Mugwort is

also applied externally in the form of small, compressed, rice-sized pieces that are burned over acupuncture points to help alleviate internal cold.

There are many grades of mugwort. When shopping for this herb, look for light olive-green- to gray-colored dried leaf that is grayish-white on the underside. It will have a thick velvety covering and should have a strong fragrance.

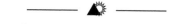

Healing Qualities of Mugwort

Bitter, Spicy and Warm Energy
Treats Spleen, Liver, and Kidney Organ Systems
Category: Herb that Stops Bleeding (see page 350)

A. vulgaris is a digestive stimulant that also acts as a gentle nerve tonic and diuretic. Mugwort is taken internally to relieve depression with lack of appetite, for dyspepsia, and to relieve menstrual cramps due to Cold. Its warming effect helps stop uterine bleeding due to Cold from Deficiency and can aid in preventing miscarriage.

Important Note: Another member of this genus, *Artemisia anomala*, has the opposite effect from *A. vulgaris*. *A. anomala* is an herb that Invigorates the Blood and helps to alleviate menstrual cramping due to blood stasis. *A. anomala* should never be used during pregnancy. When purchasing mugwort, be certain to specify that you want *A. vulgaris*. *A. anomala* is different in appearance; it has green leaves with abundant yellow flowers. *A. vulgaris*, on the other hand, is characteristically light grayish-white on the underside.

Contraindications: A. vulgaris should not be used with Heat symptoms or in case of Yin Deficiency.

Herbal Combinations Using Mugwort Leaf

Ginger root and mugwort are combined to alleviate menstrual pain due to Cold.

Cyperus and mugwort treat abdominal pain due to Congestion of Qi and Deficiency Cold conditions.

Other Herbs that Regulate the Blood or Stop Bleeding

If the healing properties of mugwort are not quite right for your condition, please see the herbs in this category: *Agrimony, Pseudoginseng (see "Ginseng"), Sanguisorba, Sophora*

Maximum Daily Dosage: 3 to 5 grams
1/10 ounce to 1/5 ounce

Mulberry Root Bark
Stops Coughing and Wheezing
Botanical Name: *Morus alba*

A Brief History of Mulberry Root
Mandarin: Sang bái pí; **Japanese:** Sohakuhi; **Korean:** Sangbaekpi

The empress Si-Ling of China is credited with starting the production of silk by using mulberry leaves to feed the silkworms around 2960 B.C.—that's nearly five thousand years ago. There are seven species belonging to the deciduous Morus genus. Valued for their edible fruits as well as their medicinal properties, mulberry trees have been cultivated for centuries. They are found growing mainly in subtropical regions of North and South America, Asia, and Africa. Mulberry wood is used in the manufacture of sports equipment, and its leaves are still fed to silkworms. Mulberry fruits are frequently made into syrups, jams, jellies, and wine.

Mulberry-root bark has the cork removed. It is white in color and tends to rip rather than snap. It has a rather unpleasant odor, somewhat similar to that of soybean flour. When shopping for root bark, look for thick, dry, white powdery pieces without impurities.

———— ● ————

Healing Qualities of Mulberry Root Bark
Sweet, Cold Energy
Treats Lung and Spleen Organ Systems
Category: Herb that Relieves Coughing and Wheezing (see page 348)

Mulberry leaves are used to treat colds and flu, nosebleeds, and eye infections, while the fruits are reputed to stop premature graying of the hair, urinary incontinence, thirst, and constipation in the elderly. The sweet, cold energy of mulberry-root bark has been found useful in treating asthma, coughs accompanied by thick yellow phlegm, bronchitis, diabetes, hypertension, and edema.

Contraindications: Mulberry-root bark should not be used in cases of excessive urination or coughing accompanied by clear or white phlegm.

Herbal Combinations Using Mulberry Root Bark
Lycii-root cortex and *licorice root* are combined with mulberry-root bark to treat fever, irritability, coughs, and thirst due to Lung Heat conditions such as bronchitis.

Other Herbs that Relieve Coughing and Wheezing

If the healing properties of mulberry bark are not quite right for your condition, please see the others herb in this category: *Apricot Kernel, Coltsfoot*
Maximum Daily Dosage: 5 to 10 grams
1/5 ounce to 1/3 ounce

Mung Bean
Clear Pesticide Poisoning
Botanical Name: *Phaseolus radiatus,* also known as *Phaseolus mungo*

A Brief History of Mung Bean
Mandarin: Lù Dòu; **Japanese:** Ryokuzu; **Korean:** Noktu

A member of the legume family, mung bean is a small, round, green-colored bean that is similar to the red aduki bean in size and shape. Native to India, and a member of the kidney-bean family, mung beans have become a traditional part of Oriental cuisine. Mung beans are now grown throughout India and China. Research has shown that mung bean counteracts poisoning from pesticides and can antidote aconite and fava-bean toxins.

Like aduki bean, soak mung beans for 18 to 24 hours prior to cooking with a piece of kombu seaweed, just long enough to start the sprouting process, which greatly increases the protein levels.

Sprouted mung beans are available at most grocery stores and are traditionally used in stir-fries. Mung-bean sprouts help detoxify the body and treat alcoholism. Look for plump, clean, olive-green beans.

———— ❋ ————

Healing Qualities of Mung Bean
Sweet, Cool Energy
Treats Heart and Stomach Organ Systems
Category: Herb that Clears and Relieves Summer Heat (see page 346)

The sweet, cool energy of mung bean is perfect for clearing what is known as Summer heat in Oriental medicine. When a person is subjected to too much heat in the summertime, symptoms can include fever, irritability, and thirst. People living in the Orient will often drink a tea made of mung beans during heat spells to prevent an occurrence of Summer heat.

Contraindications: Mung bean should not be used by persons with diarrhea due to Spleen/Stomach weakness (or Cold due to Deficiency).

Herbal Combinations Using Mung Bean

Coptis, licorice root, and mung beans treat irritability, fever, and thirst associated with Summer heat.

To counteract the toxic effects of aconite, 60 grams of licorice root is cooked with 120 grams of mung beans (or, take approximately 2 ounces of licorice root, 4 ounces of mung beans, and 6 cups of spring water; simmer on low heat for 2 hours; strain and sip the liquid throughout the day).

You can make a delicious, healthful mung-bean soup during the hot months by simmering a cup of rinsed and soaked mung beans and kombu seaweed in 8 cups of water for 1-1/2 to 2 hours. Add your favorite veggies and spices (scallions, onion, parsley, and fresh summer veggies) during the last 20 to 30 minutes of cooking time. Remove the soup from the heat and stir in a couple of tablespoons of your favorite miso.

The healthful, detoxifying effects of mung beans can also be enjoyed during cooler months by adding more warming spices, such as ginger and garlic, and root veggies and winter squash.

Other Herbs that Clear and Relieve Summer Heat

If the healing properties of mung bean are not quite right for your condition, please see the other herb in this category: *Watermelon*

Maximum Daily Dosage: 15 to 30 grams
1/2 ounce to 1 ounce

Ophiopogon
Stops Dry, Hacking Coughs

Botanical Name: *Ophiopogon japonicus;* in parts of China,
Liriope spicata, platyphylla, or *L. minor* are sometimes used.

A Brief History of Ophiopogon

Mandarin: Mài Mén Dong; **Japanese:** Bakumondo; **Korean:** Maekmundong

Ophiopogon, a member of the lily family, is also known as "Japanese hyacinth." Native to Korea and Japan, ophiopogon is an evergreen perennial with glossy, grasslike foliage and tuberous roots. Spikes of violet- to white-colored flowers bloom in the springtime and produce blue or black berry-like fruits. *O. japonicus* is one of about 40 species of ophiopogon that now grow in southern and eastern Asia to Japan. Frequently, ophiopogon is used in ornamental landscaping in Hawaii and Australia.

The ophiopogon tuber is slightly translucent, whitish-yellow colored, spindle-shaped, soft, and easily broken to reveal white, sticky flesh. Look for clean, plump, chewy tubers that give off a pleasant fragrance when broken.

——— ◑ ———

Healing Qualities of Ophiopogon
Sweet, Slightly Bitter, Slightly Cold Energy
Treats Lung, Stomach, and Heart Organ Systems
Category: Herb that Tonifies the Yin (see page XXX)

Since the first century A.D., ophiopogon has been used in Oriental medicine as a Yin Tonic. It is a soothing herb with sedative qualities that controls dry coughs and expectoration of blood. It lubricates the digestive system and bronchial tracts, relieving dryness of the mouth and tongue, sore throats, mouth sores, night fever, and constipation due to dryness.

Contraindications: The moist, lubricating qualities of ophiopogon nourish the Yin in our human garden. You do not want to take this herb if you have symptoms that are Cold and Damp in nature. According to traditional sources, ophiopogon is not compatible with dandelion.

Herbal Combinations Using Ophiopogon

Ophiopogon, *pinellia*, and *codonopsis* are combined to relieve a chronic, dry cough resulting from Lung Yin Deficiency.

Rehmannia (uncooked), scrophularia, and ophiopogon treat low-grade fevers, thirst, constipation, and irritability.

Zizyphus seeds, rehmannia (uncooked), and ophiopogon are prescribed to relieve insomnia due to Yin Deficiency.

Ginseng, schisandra, and ophiopogon treat wheezing, exhaustion, profuse perspiration, and rapid heart rate associated with dehydration and Heart/Lung Deficiency.

Dang gui, schisandra, astragalus, and ophiopogon relieve irritability due to excess perspiration.

Other Herbs that Tonify the Yin

If the healing properties of ophiopogon are not quite right for your condition, please see the other herbs in this category: *American Ginseng Root (see "Ginseng"), Dendrobium, Glehnia, Lily Bulb*
    Maximum Daily Dosage: 5 to 10 grams
                             1/5 ounce to 1/3 ounce

Oyster Shell

Calms the Spirit and Relieves Anxiety

Zoological Name: *Ostrea gigas, O. rivularis,* or *O. talienwhanensis*

A Brief History of Oyster Shell

Mandarin: Mu Lì; **Japanese:** Borei; **Korean:** Monyô

Like dragon bone, oyster shell is a substance that has long been used in Oriental medicine to calm and settle the spirit. The first references to oyster shell's use in herbal prescriptions are found in the Chinese *Divine Husbandman's Classic of the Materia Medica* from the Later Han Dynasty (A.D. 25–220).

The interior surface of the oval-shaped oyster shell is smooth, shiny, and whitish-yellow or cream colored, while the rough exterior is grayish-yellow. The hard shell is not easily broken and is ground into fine powder for ease in decocting. Look for clean, large white shells with no odor. Oyster shell should be simmered alone for at least 30 to 60 minutes prior to adding other ingredients to the decoction.

——————— ◗ ———————

Healing Qualities of Oyster Shell

Salty, Astringent, Cool Energy
Treats Liver and Kidney Organ Systems
Category: Substance that Calms the Spirit (see page 355)

Oyster shell is prescribed for restlessness, irritability, insomnia, palpitations accompanied by anxiety, headaches, blurred vision, ringing in the ears (tinnitus), spontaneous sweating, night sweats, nocturnal emissions, uterine bleeding due to weakness, and vaginal discharge. It is also used for neck lumps such as goiter or scrofula.

Contraindications: Do not use oyster shell in case of a high fever without perspiration that is due to Excess conditions. According to some traditional sources, oyster shell should not be combined with ephedra, evodia, or wild ginger. However, oyster shell works synergistically with licorice, achyranthes, polygala, and fritillary.

Herbal Combinations Using Oyster Shell

Bupleurum, peony root (red), salvia, and oyster shell are combined to treat subcostal swelling and pain.

Peony root (white), dragon bone, and oyster shell treat insomnia, palpitations, and anxiety.

Other Substances that Calm the Spirit

If the healing properties of oyster shell are not quite right for your condition, please see the other herbs in this category: *Dragon Bone, Pearl*

Maximum Daily Dosage: 10 to 30 grams

1/3 ounce to 1 ounce

Panacis Quinquefolium see *Ginseng, American*

Panax Ginseng see *Ginseng, Panax*

Panax Notoginseng see *Ginseng, Pseudoginseng*

Patchouli see *Agastache*

Pearl

Brings You Peace of Mind

Zoological Name: *Pteria margaritifera* or *P. martensii*

A Brief History of Pearl

Mandarin: Zhen Zhu; **Japanese:** Shinju; **Korean:** Chinchu

Pearl has long been a healing substance utilized in Traditional Oriental Medicine. Natural pearls are harvested off the coast of Taiwan and Guangdong, Guangxi, China, while cultivated fresh-water pearls come from the Heilongjiang, Anhui, and Jiangsu provinces. Cultured pearls have more calcium and less magnesium than natural pearls.

Pearl is generally taken in pill or powdered form and applied topically in the form of eyedrops or powders. Pearls are often cooked for two hours with soybean curd prior to being ground into a fine powder.

Good-quality pearls are large, round, smooth, and lustrous.

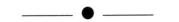

Healing Qualities of Pearl
Sweet, Salty, Cold Energy
Treats Heart and Liver Organ Systems
Category: Substance that Calms the Spirit (see page 355)

The cold, salty energy of pearl has sedative properties and is traditionally used to calm the spirit (relieving such emotions as fright and anger). Pearl also treats palpitations and childhood convulsions. Taken internally, pearl powder detoxifies and clears Liver Fire, eliminating visual obstructions that create blurred vision. Applied topically to chronic, nonhealing sores and ulcers, pearl powder promotes healing.

Contraindications: None noted.

Other Substances that Calm the Spirit

If the healing properties of pearl are not quite right for your condition, please see the other herbs in this category: *Dragon Bone, Oyster Shell*

Maximum Daily Dosage: 0.3 to 0.9 gram
1/100 ounce to 1/30 ounce

Peony Root (Red)
Increases Circulation
Botanical Name: *Paeonia obovata, P. lactiflora,* or *P. veitchii*

A Brief History of Red Peony Root
Mandarin: Chì Sháo; **Japanese:** Sekishaku; **Korean:** Chôkchak

Please see the history of peony under "Moutan Cortex" (Tree-Peony-Root Cortex, page xxx).

The use of *P. lactiflower* (cultivated root known as white peony root) can be traced back to about A.D. 500 in China. The reference to the color "white" or "red" does not apply to the appearance or coloring of the roots or flowers. Chinese herbalists classified cultivated peonies as "white peony" and those plants that were collected in the wild as "red peony." Cultivated, or *white peony,* is considered a yin tonic for the liver and circulation, while peony root collected in the wild, or *red peony,* is used as a remedy to move the blood.

Good-quality red peony root has a cortex with deep, coarse wrinkles that is easily peeled.

———— ● ————

Healing Qualities of Red Peony Root
Sour, Bitter, Slightly Cold Energy
Treats Liver and Spleen Organ Systems
Category: Herb that Invigorates the Blood (see page 350)

Red peony root is taken internally to relieve abdominal pain and menstrual complaints associated with blood stasis. As an herb that moves the blood, it helps to alleviate bruising, pain, and swelling as a result of traumatic injury, as well as to immobile abdominal masses. Red peony root clears Liver Fire that results in swollen, red, painful eyes.

Contraindications: Red peony should not be used during pregnancy or in case of anemia.

Herbal Combinations Using Red Peony Root

Chrysanthemum flower, scutellaria, and red peony root treat swelling, pain, and redness of the eyes.

Cyperus and red peony root relieve abdominal and menstrual pain due to blood and qi stasis.

Ligusticum and red peony root are combined to treat abscesses, boils, pain, and swelling due to trauma, as well as difficult menses characterized by excessive bleeding and thick purple clots of blood.

Other Herbs that Invigorate the Blood

If the healing properties of red peony root are not quite right for your condition, please see the other herbs in this category: *Ligusticum, Safflower Flower, Salvia*
Maximum Daily Dosage: 5 to 10 grams
1/5 ounce to 1/3 ounce

Peony Root (White)
Relaxes Muscle Spasms
Botanical Name: *Paeonia lactiflora*

A Brief History of White Peony Root
Mandarin: Bái Shào; **Japanese:** Byakushaku; **Korean:** Paekchak

Please see the history of peony under "Moutan Cortex" (Tree-Peony-Root Cortex, page xxx) and the discussion regarding the difference between white and red peony roots in the preceding section on red peony root.

Good-quality white peony root is straight, thick, and firm without cracks.

———— ◑ ————

Healing Qualities of White Peony Root
Bitter, Sour, Cool Energy
Treats Liver and Spleen Organ Systems
Category: Herb that Tonifies the Blood (see page 352)

White peony root is a bitter, cooling herb that reduces inflammations, lowers fevers and blood pressure, and relaxes muscle spasms. It has antibacterial properties as well as analgesic and tranquilizing effects. White peony regulates menstruation and builds blood; it is used to treat night sweats, spontaneous sweating, dizziness, and headaches.

White peony root (the cultivated root) is prescribed for liver disorders and to relieve premenstrual syndrome.

Contraindications: White peony root should not be used in case of diarrhea resulting from Coldness and Deficiency.

Herbal Combinations Using White Peony Root

White peony root, *oyster shell*, and *dragon bone* treat night sweats and spontaneous sweating due to Yin Deficiency.

Licorice and white peony root relieve abdominal pain and muscle spasms in the calf due to Blood Deficiency.

Dang gui, rehmannia (cooked), and white peony root ease menstrual cramps, dizziness, and blurred vision due to Blood Deficiency or Congestion. *Ophiopogon* is added for ringing in the ears, muscle spasms, and numbness of the extremities due to Liver Yin Deficiency.

Coptis, scutellaria, and white peony root treat Damp Heat dysenteric disorders.

Other Herbs that Tonify the Blood

If the healing properties of white peony root are not quite right for your condition, please see the other herbs in this category: *Dang Gui, Longan Berries, Lycii Fruit, Rehmannia (Cooked)*
Maximum Daily Dosage: 5 to 15 grams
1/5 ounce to 1/2 ounce

Peppermint
Eases Pain and Itching
English Name: Field Mint
Botanical Name: *Mentha haplocalyx* or *M. arvensis*

A Brief History of Peppermint
Mandarin: Bò Hé; **Japanese:** Hakka; **Korean:** Pakha

Most gardens have a place for at least one of the 25 species of aromatic perennials or few annuals that compose this genus. Mints grow in Eurasian and African temperate zones and flower from summer through early fall. Two of the world's favorite flavors—peppermint and spearmint—are widely cultivated for leaf and oil production in Asia, the Middle East, Europe, and the United States. Mints are given their characteristic fragrance and flavor by menthol, a volatile oil. This phytochemical has antiseptic, decongestant, analgesic, and anesthetic qualities. You often find the mint flavor used in sweet foods such as candy, ice cream, or chocolate because its anesthetic effects overwhelm more subtle flavors.

Look for dry, green mint that has no roots with a good, strong, minty scent.

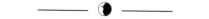

Healing Qualities of Peppermint
Spicy, Aromatic, Cooling Energy
Treats Lung and Liver Organ Systems
Category: Cool, Spicy Herb that Releases the Exterior (see page 344)

Mint is taken internally to alleviate fevers and ease sore throat pain; it is prescribed for colds, headaches, indigestion, nausea, and the early stages of skin eruptions, such as measles. Mint reduces inflammation, increases perspiration, aids digestion, and relaxes spasms. It relieves pain and itching and has antibacterial properties.

Mint can also be applied externally to ease discomfort of skin irritations.

Contraindications: Mint may decrease milk flow in women who are breast feeding. It is not recommended in case of Yin Deficiency with Heat signs.

Herbal Combinations Using Peppermint

Mint is combined with *chrysanthemum* to treat Wind-Heat conditions (colds and flus with high fevers and few chills) as well as redness, pain, and swelling of the eyes.

Bupleurum, peony root (white), and mint treat chest and flank pain due to constrained Liver Qi.

Mint, *forsythia, lonicera,* and *schizonepeta* treat rashes and skin eruptions.

Other Cool, Spicy Herbs that Release the Exterior

If the healing properties of mint are not quite right for your condition, please see the other herbs in this category: *Bupleurum, Chrysanthemum, Cohosh, Kudzu Maximum Daily Dosage:* 1.5 to 5 grams
1/15 ounce to 1/5 ounce

Persimmon Calyx
Stops Hiccups
Botanical Name: *Diospyros kaki*

A Brief History of Persimmon Calyx
Mandarin: Shì Dì; **Japanese:** Shitei; **Korean:** Sije

Composed of nearly 500 species of evergreen and deciduous trees and shrubs, members of this genus are mainly found growing in the tropics. Ebony, a beautiful hardwood, comes from trees in this genus; other species produce the familiar bright reddish-orange persimmon fruit. The Japanese persimmon produces delicious, round, flattened fruits commonly sold in the supermarket. The pulp of unripe persimmon has firming qualities and forms the base for face packs sold by the cosmetic industry. The unripe fruit is also used in the manufacture of pharmaceuticals that treat high blood pressure as well as piles, typhoid, and typhus.

D. kaki is first mentioned in traditional Chinese medical texts from A.D. 720. Combined with fresh ginger and clove, persimmon calyx is a famous cure for hiccups. The hard, brittle, dried calyx is lid-shaped, with a stalk at its tip or a hole if the stalk is missing. Look for thick, reddish-brown calyces that have no odor.

——— 🜨 ———

Healing Qualities of Persimmon Calyx

Bitter, Astringent, Neutral Energy
Treats Lung and Stomach Organ Systems
Category: Herb that Regulates the Qi (see page 349)

Persimmon calyx is an astringent herb used to direct the qi downward and stop hiccups and belching. Because of its neutral energy, persimmon calyx is used for both Hot and Cold patterns.
Contraindications: None noted.

Herbal Combinations Using Persimmon Calyx

Fresh ginger juice, a dash of clove, and persimmon calyx treat a stubborn case of hiccups or vomiting due to Stomach Cold.
Persimmon calyx, *bamboo shavings,* and *phragmitis* treat belching and vomiting due to Stomach Heat.

Other Herbs that Regulate the Qi

If the healing properties of persimmon calyx are not quite right for your condition, please see the other herbs in this category: *Cyperus, Tangerine Peel*
Maximum Daily Dosage: 5 to 10 grams
1/5 ounce to 1/3 ounce

Phellodendron

Is a Famous Infection Fighter
English Name: Amur Cork-tree Bark
Botanical Name: *Phellodendron amurense* or *P. chinense*

A Brief History of Phellodendron

Mandarin: Húang Bai or Húang Bó; **Japanese:** Obaku; **Korean:** Hwangbaek

There are only ten species of deciduous trees belonging to the *Phellodendron* genus found growing in eastern Asia. *P. Amurense,* native to northern China and Manchuria, has aromatic, dark, glossy green leaves that turn yellow in fall. The yellow-green colors of this ornamental tree give off the odor of turpentine when bruised. Its pale, deeply fissured gray bark has a corklike appearance. The medicinal use of Amur Cork-tree bark is first described in Chinese medical texts around 1578 A.D.

In conjunction with scutellaria and coptis, phellodendron comprises what is known as "the three yellow herbs" in Oriental medicine—three superior antibacterial herbs, all yellowish in color. In China, phellodendron is known as the poor man's "cure-all."

When shopping for phellodendron bark, look for flat pieces, bright yellow in color, that are thick, dry, solid, and finely grained. The rough outer layer of cork should already be removed.

--------- ● ---------

Healing Qualities of Phellodendron
Bitter, Cold Energy
Treats Kidney Elements and Bladder Organ Systems
Category: Herb that Clears Heat and Dries Dampness (see page 345)

Phellodendron is used traditionally in Oriental medicine as a detoxicant for hot, damp conditions such as boils, abscesses, jaundice, enteritis, and skin diseases. It is particularly effective for infections affecting the lower burner with such symptoms as thick, yellow vaginal discharges, acute urinary-tract infections, foul-smelling diarrhea, or dysentery. This is a cold, bitter, diuretic herb that stimulates the liver and gall bladder, reducing fevers, blood pressure, and blood-sugar levels. Phellodendron is also used to treat swollen, red, painful knees, legs, or feet.

Contraindications: Phellodendron should not be used in case of weak digestion.

Herbal Combinations Using Phellodendron Cortex

Peony root (red) and phellodendron are combined to treat hot, dysenteric disorders.

Phellodendron and *wild ginger* treat frequent urination accompanied by pain and discomfort.

Other Herbs that Clear Heat and Dry Dampness

If the healing properties of phellodendron are not quite right for your condition, please see the other herbs in this category: *Coptis, Gentian, Scutellaria*
Maximum Daily Dosage: 5 to 10 grams
1/5 ounce to 1/3 ounce

Pinellia

Controls Nausea and Vomiting

Botanical Name: *Pinellia ternata*

A Brief History of Pinellia

Mandarin: Bàn Xìa; **Japanese:** Hange; **Korean:** Panha

Pinellia gets its name from that of Giovanni Pinelli, who owned a botanic garden in Naples, Italy, sometime in the late 1500s. There are only six species of small tuberous perennials belonging to the Pinellia genus. This herb is commonly cultivated along roadsides and in fields in Japan, Korea, and southern China. Pinellia is an attractive, tuberous, shade-loving plant whose leaves are composed of three leaflets. It sends out a long stem with small flowers that develop into green fruits.

The tubers of the pinellia plant have been utilized medicinally in Chinese medicine since the Han dynasty (A.D. 25–220). However, they are poisonous and need special preparation before ingestion. The process includes soaking and boiling in ginger and then alum to eliminate the toxins. The irregularly roundish-shaped tubers are roughly marble sized. Look for firm, dry, round tubers with the skins completely removed. Processed tubers are slightly shiny or semitranslucent. Do not use tubers that are somewhat opaque—they have not been processed.

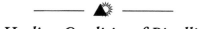

Healing Qualities of Pinellia

Spicy, Warm, Poisonous Energy
Treats Lung, Spleen, and Stomach Organ Systems
Category: Herb that Transforms Cold Phlegm (see page 348)

Pinellia's reputation as an excellent herbal ally to make Rebellious Qi Descend (or control nausea and vomiting) has been validated scientifically.

The Chinese also use it as part of an herbal prescription to remove gallstones without surgery. The expectorant and antimucus properties of pinellia help control coughs and bronchitis with copious clear or white phlegm. Pinellia aids weak digestion and eliminates lymphatic swellings or nodules, particularly in the neck.

Note: Pinellia should always be combined with either a few slices of ginger or licorice to reduce its toxicity. Never combine pinellia with aconite.

Contraindications: Do not use pinellia when any bleeding is present or in case of cough due to Yin Deficiency.

Herbal Combinations Using Pinellia

Ginger (fresh or dried) and pinellia control vomiting.

Tangerine peel, coptis, scutellaria, and pinellia treat coughs, nausea, and vomiting.

Trichosanthes and pinellia treat cough, distended chest, and vomiting due to phlegm-heat.

Magnolia bark is combined with pinellia to treat vomiting resulting from phlegm-induced coughs.

Other Herbs that Transform Cold Phlegm

If the healing properties of pinellia are not quite right for your condition, please see the other herb in this category: *Platycodon*

Maximum Daily Dosage: 5 to 10 grams
1/5 ounce to 1/3 ounce

Platycodon

Eliminates Coughing and Hoarseness
English Name: Balloon Flower
Botanical Name: *Platycodon grandiflorum*

A Brief History of Platycodon

Mandarin: Jíe Geng; **Japanese:** Kikyó; **Korean:** Kilgyong

The roots of Chinese balloon flowers, or platycodon, have been used medicinally in Chinese medicine since the Han dynasty (206 B.C.–A.D. 23). A single species, native to eastern Asia, composes this genus. The lovely perennial platycodon plant graces many gardens with single or double bell-shaped flowers in shades of white and pink to deep periwinkle blue, but relatively few people realize that its roots are edible. In Korea, platycodon roots are eaten in soups as a tonic vegetable; sometimes they are pickled or preserved in sugar.

Look for clean, dry roots with brown skin and pale-yellowish flesh; those without any fine roots attached are best.

——— 🜚 ———

Healing Qualities of Platycodon

Bitter, Spicy, Neutral Energy
Treats Lung Organ System
Category: Herb that Transforms Cold Phlegm (see page 348)

Platycodon is an excellent expectorant herb that is effective against numerous disease-causing germs. Because of its neutral energy it is used for coughs resulting from either wind-heat or wind-cold. Platycodon dilates the bronchial vessels and is prescribed for coughs with profuse phlegm, colds, bronchitis, pleurisy, throat infections, and lung or throat abscess.

Contraindications: Do not use platycodon in case of blood expectoration. It should not be combined with gentian.

Herbal Combinations Using Platycodon

Coix, trichosanthes, and platycodon treat Lung abscess.

Pinellia, platycodon, and *ginger* are combined for stubborn colds and flu characterized by copious amounts of clear or white phlegm.

Licorice and platycodon treat hoarseness and sore, swollen throats resulting from Wind-Heat.

Other Herbs that Transform Cold Phlegm

If the healing properties of platycodon are not quite right for your condition, please see the other herb in this category: *Pinellia*
Maximum Daily Dosage: 5 to 10 grams
1/5 ounce to 1/3 ounce

Polyporus see *Zhu Ling*

Polygala
Calms the Heart
English Name: Chinese Senega Root, Polygala, Siberian Milkwort
Botanical Name: *Polygala tenuifolia*

A Brief History of Polygala
Mandarin: Yuan Zhì; **Japanese:** Onji; **Korean:** Wôji

Polygala has always been one of my favorite herbs—it makes me happy just to think about it. Uses of polygala through the ages have been varied and quite interesting. *P. senega,* a relative of *P. tenuifolia* (utilized in Oriental medicine) was used by the North American Seneca people to treat rattlesnake bites. In 1735, a Scottish physician by the name of John Tennent discovered how it was being used and noted that snake-bite symptoms were similar to those of pleurisy, as well as the later stages of pneumonia. Experiments revealed that it was, indeed, incredibly effective in treating respiratory diseases. By 1740, polygala was being cultivated in Europe and used medicinally. *P. vulgaris,* the European species, also known as common milkwort, gets its folk name from the erroneous belief that it increases lactation. This variety is less potent than *P. senega* or *P. tenuifolia.*

There are approximately 500 species of annuals, perennials, shrubs, and trees growing throughout the world that make up this genus. Only a few make it into ornamental gardens for their pea flowers; the medicinal species, however, are not considered garden-worthy.

P. tenuifolia is first mentioned in traditional Chinese medical records sometime during the early Han dynasty (206 B.C.–A.D. 23). It thrives on stony slopes and in dry meadowlands in Mongolia, Siberia, and China. This small plant reaches only about 10 inches in height and spread and produces lavender to blue flowers. When shopping for polygala root, look for thick, soft, cylindrical roots with a thin, pale, light-brown skin. The exterior surface of this root is quite rough and bears the scars of branch roots that have been removed.

————— ▲ —————

Healing Qualities of Polygala
Bitter, Spicy, Slightly Warm Energy
Treats Heart and Lung Organ Systems
Category: Herb that Nourishes the Heart and Calms the Spirit (see page 355)

Polygala is particularly effective in relieving pent-up emotions due to excessive brooding. It calms the spirit, treating restlessness and palpitations with anxiety and insomnia. This herb helps clear phlegm from the Heart and Lungs. It treats coughs accompanied by copious mucus as well as painful, swollen breasts. This herb, in dry powdered form, is applied topically to boils, abscesses, and sores.

Contraindications: Do not use this herb in the presence of Deficient Heat symptoms, ulcers, or gastritis.

Herbal Combinations Using Polygala

Fritillary, pinellia, and polygala are combined to treat coughing and wheezing due to Cold (clear or white) phlegm.

Zizyphus seeds, poria cocos, and polygala treat palpitations with anxiety, irritability, and insomnia due to Heart Blood Deficiency or pent-up emotions.

Other Herbs that Nourish the Heart and Calm the Spirit

If the healing properties of polygala are not quite right for your condition, please see the other herbs in this category: *Biota, Zizyphus Seed*

Maximum Daily Dosage: 3 to 9 grams

1/10 ounce to 1/3 ounce

Polygonum
Is Reputed to Restore Graying Hair to its Natural Color
Botanical Name: *Polygonum multiflorum*

A Brief History of Polygonum
Mandarin: Hé Shou Wu; **Japanese:** Kashuu; **Korean:** Hasuo

Translation of hé shou wu's name in Chinese, "black-haired Mr. He," alludes to its rejuvenative fame of restoring prematurely gray hair to the natural color if taken for years. Dentists beware! Another folktale claims that a 150-year-old root will actually make new teeth appear in mouths of senior citizens. Polygonum's botanical name comes from the Greek words *polys* and *gony,* meaning "many knees." The jointed stems of these plants look like knots or "knees," also giving it the common name of knotweed. Brittle polygonum stems snap easily at the joint (or knee) when collected.

Related to buckwheat, approximately 150 species make up this genus composed of annuals, perennials, and deciduous shrubby climbers. Many of the members of this species are considered weeds that populate roadsides and wastelands. Others have small, attractive red, white, or green flowers and are kept as ornamentals. Polygonum is a major Oriental tonic herb. Its use was first recorded in traditional Chinese medical literature in A.D. 713.

The hard polygonum root is difficult to break. Look for clean, solid roots that are black on the exterior and reddish-colored on the inside.

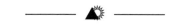

Healing Qualities of Polygonum
Bitter, Sweet, Astringent, Slightly Warm Energy
Treats Liver and Kidney Organ Systems
Category: Herb that Tonifies the Blood (see page 352)

Valued by herbalists as a blood, liver, and kidney tonic, polygonum is considered a longevity herb in the Orient. Polygonum (also known as Fo-Ti, or hé shou wu) is reputed to preserve youthful energy and sexual potency as well as reduce wrinkles. In Oriental medicine, polygonum is frequently used to Tonify the Kidney and Liver Organ Systems because it is neither too drying, cold, or hard on the digestion. Fo-Ti is a whole-body tonic also credited with the ability to reduce cholesterol. It lowers blood-sugar levels, clears toxins, has antibacterial properties, and is used to treat malaria. Polygonum is taken internally for menstrual and menopausal complaints, constipation in the elderly, swollen lymph glands, and is reputed to eliminate Evil Wind (intestinal gas). The root is applied externally for bleeding sores and wounds.

Contraindications: Taken in excess, this herb can cause skin rash and numbness of the extremities. Polygonum should not be taken by those persons with weak digestion or diarrhea. Some traditional sources indicate polygonum should not be ingested with chives, onions, or garlic.

Herbal Combinations Using Polygonum

Scrophularia, forsythia, and polygonum treat abscesses and other toxic swellings.

Dang gui, Panax ginseng, tangerine peel, and polygonum treat chronic malarial disorders and fatigue.

Lycii fruit, psoralea, cuscuta, and polygonum are combined for weak and sore back and knees, dizziness, premature graying, and blurred vision.

Polygonum is combined with *Panax ginseng* and *dang gui* as a tonic formula.

Other Herbs that Tonify the Blood

If the healing properties of polygonum are not quite right for your condition, please see the other herbs in this category: *Dang Gui, Longan Berries, Lycii Fruit, Peony Root (White), Rehmannia (Cooked)*
Maximum Daily Dosage: 10 to 15 grams
1/3 ounce to 1/2 ounce

Polyporus see *Zhu Ling*

Pomegranate Husk
Bids Farewell to Unwanted Visitors
Botanical Name: *Punica granatum*

A Brief History of Pomegranate Husk
Mandarin: Shí Líu Pí; **Japanese:** Sekiryuhi; **Korean:** Sôngnyup'i

Grenadine, a flavoring often used in cocktails, comes from delicious ruby-red pomegranate juice. Only two species of small trees or shrubs belong to this genus. Deciduous in temperate zones, *P. granatum* is evergreen in the subtropics and grows in the eastern Mediterranean to the Himalayas. Spiny branches bear reddish-orange flowers, followed by round, leathery-skinned fruits that are filled with a multitude of small seeds encased in a tasty reddish-pink juicy pulp.

As early as 1500 B.C., pomegranate was mentioned as a cure for tapeworms in the Egyptian Ebers papyri. This herb contains certain phytochemicals, alkaloids known as pelletierines, which paralyze tapeworms and roundworms (unwanted visitors!) so that, in conjunction with a laxative, they can be expelled from the system. Pomegranate is first mentioned in traditional Chinese medical texts around A.D. 470.

Look for dry, thick, solid, red pomegranate husks.

———— ▲ᨏᨏ ————

Healing Qualities of Pomegranate Husks
Sour, Astringent, Warm, Poisonous Qualities
Treats Kidney, Large Intestine, and Stomach Organ Systems
Category: Herbs that Stabilize and Bind—Astringent Herb (see page 354)

Besides eliminating those unwanted visitors—intestinal parasites—pomegranate has antiviral properties. It also controls diarrhea. Powdered pomegranate husk is applied externally for ringworm and is used in gargle form for mouth sores and throat infections.

Note: This herb, particularly in the form of bark extracts, is legally restricted in some countries.

Contraindications: This herb *should not* be mixed or taken with fats or oils to prevent its absorption into the system. Pomegranate husks should not be taken by persons experiencing early stages of diarrhea.

Herbal Combinations Using Pomegranate Husk

Coptis, phellodendron, dang gui, and pomegranate husk are combined to treat chronic dysenteric disorders.

Other Astringent Herbs that Stabilize and Bind

If the healing properties of pomegranate husk are not quite right for your condition, please see the other herbs in this category: *Cornus, Ginkgo, Schisandra*

Note: Please see other antiparasitic herbs: *Garlic, Pumpkin Seeds and Husks*

Maximum Daily Dosage: 3 to 9 grams
1/10 ounce to 1/4 ounce

Poria Cocos

Calms the Heart and Relieves Edema

English Name: Sclerotium of Tuckahoe, China-root, or Hoelen
Botanical Name: *Poria cocos*

A Brief History of Poria Cocos

Mandarin: Fú Líng; **Japanese:** Bukuryo; **Korean:** Pongnyông

Found as deep as 2 feet below the ground, growing on the roots of conifers and hardwood trees, poria cocos is a subterranean fungus. It was called tuckahoe by the American settlers, who would harvest it by simply "tucking a hoe" under the roots of trees and giving a yank. A typical fungus can be 2 to 6 inches high by 4 to 12 inches wide. Its tuberlike, round- to elliptic-shaped body has a hard, wrinkled, dark-brown covering. Inside, you find a pale-pinkish granular substance that often served as a food source for Native Americans and pioneers alike.

Ask for "sclerotium" of poria cocos. It should be solid, heavy, and white in color with a touch of light yellow at the outer margins.

———— (⚘) ————

Healing Qualities of Poria Cocos
Sweet, Bland, Neutral Energy
Treats Heart, Spleen, and Lung Organ Systems
Category: Herb that Drains Dampness (see page 347)

This wonderful diuretic herb food regulates fluid metabolism and calms the heart. Poria is taken internally for insomnia, emotional disturbances, abdominal bloating, urinary dysfunction, and palpitations.

Contraindications: Poria should not be taken in cases of frequent, copious urination due to Cold from Deficiency. Large doses or long-term usage of poria is discouraged.

Herbal Combinations Using Poria Cocoa

Poria can be purchased in very thin curled slices and added to healthful soups and stews to treat chronic edema due to dampness or stagnation of fluids.

Up to 60 grams, or 2 ounces, of poria cocos may be ingested over a 24-hour period to treat acute facial edema.

Licorice root and poria cocos treat facial edema, shortness of breath, and palpitations due to Spleen and Heart Deficiency.

Zizyphus seeds, schisandra, polygala, and poria cocos are combined to treat insomnia and palpitations.

Pinellia, tangerine peel, fresh ginger, and poria cocos are combined to expel phlegm and stop vomiting, nausea, and poor appetite due to fluid congestion in the Stomach.

Other Herbs that Drain Dampness

If the healing properties of poria cocos are not quite right for your condition, please see the other herbs in this category: *Aduki Bean, Alisma, Coix, Stephania, Zhu Ling*

Maximum Daily Dosage: 9 to 15 grams
1/4 ounce to 1/2 ounce

Pueraria see Kudzu Root

Prune Seeds

Promote Bowel Regularity

English Name: Oriental Bush Cherry Pit or Chinese Plum
Botanical Name: *Prunus japonica* or *P. humulis*

A Brief History of Prune Seeds

Mandarin: Yù Li Rén; **Japanese:** Ikurinin; **Korean:** Ungniin

Many of our favorite fruits and nuts come from the rose family, including cherries, apricots, plums, peaches, and almonds. There are more than 430 species of deciduous, occasionally evergreen trees and shrubs that belong to this genus. The Oriental Bush Cherry, or Chinese Plum, grows in wooded areas from central China through Japan and Korea.

Cultivated in China for well over 2,500 years, *P. armeniaca* (wild apricot) and *P. persica* (peach) reached Greece around the fourth century B.C. and were grown in Italy during Roman times according to historical texts. Many species of *Prunus* have been used medicinally throughout history. They are first mentioned in Chinese medical texts dating around A.D. 500.

When shopping for Chinese plum seeds, look for plump seeds, light-yellow in color, that do not exude oil. They must be ground with a mortar and pestle before use.

--------- 🜨 ---------

Healing Qualities of Prune Seeds

Spicy, Bitter, Sweet, Neutral Energy
Treats Large Intestine, Small Intestine, and Spleen Organ Systems
Category: Downward Draining Herb—Moist Laxative (see page 346)

Prune seeds lubricate or moisten the intestines, moving the bowels. They also reduce edema and promote urination.

Contraindications: Do not use prune seeds during pregnancy or in case of Yin Deficiency accompanied by depleted body fluids.

Herbal Combinations Using Prune Seeds

Prune seeds, combined with *hemp seeds,* are effective in eliminating chronic constipation due to dry intestines or Qi Deficiency.

Coix, poria cocos, talcum, and prune seeds are used to treat constipation, retention of urine, and edema accompanied by abdominal distention.
Maximum Daily Dosage: 3 to 9 grams
1/10 ounce to 1/4 ounce

Pumpkin Seeds and Husks
Eliminate Parasites
Botanical Name: *Cucurbita moschata*

A Brief History of Pumpkin Seeds and Husks
Mandarin: Nán Gua Zi; **Japanese:** Nankashi; **Korean:** Namgwacha

Think of the fragrance of a perfectly spiced pumpkin pie browning in the oven for your Thanksgiving feast. *C. pepo,* a cousin of the species used to make our pumpkin pie, has been grown in southern parts of North America for well over 8,000 years. *C. maxima* made its way to Europe from Peru as a result of the Spanish conquest of 1532. There are a total of 27 species of annual and perennial plants in this genus, all native to tropical and subtropical America. Summer and winter squashes, as well as pumpkins and marrows pertain to several different species with interchangeable common names.

Pumpkin and squash seeds are packed with valuable vitamins, oil, and minerals. They are high in zinc, a mineral that aids the healing process and is useful in treating an enlarged prostate gland. After carving that Halloween pumpkin, don't throw out the seeds. Let them dry—they are delicious raw or baked in a low oven until slightly brown (lightly salted with soy sauce, tamari, or sea salt). The medicinal use of pumpkin seeds was adopted by Oriental healers sometime in the seventeenth century.

Look for full, dry seeds with a yellowish-white husk.

———— 🌐 ————

Healing Qualities of Pumpkin Seeds and Husks
Sweet, Neutral Energy
Treats Large Intestine and Stomach Organ Systems
Category: Herb that Expels Parasites (see page 356)

This delicious, nutritious, nutty-flavored seed has diuretic properties; it soothes irritated tissues, eliminates pain, and expels parasites. It is effective against tapeworms and roundworms. It is a good preventative against schistosomiasis since it kills young schistomsomes (but not mature ones). Pumpkin seeds and husks aid milk production in lactating mothers and are used to reduce postpartum swelling of the hands and feet.

Contraindications: Do not exceed recommended dosage; taken in excess this herb might produce adverse effects on liver function.

Herbal Combinations Using Pumpkin Seeds and Husks

Pumpkin seeds and husks are often used in conjunction with Semen Arecae Catechu to dislodge and expel tapeworms. Usually, for a 150-pound adult, 2 to 4 ounces of powdered pumpkin seeds and husks are taken with water. Two hours later, a tea made with 2 to 4 ounces of Semen Arecae is ingested, followed 30 minutes later by 1/2 ounce of Mirabilitum (a purgative substance, also known as glauber's salt).

Other Herbs that Expel Parasites

If the healing properties of pumpkin seeds and husks are not quite right for your condition, please see the other herbs in this category: *Garlic,* (though not in this herbal healing category; also see *Pomegranate Husks)*

Maximum Daily Dosage: 30 to 60 grams

1 to 2 ounces

Radish Seed

Aids Digestion

Botanical Name: *Raphanus sativus*

A Brief History of Radish Seed

Mandarin: Lái Fú Zi; **Japanese:** Raifukushi; **Korean:** Naebokcha

There are a total of eight annual and perennial plants pertaining to this genus found growing in western and central Europe to central Asia. *R. sativus* was cultivated in Egypt at least 4,500 years ago and in China about 2,000 years ago. It is believed that black radishes originated in Spain sometime during the Middle Ages. By 1548, the radish had reached England. *R. sativus* contains an herbal antibiotic, called raphinin, which inhibits the growth of a number of pathogenic fungi as well bacteria, including *Strep, Staph,* and *E. coli.*

One variety of radish, *macropodus,* has roots weighing up to 44 pounds. The white daikon radish belongs to this variety and is featured in Oriental cuisine. Pickled or fresh shredded daikon is frequently served with Korean and Japanese meals as an effective digestive aid.

When shopping, look for large, plump, oily radish seeds.

————— 🜨 —————

Healing Qualities of Radish Seeds
Spicy, Sweet, Neutral Energy
Treats Lung, Stomach, and Spleen Organ Systems
Category: Herb that Relieves Food Stagnation (see page 349)

The spicy flavor of radish seed makes it a great expectorant and digestive aid. As noted earlier, it is effective against many bacterial and fungal infections. The seed is taken internally for indigestion, to alleviate food congestion, flatulence, belching accompanied by a rotten smell, abdominal bloating, and acid regurgitation. It also controls diarrhea, coughing with phlegm, wheezing, and bronchitis.

Contraindications: Do not use radish seed if you are tired or weak.

Herbal Combinations Using Radish Seed

Pinellia and radish seeds treat coughing accompanied by phlegm and wheezing. This combination also treats abdominal fullness, and vomiting due to food congestion.

Apricot kernels and radish seeds are combined for chronic coughs with mucus.

Other Herbs that Relieve Food Stagnation

If the healing properties of radish seeds are not quite right for your condition, please see the other herbs in this category: *Hawthorn Fruit*

Maximum Daily Dosage: 5 to 10 grams
1/5 ounce to 1/3 ounce

Red Peony Root see Peony Root, Red

Rehmannia (Cooked)

Builds the Blood

English Name: Chinese Foxglove Root Cooked in Wine
Botanical Name: *Rehmannia glutinosa*

A Brief History of Rehmannia

Mandarin: Shú Dì Huáng; **Japanese:** Jukujio; **Korean:** Sukchihwang

Rehmannia is named after Joseph Rehmann, a German physician (1799–1831). A total of ten rehmannia species, all perennials, are native to eastern Asia with heights averaging between 6 and 12 inches. Rehmannia, also known as Chinese foxglove, has velvety purplish-green leaves, an orange-colored tuberous root, and flowers ranging in color from dull yellow to mauvish-purple.

Rehmannia, a common ingredient in many herbal prescriptions, could be considered one of the 50 most popular herbs in the Orient. Mention of the use of fresh dried (raw) root is found in Chinese medical texts from the Han dynasty (206 B.C. to A.D. 23). The use of cooked root appears later—around A.D. 1061. Raw root is orangish-black in color, while the cooked root is totally black, moist, and sticky. The cooking process involves repeated steaming and drying of the root with various ingredient such as millet or yellow rice wine, tangerine peel, and cardamom. When shopping for rehmannia roots, look for plump, heavy roots that are moist and dark in color, with an oily texture.

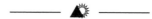

Healing Qualities of Rehmannia

Sweet, Slightly Warm Energy
Treats Heart, Kidney, and Liver Organ Systems
Category: Herb that Tonifies the Blood (see page 352)

In Traditional Oriental Medicine, cooked rehmannia belongs to a category of herbs that build, or "tonify the blood." This herb regulates menstruation and uterine and postpartum bleeding. It is also used to treat night sweats, insomnia, low-back pain, infertility, impotence, ringing in the ears, loss of hearing, lightheadedness, palpitations, and premature graying of hair.

Contraindications: Do not use rehmannia in case of digestive weakness; excessive phlegm, or congestion. Overuse can lead to abdominal fullness and diarrhea.

Herbal Combinations Using Cooked Rehmannia Root

Peony root (white), dang gui, and cooked rehmannia root treat palpitations, dizziness, anemia, insomnia, and menstrual irregularities associated with Blood Deficiency.

Cooked rehmannia is combined with *cardamom* for persons suffering from both Blood and Spleen Deficiency (weak digestion).

Other Herbs that Tonify the Blood

If the healing properties of cooked rehmannia are not quite right for your condition, please see the other herbs in this category: *Dang Gui, Longan Berries, Lycii Fruit, Peony Root (White), Polygonum*
Maximum Daily Dosage: 5 to 20 grams
1/5 ounce to 2/3 ounce

Rehmannia (Raw)

Replenishes Depleted Body Fluids
English Name: Chinese Foxglove Root—Uncooked
Botanical Name: *Rehmannia glutinosa*

A Brief History of Rehmannia

Mandarin: Shen Dì Huáng; **Japanese:** Shojio; **Korean:** Saengjihwang

Please see the preceding history of Rehmannia (Cooked).

———— ● ————

Healing Qualities of Raw Rehmannia Root

Sweet, Bitter, Cold Energy
Treats Heart, Kidney, and Liver Organ Systems
Category: Herb that Clears Heat and Cools the Blood (see page 345)

Raw rehmannia root has therapeutic properties different from cooked root. It is a specific remedy for high fevers or continuous low-grade fevers that deplete body fluids. Raw rehmannia treats thirst, dry mouth, constipation, mouth and tongue sores, irritability, insomnia, and malar flush.

Contraindications: Do not ingest raw rehmannia root if you have weak digestion with edema; pregnant women with digestive weakness or anemia should not take this herb.

Herbal Combinations Using Raw Rehmannia Root

Scrophularia and raw rehmannia are combined to treat depleted body fluids resulting from very high fevers. Symptoms include excessive thirst, dry mouth and throat, a bright red tongue, and irritability.

Ophiopogon, glehnia, and raw rehmannia treat Stomach Yin Deficiency with such symptoms as thirst, dry mouth, and red tongue.

Cooked rehmannia is often combined with raw rehmannia to treat Heat symptoms due to Yin Deficiency.

Cardamom seed is frequently added to herbal prescriptions containing raw rehmannia to aid digestion and avoid side effects such as nausea, diarrhea, or abdominal pain.

Other Herbs that Clear Heat and Cool the Blood

If the healing properties of foxglove are not quite right for your condition, please see other herbs in this category: *Lycii Root Cortex, Moutan Cortex, Scrophularia*

Maximum Daily Dosage: 5 to 20 grams
1/5 ounce to 2/3 ounce

Rhubarb Rhizome

Is Nature's Purgative

Botanical Name: *Rheum tanguticum, R. palmatum,* or *R. officinale*

A Brief History of Rhubarb Rhizome

Mandarin: Dà Húang; **Japanese:** Daio; **Korean:** Taehwang

Rhubarb belongs to a genus composed of about 50 perennial plants. Native to Northwest China and Tibet, rhubarb has been used medicinally for well over 2,000 years. Monopolies to prevent the international trade of rhubarb were fairly successfully maintained by the Chinese and Russians until 1782. In fact, the sole purpose of the Kiakhta Rhubarb Commission (or Rhubarb Office), located on the border between Mongolia and Siberia, was to prevent the exportation of this healing herb. However, *R. palmatum* made its way into Europe by 1762 with *R. palmatum* following in 1867. A large area of the Royal Botanic Garden Edinburgh was dedicated to the cultivation of rhubarb (according to a map dated 1777).

The Chinese cultivated various species that have been used medicinally for over 2,000 years. An ancient Chinese medical text known as the *Shen Nong*

Canon of Herbs, dating back to the Han dynasty (206 B.C.–A.D. 23), contains the first written reference to the medicinal use of rhubarb. Medicinal rhubarb is quite different from the familiar edible rhubarb frequently used in pies. Edible rhubarbs (developed through hybridization sometime in the nineteenth century) are not utilized for medicinal purposes. It's important to note that only the roots of medicinal varieties are used because the leaves are poisonous.

When shopping for rhubarb root, look for solid, hard, heavy root pieces that are bitter (but not astringent), oily, and golden-brown in color.

Healing Qualities of Rhubarb Rhizome

Bitter, Cold Energy
Treats Heart, Large Intestine, Liver, and Stomach Organ Systems
Category: Downward Draining—Purgative Herb (see page 346)

Rhubarb contains phytochemicals known as anthraquinone glycosides, which have extremely strong laxative qualities. Besides its laxative effect, rhubarb improves digestion. It is taken internally to relieve chronic constipation and for Heat-related symptoms such as high fever, profuse sweating, dysentery, jaundice, swollen and painful eyes, nosebleed, and skin eruptions due to the accumulation of toxins. It is also taken for liver and gall-bladder complaints and hemorrhoids. Rhubarb is applied externally for burns.

Contraindications: Do not take rhubarb if you have Cold symptoms, weakness, anemia, or diarrhea. Rhubarb should not be used by pregnant or lactating women or by persons with intestinal obstruction.

Herbal Combinations Using Rhubarb Rhizome

Rhubarb is combined with *cinnamon bark* for chronic constipation.

Coptis is combined with rhubarb to treat a feeling of fullness and distension due to accumulation of Heat; *scutellaria* is added if nosebleed or vomiting of blood is present.

Dang gui is combined with rhubarb to treat blood stasis.

Other Purgative Herbs

If the healing properties of rhubarb are not quite right for your condition, please see the other herb in this category: *Aloe*

Maximum Daily Dosage: 3 to 10 grams
1/10 to 1/3 ounce

Safflower Flower
Lowers Cholesterol
Botanical Name: *Carthamus tinctorius*

A Brief History of Safflower Flower
Mandarin: Hóng Hua; **Japanese:** Koka; **Korean:** Honghwa

Long an herbal ally to human beings, remains of safflower flowers were discovered in Egyptian tombs dating back to 3500 B.C. Introduced in 1551 from Egypt to Europe, Carthamus gets its name from the Arabic word *qurtom* or Hebrew *qarthami*—both mean "to paint." Carthamus flowers contain a pigment (carthamin) that turns yellow in water and red in alcohol. This coloring agent has been used for thousands of years to dye fabrics, feathers, and foods. Safflower flowers were traditionally used to dye the robes of Buddhist nuns and monks. Today, carthamus is grown mostly for the manufacture of safflower oil.

There are 14 annuals and a few perennials pertaining to this thistlelike genus, all natives of the Mediterranean and Asian regions. *C. tinctorius,* a tall annual with strikingly yellow florets, is first mentioned in traditional Chinese medical texts in the year A.D. 1061. From June through July, the color of the carthamus flower gradually changes from yellow to red.

Look for large, soft, brightly colored dried flowers that do not contain any stalks.

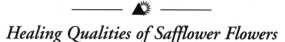

Healing Qualities of Safflower Flowers
Spicy, Warm Energy
Treats Heart and Liver Organ Systems
Category: Herb that Invigorates the Blood (see page 350)

Carthamus stimulates circulation, the heart, and the uterus. It helps lower cholesterol levels and is used to relieve pain and reduce fevers and inflammation. This herbal ally is taken internally for coronary artery disease, jaundice, measles, menstrual complaints (such as absent menses), and menopausal problems. Externally, carthamus is applied to painful or paralyzed joints, bruises, sprains, wounds, and inflammations of the skin.

Contraindications: Do not ingest this herb during pregnancy.

Herbal Combinations Using Safflower Flower

Ligusticum and safflower flower relieve chest and abdominal pain due to Stagnant Qi and blood stasis.

Forsythia, peony root (red), raw rehmannia root, and safflower flower treat red, painful, swollen eyes.

Other Herbs that Invigorate the Blood

If the healing properties of safflower flower are not quite right for your condition, please see the other herbs in this category: *Achyranthes, Ligusticum, Peony Root (Red), Salvia, Turmeric*
Maximum Daily Dosage: 3 to 5 grams
1/10 ounce to 1/5 ounce

Salvia

Stimulates Circulation
Botanical Name: *Salvia miltiorrhiza*

A Brief History of Salvia
Mandarin: Dan Shen; **Japanese:** Tanjin; **Korean:** Tansam

Common sage, traditionally ingested to enhance memory and ensure longevity, was once strewn on graves because of its reputed ability to soothe grief. Sage leaves were consulted by young English maidens as a means of catching a glimpse of their future husband. Sage—also that wonderful seasoning that gives Thanksgiving stuffing its delicious flavor—comes from a genus composed of more than 900 species of aromatic annual, biennial, and perennial plants. The tender and half-hardy evergreen shrubs and subshrubs in this genus grow all over the world, favoring open ground and dry, sunny hillsides in warmer temperate regions. Salvia gets its name from the Latin word *salvere*, which means "to be well." About 80 species of these health-enhancing herbal allies have medicinal and culinary uses. Salvias, often grown as ornamentals, come in an incredible array of aromas, colors, and textures. Salvia blossoms secrete abundant nectar, making them a favored species in honey-bee communities.

S. officinalis was used by the ancient Egyptians to promote fertility. This species has been cultivated in northern Europe since the Middle Ages and during the Classical times got a reputation for promoting longevity. *S. officinalis* reached North America sometime during the seventeenth century. One species from Mexico, *S. hispanica,* is used to make a drink called *chia*—its mucilaginous seeds are mixed with lemon juice, water, and sugar. *S. miltiorhiza,* also known as red sage, Chinese sage, or Dan Shen, has been an important herb in traditional Chinese medicine since 206 B.C. Dan Shen is known as "red ginseng" by the Chinese because of the brick red color of its roots.

When shopping for salvia roots, look for large, clean, dry roots that are solid and have reddish-colored outer bark.

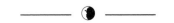

Healing Energies of Salvia
Bitter, Slightly Cold Energy
Treats Heart, Pericardium, and Liver Organ Systems
Category: Herb that Invigorates the Blood (see page 350)

Salvia root stimulates circulation and strengthens the immune system. At the same time, it controls bleeding. It may lower cholesterol levels and inhibits the growth of many disease-causing organisms. Salvia is taken internally for poor circulation, palpitations, coronary heart disease, breast abscesses, mastitis, boils, sores, bruises, menstrual problems (such as dysmenorrhea and amenorrhea) and postnatal pain, irritability, and insomnia.

Contraindications: This herb should be used cautiously in cases where blood stasis is not the issue.

Herbal Combinations Using Salvia

Dang gui and salvia treat irregular menses and are given after childbirth for lochioschesis.

Moutan peony, raw rehmannia, and salvia treat high fevers, irritability, subcutaneous bleeding, nosebleed, and pitting of blood associated with warm-febrile diseases.

Zizyphus seeds, biota seed, and salvia treat insomnia and palpitations due to Heart Blood Deficiency.

Other Herbs that Invigorate the Blood

If the healing properties of salvia are not quite right for your condition, please see the other herbs in this category: *Achyranthes, Ligusticum, Peony Root (Red), Safflower Flower, Turmeric*

Maximum Daily Dosage: 5 to 10 grams
1/5 ounce to 1/3 ounce

Sanguisorba

Stops Bleeding

English Name: Burnet-bloodwort Root
Botanical Name: *Sanguisorba officinalis*

A Brief History of Sanguisorba

Mandarin: Dì Yú; **Japanese:** Jiyu; **Korean:** Chiyu

In Latin, *sanguis* means "blood," while *sorbe* means "to absorb or soak up"—referring to this herb's ability to stop or control bleeding. A member of the rose family, sanguisorba belongs to a genus composed of approximately 20 species of rhizomatous perennials that grow in northern temperate regions. Sanguisorba favors damp grasslands throughout Europe, China, and Japan. In summer, the hardy sanguisorba rootstock supports elegant foliage and maroon-colored bottlebrush blossoms. The leaves of *S. minor*, or burnet, are added to salads, vinegar, and tomato juice for a hint of cucumber flavor.

S. officinalis was first mentioned in Chinese medicine during the Han dynasty (206 B.C.–A.D. 23) in the *Shen Nong Canon of Herbs*. When shopping for sanguisorba, look for hard, thick, dry roots that are reddish in color.

———— ◐ ————

Healing Qualities of the Sanguisorba

Bitter, Sour, Slightly Cold Energy
Treats Liver, Large Intestine, and Stomach Organ Systems
Category: Herb that Regulates the Blood—Stops Bleeding (see page 350)

Sanguisorba controls bleeding, reduces inflammation, and destroys many disease-causing organisms (including *Staph, Strep*, and some flu viruses). It is taken internally to stop hemorrhage, abnormal uterine bleeding, nosebleed, coughing of blood, blood in the stool, diarrhea, dysentery, hemorrhoids, and ulcerative colitis. It is applied externally for burns, sores, and skin diseases. It is also applied as a dentifrice for periodontal disease.

Contraindications: Do not take in case of digestive weakness due to Cold from Deficiency.

Herbal Combinations Using Sanguisorba

Phellodendron and sanguisorba are combined and applied topically as a plaster for burns and eczema.

Sophora and sanguisorba treat bleeding hemorrhoids due to Heat conditions.

Prune seeds and sanguisorba treat bloody stool, bleeding hemorrhoids, bleeding dysenterial disorders, and vaginal leukorrhea due to chronic Damp-Heat (thick, yellow discharge).

Other Herbs that Regulate the Blood

If the healing properties of sanguisorba are not quite right for your condition, please see the other herbs in this category: *Agrimony, Mugwort, Pseudoginseng (see "Ginseng"), Sophora*
Maximum Daily Dosage: 5 to 10 grams
1/5 to 1/3 ounce

Schisandra

Rejuvenatives and Moistens Dry Tissues
Botanical Name: *Schisandra chinensis*

A Brief History of Schisandra
Mandarin: Wu Wèi Zi; **Japanese:** Gomishi; **Korean:** Omicha

There are 25 species of deciduous and evergreen climbers in this genus that grow in eastern North America and eastern Asia. The Northeastern Chinese and Japanese variety, *S. chinensis,* made its way into Western botanic gardens some time in the late 1850s. Frequently planted as ornamentals, female schisandra plants produce fragrant, solitary, cream-to-pink colored flowers in late spring followed by glossy scarlet fruits. The red-flowered *S. sphenanthera* used in southern China is seldom exported, while the *S. chinensis* species is used in the north.

Historically, Chinese references to the use of schisandra first appear in medical texts from the later Han dynasty (A.D. 25–220). "Wu Wèi Zi," the Mandarin name for schisandra, means "five-flavor fruit." The peel is both sweet and sour while the pulp and seeds contain spicy, bitter, and salty flavors. Chinese women use schisandra to improve their complexion and it's ingested by both women and men due to the reputation of being a rejuvenative for sexual energy.

Look for large, plump, shiny, purplish-red, oily berries with marked wrinkles.

———— ▲ ————

Healing Energies of Schisandra

Sour, Warm Energy
Treats Lung and Kidney Organ Systems
Category: Astringent Herb that Stabilizes and Binds (see page 354)

Schisandra is a warm, astringent herb that moistens dry and irritated tissues, regulates the secretion of body fluids, and helps control chronic coughing and wheezing. It is used as an herbal tonic for the nervous system and the Kidney and Heart Organ Systems. Schisandra is taken internally to relieve irritability, insomnia, diabetes, hepatitis, urinary disorders, night sweats, chronic diarrhea, asthma, dry coughs, and involuntary ejaculation. It is applied externally for skin irritations and allergies.

Contraindications: This herb may cause heartburn. Do not take schisandra in the presence of fevers, colds, flu, or the early stages of coughs or rashes.

Herbal Combinations Using Schisandra

Ephedra, oyster shell, and schisandra are taken to relieve night sweats due to Yin Deficiency.

Astragalus, trichosanthes, ophiopogon, and schisandra are combined to treat wasting and thirsting syndromes.

Zizyphus seeds, raw rehmannia root, and schisandra treat irritability, insomnia, and forgetfulness (symptoms associated with Heart Deficiency).

Dried ginger root, wild ginger, and schisandra treat cough and wheezing due to Cold in the Lungs.

Panax ginseng, ophiopogon, and schisandra are combined to treat loss of Qi and Yin in the aftermath of febrile diseases (symptoms include depleted body fluids, shortness of breath, cough, and thirst).

Note: Crush schisandra berries before adding to decoctions.

Other Herbs that Stabilize and Bind

If the healing properties of schisandra are not quite right for your condition, please see the other herbs in this category: *Cornus, Ginkgo, Pomegranate Husk*

Maximum Daily Dosage: 1.5 to 3 grams for chronic cough
1/20 ounce to 1/10 ounce
3 to 5 grams as a tonic
1/10 ounce to 1/5 ounce

Schizonepeta

Treats Rashes and Alleviates Itching

Botanical Name: *Schizonepeta tenuifolia*

A Brief History of Schizonepeta

Mandarin: Jing Jiè; **Japanese:** Keigai; **Korean:** Hyôngkae

Like mint, schizonepeta belongs to the Labiatae family; so, you might say they're cousins. Most schizonepeta comes to us from five provinces in China— Zhejiang, Jiangsu, Jiangxi, Hunan, and Hubei. The squared purplish-colored stem of schizonepeta has a long furrow on each side and is covered with short hairs. The light stem snaps easily to reveal a yellowish-white, fibrous center.

When shopping for schizonepeta, look for light-purple colored herbs with fine stems and dense flower spikes.

──────── ▲☀ ────────

Healing Qualities of Schizonepeta

Spicy, Aromatic, Slightly Warm Energy
Treats Lung and Liver Organ Systems
Category: Warm, Spicy Herb that Releases the Exterior (see page 344)

Schizonepeta is used for the initial stage of measles and pruritic skin eruptions to help bring them to the surface and alleviate itching. (Pruritus is defined as severe itching which can be the result of an allergic or emotional response or other disease factors.) Schizonepeta treats boils and carbuncles when they first erupt, particularly in cases where they are accompanied by fever and chills. It is utilized as an auxiliary herb to stop bleeding such as uterine bleeding or blood in the stool. Schizonepeta is also used to treat colds and flu and sore throats.

Contraindications: Do not use schizonepeta in cases where the measles are fully erupted. Schizonepeta should be avoided in case of open sores.

Herbal Combinations Using Schizonepeta

Mint and schizonepeta are combined to alleviate itching due to rashes and for beginning stages of measles and other skin eruptions. Add the following herbs for symptoms indicated with each entry:

- *Chrysanthemum flower, honeysuckle flower, forsythia fruit, and mulberry leaves* are added to treat colds and flu accompanied by fevers.

- *Scutellaria and chrysanthemum flower* are added to mint and schizonepeta to treat inflammations of the eye.
- *Platycodon* and *licorice,* added to *mint* and schizonepeta, treat acute coughs accompanying colds and flu.

To stop bleeding, schizonepeta is toasted to ash and applied directly to the wound.

Note: Schizonepeta and mint should both be added to herbal decoctions during the last 10 minutes of simmering.

Other Herbs that Release the Exterior

If the healing properties of schizonepeta are not quite right for your condition, please see the other herbs in this category: *Cinnamon Twigs, Ephedra, Ginger (Fresh), Magnolia Flower, Siler*

Maximum Daily Dosage: 5 to 10 grams

1/5 ounce to 1/3 ounce

Scrophularia

Treats Rashes and Throat Infections

English Name: Ningpo Figwort Root, Scrophularia
Botanical Name: *Scrophularia ningpoensis*
S. buergeriana is used in northeastern China
Pharmaceutical Name: Radix Scrophulariae Ningpoensis

A Brief History of Scrophularia

Mandarin: Xuán Shen; **Japanese:** Genjin; **Korean:** Hyônsam

Tuberculosis of lymph glands in the neck is a disease called scrofula (also known as "King's Evil" due to the belief that the king's touch could cure the malady). Scrophularia gets it name from this disorder since it was used as an early cure for scrofula. Tubers of the European species, *S. nodosa,* were consumed by starving French troops in 1627–1628 during the siege of La Rochelle. The stems, leaves, and flowers (aerial parts) of this species are used to treat skin problems, gout and rheumatic disorders, cleanse the lymphatic system, and relieve constipation accompanied by sluggish digestion.

Approximately 200 species of annuals, perennials, and subshrubs found growing in northern temperate zones compose this genus. *S. ningpoensis,* the species native to China, has been used medicinally since the later Han dynasty (A.D. 25–220). Its healing properties are different from those of its European cousin, *S. nodosa.* To enhance its yin nourishing properties, the scrophularia root is dry-fried with salt. Look for big, thick root slices, black in color (with light flecks), and a thin skin.

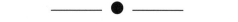

Healing Qualities of Scrophularia

Salty, Sweet, Bitter, Cold Energy
Treats Kidney, Lung, and Stomach Organ Systems
Category: Herb that Clears Heat and Cools the Blood (see page 345)

Scrophularia is prescribed to treat feverish illnesses (associated with Excess Heat in Oriental medicine) with such symptoms as dry cough, throat infections, red and swollen eyes, insomnia, rashes, delirium, constipation, irritability, carbuncles, and abscesses.

Contraindications: According to traditional sources, scrophularia should not be combined with ginger, zizyphus seeds, cornus, or astragalus. Do not ingest scrophularia if symptoms include diarrhea due to Spleen Deficiency (digestive weakness) or Spleen and Stomach Dampness.

Herbal Combinations Using Scrophularia

Oyster shell and *fritillary* are combined with scrophularia to treat scrofula, goiter, and other lymphatic swellings.

Dang gui, honeysuckle, and scrophularia treat painful, ulcerated sores.

Moutan peony root cortex and scrophularia treat erysipelas (localized skin rashes due to strep infection) and purpuric rashes (characterized by hemorrhages into the skin due to various reasons including bacteria and reactions to food or drugs).

Other Herbs that Clear Heat and Cool the Blood

If the healing properties of scrophularia are not quite right for your condition, please see the other herbs in this category: *Lycii Root Cortex, Moutan Cortex, Rehmannia (Raw)*

Maximum Daily Dosage: 5 to 20 grams

1/5 ounce to 2/3 ounce

Scutellaria

Possesses Broad Antimicrobial Action

English Name: Scutellaria, Scute, Baical Skullcap Root
Botanical Name: *Scutellaria baicalensis.*
S. Amoena is used in southwestern China
while *S. viscidula* is used in northeastern China.

A Brief History of Scutellaria

Mandarin: Huáng qín; **Japanese:** Ogon; **Korean:** Hwanggum

More than 300 species of plants belong to the Scutellaria genus. *S. baicalensis,* the medicinal variety used in Oriental herbal medicine, is native to eastern Asia, while *S. lateriflora* is commonly found growing in North American nurseries and gardens. The later variety was used by the Native American Cherokee people to promote menstruation. In 1772, the healing properties of this species were studied by Dr. Van Deveer, who found it useful in treating rabies. For this reason, scutellaria's common name is "mad-dog skullcap."

When shopping for "scute," look for long, hard, yellow roots without a cortex and with a hard core.

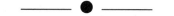

Healing Qualities of Scutellaria

Bitter, Cold Energy
Treats Gallbladder, Large Intestine, Lung, and Stomach Organ Systems
Category: Herb that Clears Heat and Dries Dampness (see page 345)

Besides possessing superior antimicrobial properties, scutellaria lowers cholesterol, blood pressure, and fevers. It stimulates the liver, improves digestion, controls bleeding, and has diuretic effects. Scutellaria has the reputation of calming a restless fetus during pregnancy. Scutellaria is particularly useful in treating urinary-tract infections, enteritis, dysentery, chronic hepatitis, jaundice, hypertension, coughing accompanied by thick, yellow mucus; hot sores and swellings, nosebleeds, bloody stools, irritability, reddened eyes, and a flushed face.

Contraindications: According to traditional sources, scutellaria should not be used with moutan peony root cortex. Do not ingest scutellaria if symptoms pertaining to Coldness exist or in case of Deficient Lung Heat.

Herbal Combinations Using Scutellaria

Coptis and scutellaria are combined to treat high fever and irritability associated with warm-febrile diseases.

Peony root (white), gardenia fruit, artemisia, phellodendron, and scutellaria treat Damp-Heat jaundice.

Anemarrhena and scutellaria are combined to relieve acute and chronic coughs due to Lung Heat (symptoms could include spitting up of thick yellow or greenish-colored phlegm).

Scutellaria and *sanguisorba* are combined to relieve fever, abdominal pain, and bloody stool associated with Intestinal abscess.

Other Herbs that Clear Heat and Dry Dampness

If the healing properties of scutellaria are not quite right for your condition, please see the other herbs in this category: *Coptis, Gentian, Phellodendron*
Maximum Daily Dosage: 5 to 10 grams
1/5 ounce to 1/3 ounce

Sea Vegetables
Reduce Tumors and Neutralize Heavy Metals

A Brief History of Sea Vegetables

Sea veggies have been consumed around the globe since antiquity. The archaeological record provides indications of sea-veggie foraging wherever humankind has lived near an ocean. Ten-thousand-year-old Japanese burial mounds yield evidence of seaweed consumption, while Iceland's oldest law book, dated 961 B.C., outlines rights regarding harvesting dulse on a neighbor's property. Ancient Chinese and Egyptians used seaweed to treat cancer. From the high Andes to the South Pacific and throughout Northern Europe, Russia and the Arctic, sea veggies have always found a place on the table and in the diet.

According to scientists, ocean water contains all 56 minerals and essential trace elements. Constantly bathed in the ocean's nutrient-rich broth, sea vegetables naturally offer our human cells important building blocks in the exact proportion they inherently understand. Approximately 70 percent of the human body and 90 percent of the brain are composed of water, nearly identical to that found in our world's oceans. While boasting a high mineral content, most seaweed varieties possess less than 2 percent fat. A half-cup of cooked hijiki seaweed contains more iron than a couple of eggs and just about the same amount of calcium as a half cup of milk. Nori seaweed contains nearly 30 percent protein while other varieties range from 12 to 18 percent.

Sea veggies possess the ability to lower serum cholesterol, aid digestion and metabolism, and help the body eliminate common radioactive contaminants and heavy toxic metals such as lead, barium, radium, plutonium, and cadmium. According to studies conducted at McGill University in Montreal, Canada, a compound found in members of the kelp family, called sodium alginate, binds with heavy metals in the intestinal tract, forming an insoluble gel-like salt that is excreted in the feces. These same studies indicate that absorption of radioactive strontium was reduced by 50 to 80 percent with the consumption of sea veggies.

Believe it or not, sea vegetables are actually quite delicious once you become accustomed to their flavor, which ranges from extremely mild to a strong sea tang. Remember the first artichoke heart, mushroom, oyster, or olive you ate? You might have disliked it at first, but something kept calling you back until it became a favorite. Sea veggies are much the same. When we taste something new, it always takes a period of adjustment. Susan, one of my patients, reported that when she accidentally dropped a kelp tablet, it was immediately gobbled up by her kitten. Susan now gives four kelp tablets a day to "Jewels" when she takes her own.

Sea vegetables come in a great variety of flavors, colors, and textures. They can be sprinkled on popcorn, added to soups, stews, stir-fries, grain dishes, salads, used as thickener for desserts (agar is tasteless)—the list goes on and on. You'll find some great recipes in Chapter 5. Luckily, these days you can find sea veggies in almost all health-food stores and in many supermarkets. Responsible harvesters collect sea veggies in clean ocean water, and frequent tests are performed to detect any chemical pollutants. Kelp has long been used in Oriental medicine to help dissolve tumors. While not a panacea to cure all disease, sea vegetables should form a part of our daily diet, just as do broccoli, cauliflower, or kale.

Meet the Three Sea-Vegetable Families

There are three divisions of sea veggies: Green Algae *(Chlorophyta)*, Brown Algae *(Phaeophyta)*, and Red Algae *(Rhodophyta)*. All three divisions offer us some wonderful, nutrient-packed sea veggies.

Green Algae: Nori

Green algae form the link between plants that grow on the land and those that remained in the sea. Most of us are now familiar with Nori; it's the sea veggie used to make sushi and other wrapped delicacies. Be sure to try my recipe for Summer Sushi Rolls in Chapter 5. Cakes made from oatmeal and nori are sauteed to create laver bread, a favorite dish on the British Isles. Nori is higher in protein than lentils and contains significant quantities of beta carotene, the B vitamins, manganese, copper, and zinc.

Brown Algae: Alaria, Arame, Hijiki, Kombu, Wakame

The largest sea vegetables belong to this division; they live in cooler water at medium depths. Kelp, a brown algae, grows up to 1,500 feet long—compare that to a Douglas fir (the tallest land plant) that reaches only 400 feet in height.

Alaria is harvested along the Atlantic and Pacific coasts of North America and is a cousin of wakame, a popular Japanese sea veggie. An almost transparent pale green sea veggie, Alaria should be cooked a minimum of 20 minutes for the best texture and taste. It can be added to soups, grain dishes, or (after a brief soaking) to salads. Alaria is high in vitamins A, B, and E.

Arame is one of my favorite sea veggies and probably the best one for first-time consumers to try since it is very mild flavored. Arame is almost black in color and comes in long, thin strands. Most arame is harvested in Japan where it is first simmered and then dried before being sold. Since no further cooking is required, arame can be soaked (it will double in size) and added to salads. Arame's flavor is so mild, I throw a handful into almost all soups, stews, or grain dishes while they are simmering away. Arame is high in vitamins A and B, potassium, iron, and calcium.

Hijiki is similar to arame, but possesses a somewhat stronger flavor and thicker strands. When soaked, hijiki expands up to three or four times its original size. Always soak and cook hijiki briefly before using. Hijiki is known for its high calcium levels.

Kombu is a variety of kelp that comes to us from Japan. A similar variety is harvested off American shores that cooks much faster than its Japanese cousin—it will dissolve and disappear if cooked longer than 30 minutes. Always soak beans or lentils with a piece of kombu for at least 24 hours before cooking. Kombu helps bean dishes cook more quickly and increases their digestibility. Members of the kelp family contain natural MSG, called glutamic acid; this form does not cause any side effects. MSG was originally synthesized from kelp. It's naturally high in calcium, magnesium, potassium, iron, and iodine.

Wakame is quite similar to alaria. Use it as a vegetable, in salads, or in soups. It can be toasted in the oven and crumbled over foods as a condiment.

Red Algae: Dulse, Purple Nori, Irish Moss (Carrageen), Agar

Dulse is delightfully delicious. Brick-red in color, this mild, sweet sea vegetable remains soft and pliable after it is dried. Considered a snack food in Ireland, dulse can be pan-toasted and served like chips or, after rinsing, added to sandwiches or salads. Dulse cooks in about five minutes and is commonly added to soups or chowders. Dulse is used as a substitute for chewing tobacco in Alaska and fermented to make an alcoholic beverage in Russia. In the 1920s dulse was toasted and served in New England taverns to increase beer sales (because of its natural saltiness). This sea vegetable, indigenous to our waters, remains relatively unknown in Asia.

Purple nori can be used in place of green nori. It has a purplish hue and is not as delicate in flavor as the green variety.

Irish moss or *carrageen* grows in the coastal waters of the North Atlantic. It can be soaked and eaten as a vegetable but more commonly is used as a thickener (like gelatin) in desserts, soups, or stews.

Agar has the unique ability to enhance the flavor of other foods. It is commonly used as a thickener that quickly sets at room temperature. Simply dissolve it in hot water and then add it to your favorite fruit juice to create a sugar-free, health-packed gelatin for the kids. It can also be combined with other liquids such as amazake (a delicious almond drink), rice milk, or soy milk. Agar provides bulk, acting as a mild laxative. It soothes the digestive tract and is a great food for recovering from illness as well as for infants and children. Agar is available in flaked, powdered, or bar form (known as kanten).

Carrageen and agar are used as stabilizers in many foods we currently consume including marshmallows, yogurt, and ice cream.

For first-time consumers, I recommend purchasing and trying sea veggies in the following order: *First, buy arame,* rinse and crumble it into your favorite soup or stew as it is simmering. The delicate flavor of arame usually goes unnoticed even by those who have never had sea vegetables. *Second, buy kombu.* Soak your beans with it overnight. Throw out the rinse water; then cook the beans and kombu the required amount of time. If it cooks long enough, the kombu will disintegrate into your soup. It actually enhances the flavors and aids digestibility. *Third buy, dulse.* Rinse it lightly and place it in your favorite sandwich or toast it lightly by laying it on a cookie sheet in a high oven for a few minutes (be sure not to scorch it). Enjoy dulse's wonderful flavor as a snack food. You can crumble it over popcorn. *Fourth, buy nori sheets* and make some delicious sushi rolls.

Siler

Relieves Body Aches and Migraine Headaches

Botanical Name: *Ledebouriella divaricata*

A Brief History of Siler

Mandarin: Fáng Feng; **Japanese:** Bofu; **Korean:** Bangp'ung

Like ligusticum, parsley, and celery, siler is a member of the Umbelliferae family. It grows wild in a number of Chinese provinces, including Shanxi, Hebei, Shandong, Heilongjiang, Jilin, and Inner Mongolia.

The cylindrical ledebouriella, or siler root, is long, soft, and spongy when broken. The outside of the root is brown with wrinkles while the inner wood is pale yellow. Look for strong roots with a thin, tight cortex.

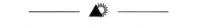

Healing Qualities of the Siler

Spicy, Sweet, Slightly Warm Energy
Treats Bladder, Liver, and Spleen Organ Systems
Category: Herb that Releases the Exterior (see page 344)

The slightly warm siler root treats headaches, chills, and body aches due to colds and flu. It is also used for trembling of the hands and feet, migraine headaches, and muscle cramps or spasms.

Contraindications: According to traditional texts, siler should not be combined with ginger. Do not use this herb in case of anemia or Yin Deficiency with Heat signs. Do not use in cases of anemia accompanied by muscle spasms.

Herbal Combinations Using Siler

Du huo, clematis, notopterygii, and siler treat pain due to obstruction. *Arisaematis* and siler are used for headaches, numbness, and generalized body aches.

Other Herbs that Release the Exterior

If the healing properties of siler are not quite right for your condition, please see the other herbs in this category: *Cinnamon Twigs, Ephedra, Ginger (Fresh), Magnolia Flower, Schizonepeta*
Maximum Daily Dosage: 5 to 10 grams
1/5 ounce to 1/3 ounce

Sophora Flower
Treats Bleeding Hemorrhoids
English Name: Pagoda Tree Flower Bud
Botanical Name: *Sophora japonica*

Brief History of Sophora Flower
Mandarin: Huái Hua Mi; **Japanese:** Kaikamai; **Korean:** Koehwami

A member of the legume family, the deciduous Japanese pagoda tree produces fragrant creamy white pealike flowers in late summer, followed by 2- to 3-inch-long seed pods. There are approximately 50 species of deciduous and evergreen trees, shrubs, and subshrubs that make up the Sophora genus. The red coral or mescal beans produced by *S. secundiflora* were used by Native Americans living in southwestern United States and Mexico in tribal initiation rites. Native people living in Wisconsin used the beans as an external treatment for earache.

Medicinal use of *S. flavescens* (yellow pagoda tree) was first mentioned in Chinese medical texts written during the later Han dynasty (A.D. 25–220) while the use of *S. japonica* can be traced back to about A.D. 600. The flower buds of this last species are used in brewing beer as well as being an important commercial source for yellow-dye crystals called quercetin.

When shopping for flower buds of *S. japonica,* look for those that are the size of a grain of rice. Crude buds are greenish-yellow in color and if soaked in water, color it bright yellow. However, charred buds are used to stop bleeding; they are dark-brown to black in color.

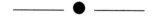

Healing Qualities of Sophora Flower
Bitter, Cool Energy
Treats Liver and Large-Intestine Organ Systems
Category: Herb that Regulates the Blood and Stops Bleeding (see page 350)

This cooling, antibacterial herb controls bleeding, lowers cholesterol and blood pressure, reduces inflammation, strengthens capillaries, and relaxes spasms. Sophora flower buds are particularly important in treating bleeding hemorrhoids and dysenterial disorders. This herb Cools the Liver, relieving such symptoms as headache, dizziness, and red eyes.

Contraindications: This herb is not prescribed during pregnancy or in case of digestive weakness (Spleen or Stomach Cold due to Deficiency).

Herbal Combinations Using Sophora Flower

Biota and sophora treat uterine bleeding, bloody stool, bloody urine, and nosebleed.

Other Herbs that Regulate the Blood and Stop Bleeding

If the healing properties of sophora are not quite right for your condition, please see other the herbs in this category: *Agrimony, Mugwort, Pseudoginseng (see Ginseng), Sanguisorba*

Maximum Daily Dosage: 5 to 10 grams
1/5 ounce to 1/3 ounce

Stephania
Reduces Lower Body Edema
Botanical Name: *Stephania tetrandra*

A Brief History of Stephania
Mandarin: Hàn Fáng Ji; **Japanese:** Kanboi; **Korean:** Hanbanggi

Two different herbs with similar properties, *Aristolochia fangchi* and *Stephania tetrandra,* are referred to as stephania root. These herbs come from different families; however, both are used to drain dampness. Aristolochia is most often used to treat upper-body edema while *S. tetrandra* treats edema in the lower body.

Stephania tetrandra grows in the Zhejian, Anhui, Jiangxi, and Hubei provinces of China and belongs to the Menispermaceae family. If the type of stephania is not specified when herbal prescriptions are written, most pharmacists will automatically dispense this species. Look for hard, cylindrical roots. Slices of stephania are whitish-yellow in color, firm, and slightly powdery in texture. Grayish-brown ducts originate near the center of the slice and radiate out to about one eighth inch from the outside edge.

———— ● ————

Healing Qualities of Stephania

Bitter, Spicy, Cold Energy
Treats Bladder, Spleen, and Kidney Organ Systems
Category: Herb that Drains Dampness (see page 347)

Stephania tetrandra promotes urination and treats edema, particularly of the lower body. It relieves abdominal distension, intestinal gurgling, swollen legs, knee inflammation, and red, swollen, hot, painful joints.

Contraindications: Stephania should not be used in the presence of Deficient Heat.

Herbal Combinations Using Stephania

Poria cocos, cinnamon twigs, and stephania are often combined to treat lower-body edema in weak patients.

Other Herbs that Drain Dampness

If the healing properties of stephania are not quite right for your condition, please see the other herbs in this category: *Aduki Bean, Alisma, Coix, Poria Cocos, Zhu Ling*

Maximum Daily Dosage: 3 to 10 grams
1/10 ounce to 1/3 ounce

Sweet Flag Rhizome see Acorus Rhizome

Tangerine Peel
Stimulates Digestion
Botanical Name: *Citrus reticulata, C. tangerina,*
or *C. erythrosa*

A Brief History of Tangerine Peel
Mandarin: Chén Pí; **Japanese:** Chinpi; **Korean:** Chinp'i

There are 16 species of small evergreen trees and shrubs that make up the citrus genus including many of our favorite fruits such as lemon, lime, grapefruit, orange, and tangerine. Many of us enjoy a fresh glass of orange or
grapefruit juice for breakfast. We regularly throw out orange and tangerine
peels not knowing that many varieties have therapeutic value. Teas are made
from leaves of the lime tree to treat bilious headaches. Orange-blossom water
from the bergamot orange helps ease colic in infants, while bergamot oil flavors Earl Grey tea.

The origin of citrus plants is somewhat obscure due to their long cultivation. Originally native to Southeast Asia and the Pacific islands, the first
member of the citrus family to make it to Europe was the bitter orange, *C.
aurantium,* probably aboard a Portuguese ship returning home from the East
Indies. *C. limon* arrived sometime in the thirteenth century.

Both the dried ripe peel and dried unripe peel of *C. reticulata* (mandarin orange or tangerine) is used in Oriental medicine. When shopping for
ripe peel, look for pliable, large, thin-skinned pieces. They should be oily,
aromatic, and reddish-orange in color. When shopping for green or unripe
peel, look for large, thin-skinned pieces—the color will be dark greenish-
gray.

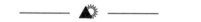

Healing Qualities of Tangerine Peel
Spicy, Bitter, Aromatic, Warm Energy
Ripe Peel Treats Lung, Spleen, and Stomach Organ Systems
Green Peel Treats Gallbladder, Liver, and Stomach Organ Systems
Category: Herb that Regulates the Qi (see page 349)

In Traditional Oriental Medicine, tangerine peel belongs to a category of
herbs that Regulate Qi. herbs in this healing category are aimed at breaking
up Qi Congestion affecting the Organ Systems. Symptoms usually involve

pain in the abdomen or chest. For example, Stagnant Stomach and Spleen Qi manifests as belching, gas, acid regurgitation, epigastric and abdominal pain, nausea, vomiting, and loose stool or constipation. Congested Liver Qi includes such symptoms as irritability, pain in the flanks, loss of appetite, and a stifling feeling in the chest. Stagnant Lung Qi is characterized by a stifling feeling in the chest that is accompanied by coughing and wheezing.

From a Western medical standpoint, it could be said that herbs in this category are aimed at correcting a gastrointestinal dysfunction responsible for creating pain.

Dried ripe tangerine peel is prescribed for indigestion, vomiting, gas and wet coughs, while dried green tangerine peel treats bronchial congestion, liver and gallbladder disorders, mastitis, and breast cancer.

Contraindications: Qi-Regulating herbs are aromatic and Dry in nature and should be used cautiously by persons with Yin or Qi Deficiency. This herb is contraindicated in cases with dry, unproductive coughs. Simmer Qi-Regulating herbs for no more than 15 minutes, since therapeutic volatile oils will be lost if they are cooked longer.

Herbal Combinations Using Ripe Tangerine Peel

Ripe tangerine peel is combined with *ginger* to treat vomiting and hiccups.

Siler, atractylodes, and ripe peel treat abdominal pain, gas, and diarrhea.

Ripe peel is combined with qi-tonifying herbs such as *astragalus* and *codonopsis* to prevent bloating.

Ripe peel is combined with *green peel* to treat abdominal bloating accompanying flank and chest pain.

Pinellia and ripe peel treat coughs with excessive white phlegm and a stifling sensation in the chest. *Magnolia bark* and *poria cocos* are added to strengthen the Spleen Organ System and help move phlegm.

Herbal Combinations Using Green Tangerine Peel

Green peel is combined with *bupleurum* and *turmeric* to relieve pain and distention in the chest and flanks (area between the rib cage and the hips).

Cyperus and green peel treat flank pain due to blocked Liver Qi. Salvia and vaccaria seeds are added to alleviate pain and swelling of the breasts.

Other Herbs that Regulate the Qi

If the healing properties of tangerine peel are not quite right for your condition, please see the other herbs in this category: *Cyperus, Persimmon Calyx*
Maximum Daily Dosage: 3 to 10 grams
1/10 ounce to 1/3 ounce

Tangkuei Root (Angelica Sinensis) see *Dang Gui*

Taraxaci see *Dandelion*

Tien Qi Ginseng see *Ginseng, Pseudoginseng*

Tree Peony Root Cortex see *Moutan Cortex*

Trichosanthes

Treats Coughs and Lung Infections
Botanical Name: *Trichosanthes kirlowii* or *T. uniflora*

A Brief History of Trichosanthes
Root—**Mandarin:** Tian Hua Fen; **Japanese:** Tenkafun; **Korean:** Ch'ônhwabun
Fruit—**Mandarin:** Gua Lou; **Japanese:** Karo; **Korean:** Kwalwi
Seed—**Mandarin:** Gua Lóu Rén; **Japanese:** Karonin; **Korean:** Kwalwiin

Trichosanthes, also known as Chinese cucumber or snake gourd, is rarely found growing in the West. These tropical climbers range from the Pacific islands to Indo-Malaysia, Vietnam, Mongolia, and China. A total of 15 species of annual and perennial plants make up the genus with *T. kirilowii* being the hardiest. This particular species is cultivated in southern China for use as a medicinal herb. White-fringed female flowers bear reddish-orange fruits that contain pale-brown seeds. Male plants are preferred for root production. Native Americans used a relative of Chinese cucumber known as buffalo gourd. They crushed it in water to produce a washing agent.

Medicinal use of this herb was first described in the *Shen Nong Canon of Herbs,* a medical text from the later Han dynasty (A.D. 25–220). A protein in *T. kirilowii* called "Compound Q" is undergoing tests as a possible remedy for AIDS.

When shopping for trichosanthes, look for large, undamaged fruits with dark golden-yellow skins and plump, oily seeds. Trichosanthes root should be large, fat, and light tan in color with a white fibrous interior.

———— ● ————

Healing Qualities of Trichosanthes Fruit and Seed
Fruit: Sweet, Bitter, Cold Energy
Seed: Sweet, Cold Energy
Treat Large Intestine, Lung, and Stomach Organ Systems

Traditionally, trichosanthes fruit is used to prepare a special winter soup reputed to provide immunity from colds and flu. The fruit treats dry constipation, lung and breast tumors, and bronchial infections with thick mucus.

———— 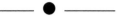 ————

Healing Qualities of Trichosanthes Root
Bitter, Slightly Sweet, Sour, Cool Energy
Treats Lung and Stomach Organ Systems
Category: Herb that Cools and Transforms Hot Phlegm (see page 348)

Trichosanthes tubers are given in the second stage of labor to speed childbirth. They also treat dry coughs, abscesses, diabetes, and tuberculosis. Trichosanthes root has anti-inflammatory properties, lowers fevers, and increases lactation.

Contraindications: Pregnant women should not ingest trichosanthes. Avoid trichosanthes if coldness, poor digestion, or diarrhea are present.

Herbal Combinations Using Trichosanthes

Trichosanthes fruit, *fritillary, platycodon,* and *tangerine peel* treat dry coughs with thick mucus that is difficult to expectorate.

Dandelion and trichosanthes fruit are used for the early stages of breast abscess.

Trichosanthes seed, *pinellia,* and *coptis* treat cough, chest pain, and thick mucus that is difficult to expectorate. *Bupleurum* and *scutellaria* are added if inflammation or infection is present.

Dandelion and trichosanthes seed are used for intestinal abscess.

Trichosanthes root, *fritillary, white mulberry root cortex,* and *platycodon* treat coughs producing thick, blood-streaked mucus.

Anemarrhena, kudzu, schisandra, and trichosanthes root are utilized to replenish moisture after long, febrile diseases.

Other Herbs that Transform Phlegm and Stop Coughing

If the healing properties of trichosanthes are not quite right for your condition, please see the other herbs in this category: *Bamboo Sap and Shavings, Fritillary, Kelp (see Seaweed)*

Maximum Daily Dosage: 10 to 12 grams

1/3 ounce to 1/2 ounce

Tussilago see *Coltsfoot*

Turmeric

Treats Menstrual Disorders and Poor Circulation

Botanical Name: *Curcuma longa* (domestic)

Curcuma aromatica (wild turmeric)

A Brief History of Turmeric

Mandarin: Jiang Húang; **Japanese:** Kyoo; **Korean:** Kanghwang

Turmeric, a member of the ginger family, is native to tropical Asia and Australia. There are a total of 40 perennial species belonging to this genus. *C. longa* has been traditionally utilized as a source of yellow and orange dyes for wool and silk. Turmeric, which means "yellow" in Sanskrit, has long been used by Hindus in body-painting rites connected with religious observances. It also gives the characteristic "orange" color to the robes of many Buddhist monks. This variety is harvested seasonally in dry, forested areas of India while *C. aromatica* grows in Indian teak forests. Recent research on *C. longa* (used abundantly in Asian cuisine as flavoring and coloring) demonstrates that this wonderful spice has significant liver-protective effects as well as anti-inflammatory properties. *C. zedoaria* is utilized in China to treat cervical cancer.

Turmeric is frequently used in East Indian Ayurvedic medicine and was first described in Chinese medical texts around the seventh century. When shopping for *C. longa*, look for dry, hard, heavy rhizomes. The exterior is a deep yellowish-brown color while the interior ranges from deep yellow to orange-brown.

Healing Qualities of Turmeric

Spicy, Bitter, Warm Energy
Treats Spleen, Stomach, and Liver Organ Systems
Category: Herb that Invigorates the Blood (see page 350)

C. aromatica (wild turmeric) stimulates circulation and the gall bladder, dissolves clots, stops bleeding, and improves digestion. It is taken internally for jaundice, painful menstruation, shock, angina, and nosebleeds. *C. longa* (domestic turmeric) stimulates digestion, circulation, respiration, and the uterus and has antibiotic and anti-inflammatory properties. It is prescribed for menstrual disharmonies, uterine tumors, liver disease, poor circulation, and for digestive and skin complaints.

Contraindications: Use turmeric with caution during pregnancy and in the presence of Deficient Heat.

Herbal Combinations Using Turmeric

Dang gui, cyperus, white peony root, and turmeric are combined for flank and abdominal pain due to painful menstruation.

Salvia is combined with turmeric to treat chest pain associated with Heat symptoms and blood congestion.

Achyranthes, moutan peony root cortex, and turmeric relieve skin with purplish blotches, nosebleed, and spitting of blood.

Bupleurum and turmeric treat lack of or irregular menstruation with pain and blood stasis.

Other Herbs that Invigorate the Blood

If the healing properties of turmeric are not quite right for your condition, please see the other herbs in this category: *Achyranthes, Ligusticum, Peony Root (Red), Safflower Flower, Salvia*

Maximum Daily Dosage: 3 to 10 grams
or 1/10 ounce to 1/3 ounce

Watermelon
Clears Summer Heat
Botanical Name: *Citrullus vulgaris*

A Brief History of Watermelon
Mandarin: Xi Gua; **Japanese:** Suika; **Korean:** Sôgwa

Who can resist a piece of sweet, cold, crisp, juicy red watermelon in the sweltering hot summer months? This tropical climbing vine fruit originated in Africa and is a member of the gourd family.

———— ● ————

Healing Qualities of Watermelon
Sweet, Cold Energy
Treats Bladder, Heart, and Stomach Organ Systems
Category: Herb that Clears and Relieves Summer Heat (see page 346)

Summer heat is a condition that occurs primarily in the hot summer months and is associated with fever, diarrhea, sweating, thirst, and irritability. Severe heat patterns include dry heaves with dark, scanty urine and significant thirst. The herbs in this group reduce fevers, eliminate thirst, and produce fluids.

According to Oriental medical thought, watermelon juice treats jaundice and reduces edema because of its diuretic properties.

Contraindications: Persons who suffer from Cold due to digestive weakness or excessive Damp-Cold should avoid watermelon.

Herbal Combinations Using Watermelon
To treat symptoms of summer heat, give the patient 8 ounces (1 cup) of watermelon juice.

Other Herbs that Clear and Relieve Summer Heat
If the healing properties of watermelon are not quite right for your condition, please see the other herb in this category: *Mung Bean*

White Cardamom Seed
see *Cardamom Seed (White)*

White Peony Root
see *Peony Root (White)*

Zhu Líng
Reduces Edema
English Name: Polyporus Sclerotium
Botanical Name: *Polyporus umbellatus*

A Brief History of Zhu Líng
Mandarin: Zhu Líng; **Japanese:** Chorei; **Korean:** Cheyyông

Polyporus has been used in Traditional Oriental Medicine since at least the first century A.D.; it is referenced in a classical Chinese text compiled during that time called the *Divine Husbandman's Classic of the Materia Medica.*

The lustrous outer skin of zhu líng is dark-red to grayish-black in color while the inner flesh should be white and powdery. Like poria cocos, zhu líng is a member of the fungus family. Its roughly spherical body should be solid, hard, and light like cork.

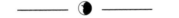

Healing Qualities of Zhu Líng
Sweet, Bland, Slightly Cool Energy
Treats Spleen, Kidney, and Bladder Organ Systems
Category: Herb that Drains Dampness (see page 347)

In Traditional Oriental Medicine, Dampness refers to (1) edema and congested fluids that have accumulated in the body, particularly below the waist and in the legs and feet, and (2) Damp-Heat with signs of Heat and Stagnation (dark or yellow secretions, fever, and burning sensations). In case of the second category, herbs that "Drain Dampness" are normally combined with herbs that "Clear Heat and Dry Damp."

Since "Draining Damp" is a matter of increasing urination to relieve the accumulation of fluids in the body, many of these herbs are diuretics. Zhu líng treats cloudy, painful urination, kidney stones, nephritis, scanty urine, vaginal discharge, jaundice, and diarrhea.

Contraindications: It is extremely important that herbs in this group not be given to persons with depleted body fluids or Yin Deficiency. Long-term use of this herb is discouraged since it can injure the Yin in our human garden.

Herbal Combinations Using Zhu Líng

Poria cocos and zhu líng are combined to treat painful urination, scanty urine, diarrhea, and edema.

Other Herbs that Drain Dampness

If the healing properties of zhu líng are not quite right for your condition, please see the other herbs in this category: *Aduki Bean, Alisma, Coix, Poria Cocos, Stephania*
Maximum Daily Dosage: 6 to 15 grams
or 1/5 ounce to 1/2 ounce

Zizyphus Seed

Helps You Catch Some Zzz's
English Name: Seed of Sour Jujube Date
Botanical Name: *Ziziphus jujuba* var. *spinosa*

A Brief History of Zizyphus Seed
Mandarin: Suan Zao Rén; **Japanese:** Sansonin; **Korean:** Sanchoin

Zizyphus seeds come from the jujube fruit, or Chinese date. This plant is native to temperate Asia and is rarely encountered outside botanic gardens today. Approximately 3,000 years ago, jujube plants were introduced to western Asia from China. There are 85 species of this deciduous tree or large shrub growing in tropical and subtropical regions with spiny twigs that reach up to 45 feet in height. Small yellow flowers develop into 1-inch long oval-shaped fruits. A dark reddish-brown-to-black skin covers the sweet, whitish pulp. Jujube has been cultivated in China for ages and was first mentioned in Chinese medical literature during the Han dynasty (A.D. 25–220). The ancient Romans and Greeks also grew jujubes; they introduced the plant to Spain, where it became naturalized.

When shopping for jujube date seeds, look for large, plump seeds that are maroon in color. They have a faint odor, a nutlike crunchiness, and an interesting toasted flavor.

———— ✿ ————

Healing Qualities of Zizyphus Seed

Sweet, Sour, Neutral Energy
Treats Heart, Spleen, Liver, and Gall Bladder Organ Systems
Category: Herb that Nourishes the Heart and Calms the Spirit (see page 355)

When someone is experiencing symptoms such as insomnia, irritability, palpitations accompanied by anxiety, or forms of mental instability, substances from this healing category are used to Calm the Spirit. In Oriental thought, the spirit resides in the Heart while the soul resides in the Liver. Disorders of both organ systems manifest with similar symptoms.

Like zizyphus seeds, most herbs that Nourish the Heart and Calm the Spirit are very gentle substances.

Contraindications: Use with caution in case of excess heat or severe diarrhea.

Herbal Combinations Using Zizyphus Seed

Zizyphus seeds are combined with *codonopsis, poria cocos,* and *longan berries* to treat insomnia, irritability, and palpitations associated with weak digestion and anemia.

Schisandra, oyster shell, astragalus, and zizyphus seeds treat night sweats and spontaneous sweating.

If you are experiencing anxiety, munch on a teaspoon of zizyphus seeds two or three times a day.

Other Herbs that Nourish the Heart and Calm the Spirit

If the healing properties of zizyphus seed are not quite right for your condition, please see the other herbs in this category: *Biota, Polygala*
Maximum Daily Dosage: 5 to 10 grams
1/5 ounce to 1/3 ounce

Chapter 4
Common Ailments and Their Simple Herbal Home Remedies

Chapter 4 is devoted to offering you practical ways to treat common, everyday complaints with healing Oriental herbs. For ease, ailments with similar symptoms have been grouped together, for example, the first section is entitled "Allergies, Rhinitis, and Sinusitis." Under each section you will find three subheadings: (1) Individual Herbal Helpers, (2) Chinese Patent Formulas, and (3) Classical Oriental Herbal Prescriptions.

The first subheading, "Individual Herbal Helpers," refers you back to individual herbs covered in Chapter 3. From this listing, you can pick and choose the herbs that best address your disharmony, and you can create your own formula. For example, if you're suffering from the beginning stages of a cold or flu and are experiencing considerable neck and shoulder tension with a high fever and no nasal stuffiness, you could opt to use kudzu root over magnolia flower (kudzu relaxes neck and shoulder muscles while magnolia flower unblocks stuffed nasal passages). Remember that each herb also has a section describing herbal combinations that are commonly used; one of these combinations might be right for you. Usually, you will want to harmonize your formula by adding two to three slices of licorice, two to three jujube dates, or three to five small pieces of dried ginger, whichever of these three herbs best suits your personal constitution.

The second subheading, "Chinese Patent Formulas," gives you another option. Chinese Patent medicines can generally be purchased in most health-food stores—they're convenient, effective, economical, can be stored for long periods of time, and are free from side effects if taken as directed. I often prescribe patent formulas in my own practice; most of them have more than 2,000 years of successful clinical application behind them. They are prepared in the age-old tradition of Oriental herbalism. Some formulas have been adulterated by Western medications, however. In this case, I have given you the name brands that are best to purchase.

The third subheading, "Classical Oriental Herbal Prescriptions," offers you two or three of my favorite formulas to treat various conditions and, if applicable, pointers as to constitutional types best suited to take them. You might even consider reading over the qualities of the herbs in such a formula and adding or substituting an herb that seems more appropriate for your particular condition. Often, this is the way formulas are individualized to address the needs of different persons. There are truly hundreds, if not thousands of wonderful classical formulas geared to meet the different needs of each individual. If you find yourself intrigued by Oriental herbal medicine and want to expand your knowledge of herbs and formulas, please see page 357 for recommended reading on this subject.

(*Note:* For chronic or serious complaints, I recommend you seek out a trained professional practitioner of Traditional Oriental Medicine; they are listed in the Yellow Pages under "Acupuncture." You can also call your State Department of Health to confirm if the practice of Oriental medicine is legal in your state. If so, request a list of licensed acupuncturists. When calling for an appointment, always ask if the practitioner is trained in Oriental or Chinese herbal medicine. You can take this book to your first appointment and ask the practitioner to mark recommended herbs or herbal prescriptions for you.)

Herbal Rules of Thumb Revisited

Herbal formulas for acute conditions such as colds, sore throats, and flus are taken for only a few days (two to three) and modified as symptoms change. If you do not experience improvement in your condition, please consult a licensed health-care professional.

Formulas for chronic conditions will be ingested for longer periods of time. Under ideal conditions, expect to take the formula one month for each year you have experienced the problem. It might take up to a month for you to start feeling the benefits of your herbal therapy. Remember, while all herbs are not safe all of the time for all people, most herbs are gentle foodlike medicines that help give your body a nudge in the right direction. They are addressing the underlying deficiencies or imbalances. It may have taken you many years to arrive at your present state of disharmony, so it's important to be patient and let your body gradually build up its natural defenses. *When taking formulas for chronic conditions, herbalists will normally recommend that you ingest the herbs only five or six days a week and rest from them for one or two days. You can take a formula that treats chronic conditions for three months, then rest from it for two weeks. The formula can be repeated or modified slightly with the change of seasons or a change in your condition. If you come down with a cold, flu, infection, or other acute disease, discontinue all Tonifying herbs until you have recovered.*

ALLERGIES, RHINITIS, SINUSITIS

Individual Herbal Helpers

See Chapter 3: Anemarrhena, chrysanthemum, cocklebur fruit, dang gui, forsythia, gypsum, honeysuckle, kudzu, magnolia flower, peppermint, phellodendron, platycodon, schisandra, schizonepta, siler

Chinese Patent Formulas

BI YAN PIAN　　This excellent patent formula treats sneezing, itchy eyes, sinus pain, and facial congestion. If you suffer from acute or chronic rhinitis, sinusitis, hay fever, stuffy nose, nasal allergies, experience thick, yellowish, foul-smelling sinus discharge, this formula could help.
　　Dosage: 4 to 6 pills, 3 to 5 times daily. Available in bottles of 100 pills.

PE MIN KAN WAN　　This patent formula specifically treats postnasal drip. It alleviates acute or chronic sinusitis, hay fever, rhinitis, itchy, watery eyes, sneezing.
　　Dosage: 3 pills, 3 times daily. Available in bottles of 50 pills. Purchase Plum Flower brand.

Classical Oriental Herbal Prescription

PUERARIA NASAL COMBINATION　　This is an excellent formula to treat rhinitis, sinusitis, and colds and flus accompanied by such symptoms as sneezing, headache, fatigue, chills, stuffy nose, and stiff neck and shoulders.

Pueraria	6.0 grams	*or* approximately 1/5 ounce
Coix	5.0	1/6 ounce
Platycodon	4.5	1/6 ounce
Magnolia Flower	4.0	1/7 ounce
Ephedra Stems	3.0	1/10 ounce

Peony Root (White)	3.0	1/10 ounce
Cinnamon Twigs	2.5	1/10 ounce
Jujube Dates	2.0	1 or 2 pieces
Gypsum	2.0	1/14 ounce
Ligusticum	1.5	1/20 ounce
Ginger	1.5	1/20 ounce
Rhubarb	1.5	1/20 ounce
Licorice	1.0	2 or 3 slices

Also see formulas listed under "Colds and Flu."

Asthma

see section entitled, "Coughs, Bronchitis, Phlegm, Asthma, Wheezing"

ANXIETY, RESTLESSNESS, AND INSOMNIA

Individual Herbal Helpers

See Chapter 3: Biota, codonopsis, cuscuta, dang gui, dragon bone, gardenia, ophiopogon, oyster shell, pearl, polygala, polygonum, poria cocos, rehmannia (raw), salvia, schisandra, scrophularia

Chinese Patent Formulas

AN MIEN PIEN   This patent treats mental agitation or exhaustion leading to insomnia, overthinking, anxiety, red or irritated eyes, dream-disturbed sleep, and poor memory.
    Dosage: 4 pills, 3 times daily. Available in bottles of 60 pills.
    Precaution: Avoid eating hot, greasy foods while taking An Mien Pien.

AN SHENG BU XIN WAN   This calming, tranquilizing formula alleviates palpitations, insomnia, anxiety, uneasiness, restlessness, dizziness, poor memory, and dream disturbed sleep.
    Dosage: 15 pills, 3 times daily. Available in bottles of 300 pills.
    Precaution: Take this formula for 2 weeks maximum time; discontinue for 2 weeks and resume ingestion for another 2 weeks.

DING XIN WAN   This patent treats insomnia, anxiety, palpitations, dizziness, hot flashes, dry mouth, and poor memory.

Dosage: 6 pills, 2 to 3 times daily. Available in bottles of 100 pills.

Precaution: Avoid eating hot, greasy foods while taking Ding Xin Wan.

Emperor's Tea (Tian Wang Bu Xin Wan)

This tea eliminates night sweats accompanied by nocturnal emissions, anxiety, insomnia, restlessness, palpitations, and vivid dreaming. Emperor's Tea is a great aid for students who are experiencing the preceding symptoms due to long hours of excessive studying. In Oriental medicine, we say that excessive mental work depletes Heart Blood and Yin resulting in the preceding symptoms.

Dosage: 8 pills, 3 times daily. Available in bottles of 200 pills.

Precaution: Ingest this tea for 2 weeks only; rest one week and repeat for another 2 weeks if desired. Avoid eating hot, greasy foods while taking Emperor's Tea.

Gui Pi Wan (Kwei Be Wan)

This formula effectively treats irregular menstruation and abnormal uterine bleeding as well as fatigue, insomnia, restless dreaming, palpitations, dizziness, night sweats, and poor memory. This formula is also great for students.

Dosage: 8 pills, 3 times daily. Available in bottles of 200 pills.

Classical Oriental Herbal Prescriptions

BUPLEURUM AND DRAGON-BONE COMBINATION   This formula comes to us from the famous doctor Chang Chung-ching who wrote the *Shang han lun* (a classical medical text compiled in A.D. 205). It treats chest and subcardiac distention (sensation of fullness), shoulder stiffness, irritability, insomnia, fearfulness, agitation, depression with a tendency toward fatigue and clumsiness that accompany such diseases as arteriosclerosis, hypertension, hysteria, uremia, chronic arthralgia, cirrhosis, and angina pectoris.

Bupleurum	5.0 grams	*or* approximately 1/6 ounce
Pinellia	4.0	1/7 ounce
Poria Cocos	3.0	1/10 ounce
Scutellaria	2.5	1/12 ounce

Jujube Dates	2.5	1/12 ounce
Ginseng, Panax	2.5	1/12 ounce
Ginger (Dried)	2.5	1/12 ounce
Oyster Shell	2.5	1/12 ounce
Dragon Bone	2.5	1/12 ounce
Rhubarb	1.0	1/30 ounce

ZIZYPHUS COMBINATION   Another formula from the Han dynasty that is well over 1,700 years old, Zizyphus Combo treats persons with delicate constitutions who are weak, fatigued, panicky, irritable, and suffering from night sweats and/or insomnia due to stress.

Zizyphus Seeds	10.0 grams	*or* approximately 1/3 ounce
Poria Cocos	5.0	1/6 ounce
Anemarrhena	3.0	1/10 ounce
Ligusticum	3.0	1/10 ounce
Licorice	1.0	2 or 3 slices

ARTHRITIS, RHEUMATISM, LUMBAGO

Individual Herbal Helpers

See Chapter 3: Achyranthes, aconite, alisma, cinnamon bark, clematis, codonopsis, coix, dang gui, du huo, eucommia, gastrodia, gentian, ginger, ginseng, ligusticum, peony root (red), polygonum, poria cocos, rehmannia, safflower flower, salvia, siler, stephania, zhu ling

Chinese Patent Formulas

DU HUO JISHENG WAN   This effective classical herbal formula treats arthritis, rheumatism, and chronic sciatica resulting from Cold. Symptoms include clear-colored urination, low-back and knee pain with weakness, stiffness and numbness, nighttime urination, sensations of cold, and aversion to cold. Purchase Plum Flower brand.

Dosage: 9 pills, 2 times daily. Available in bottles of 100 pills.

Precautions: Do not take this formula during pregnancy. Avoid cold foods, beans, and seafood while taking Du Huo Jisheng Wan.

Feng Shih Hsiao Tung Way This patent is excellent for chronic rheumatoid arthritis, osteoarthritis, and geriatric weakness of the legs. Symptoms include aching lower back and finger, shoulder, knee, or hip pain accompanied by a sensation of coldness in the limbs.

Dosage: 10 pills, 2 times daily. Available in bottles of 100 pills.

Precautions: Do not take this formula during pregnancy. Avoid cold foods, beans, and seafood while taking Feng Shih Hsiao Tung Way.

Specific Lumbaglin This formula moves congested Blood and Qi, dispelling Wind and Damp (traveling pain and edema) from your human garden. It relieves inflammation, pain and achiness, muscular strain and low-back and sciatic pain.

Dosage: 1 to 2 capsules, 3 times daily. Available in bottles of 24 capsules.

Precautions: Do not take this formula during pregnancy. Avoid beans and seafood while taking Specific Lumbaglin.

Tian Ma Wan This is an excellent formula for elderly persons experiencing rheumatic or arthritic pain accompanied by sensations of cold, Bell's palsy, migraines, and arm, leg, or facial paralysis.

Dosage: 6 to 8 pills, 3 times daily. Available in bottles of 100 pills.

Xiao Huo Luo Dan This patent treats difficult joint movement, numbness, sharp joint pain, aching muscles or joints, chronic lower-back pain due to Cold, frequent, clear-colored urination, sensations of cold, and aversion to cold.

Dosage: 6 pills, 2 to 3 times daily. Available in bottles of 100 pills.

Precautions: Do not take this formula during pregnancy. Do not ingest this formula in the presence of fever or red, swollen joints. Avoid cold foods, beans, and seafood while taking Xiao Huo Luo Dan.

Classical Oriental Herbal Prescriptions

Coix Combination Mucoid arthritis and rheumatism have long been treated with this excellent formula that comes to us from the Tang dynasty A.D. 652. It is often referenced in Chinese medical classics as a cure for muscle spasms, rheumatism, and arthralgia. It is also used to treat swelling and chronic fever in the arms and legs.

Coix	8.0 grams	*or* approximately 1/4 ounce
Ephedra	4.0	1/7 ounce
Dang Gui	4.0	1/7 ounce

Atractylodes	4.0	1/7 ounce
Peony Root (White)	3.0	1/10 ounce
Licorice	2.0	2 to 3 slices

CINNAMON AND ANEMARRHENA COMBINATION   First mentioned in medical texts from the Han dynasty, this formula treats arthralgia, rheumatism, nausea and general aches and pains as well as pain due to swelling of the joints and muscle atrophy in the legs.

Atractylodes	4.0 grams	1/7 ounce
Cinnamon Bark	3.0	1/10 ounce
Ginger (Dried)	3.0	1/10 ounce
Anemarrhena	3.0	1/10 ounce
Peony Root (White)	3.0	1/10 ounce
Siler	3.0	1/10 ounce
Ephedra Stems	3.0	1/10 ounce
Aconite	0.5 to 1.0	1/60 to 1/30 ounce
Licorice	1.5	2 slices

Bronchitis

see section entitled "Coughs, Bronchitis, Phlegm, Asthma, Wheezing"

COLDS AND FLU

Individual Herbal Helpers

See Chapter 3: Bupleurum, chrysanthemum, cinnamon twigs, cocklebur fruit, cohosh, coptis, ephedra, forsythia, ginger, gypsum, honeysuckle, kudzu, licorice ligusticum, magnolia flower, peony, peppermint, phellodendron, platycodon, schisandra, schizonepeta, scutellaria, siler

Chinese Patent Formulas

CHUAN XIONG CHAO TIAO WAN   This herbal patent formula is taken to treat sudden headaches from a cold accompanied by such symptoms as rhinitis, sinusitis, nasal congestion, and chills.

Dosage: 8 pills, 3 to 5 times daily. Available in bottles of 200 pills.
Note: You can enhance the effects of this formula by taking it with a cup of green tea.

GANMAOLING TABLETS   This patent formula treats both Wind-Heat or Wind-Cold symptoms including upper-back and neck stiffness, fevers, chills, sore throats, and swollen lymph glands. If you take minimal dosages at the first hints of a cold or flu, this formula may help to prevent the illness.
Dosage: 3 to 6 tablets, 3 times daily for acute stages of a cold or flu.
Prevention: 2 to 3 tablets, 3 times daily for 3 days. Available in bottles of 36 tablets.

HUO HSIANG CHENG CHI PIEN   This patent, also known as Lopanthus Antifebrile Pills, effectively treats colds and flu accompanied by abdominal pain, diarrhea, nausea, vomiting, gas and gurgling, chills, fever, and headaches. This formula is also effective in alleviating motion sickness, morning sickness in pregnant women, and as an aid for weak digestion accompanied by loose stools.
Dosage: 4 to 8 pills (sugar coated), 2 times daily. Available in bottles of 100 pills
or 4 to 8 tablets (uncoated), 2 times daily. Available in vials of 8 tablets each.
Precautions: Do not take this formula if you have a dry mouth, thirst, and fever without chills.

YIN CHIAO TABLETS   Similar to Ganmaoling, Yin Chiao is often used to treat colds and flu, tonsillitis, sore throats, body aches, headaches, stiff and sore neck and shoulders, swollen lymph nodes, itching skin (as in measles) accompanied by aversion to heat, and hives.
Dosage: 5 to 6 pills every 2 to 3 hours for first 9 hours of illness.
Then 5 to 6 pills every 4 to 5 hours, as needed.
Discontinue this patent by the third day of the illness.
Precautions: Do *not* purchase Superior Quality Yin Chiao Tablets. This particular brand contains antelope horn, as well as Western chemicals, and is sugar coated. Other brands are quite effective without these unwanted additions.

Classical Oriental Herbal Prescriptions

PUERARIA (KUDZU) COMBINATION   This treats the common cold accompanied by severe chills, congestion, diarrhea, neck and upper-back stiffness, and extreme muscle aches or spasms.

Kudzu Root	8.0 grams	*or* approximately 1/5 ounce
Ephedra	4.0	1/7 ounce
Jujube Dates	4.0	1/7 ounce
Cinnamon Twigs	3.0	1/10 ounce
Peony Root (White)	3.0	1/10 ounce
Licorice	2.0	2 to 4 slices
Ginger (Dried)	1.0	3 to 5 small slices

CINNAMON COMBINATION   Treats the common cold or flu in weak or delicate persons with such symptoms as severe chills, low fever, headache, and abdominal pain due to chills.

Cinnamon Twigs	4.0 grams	*or* approximately 1/7 ounce
Jujube Dates	4.0	1/7 ounce
Ginger	4.0	1/7 ounce
Peony Root (White)	4.0	1/7 ounce
Licorice	2.0	1/14 ounce

COUGHS, BRONCHITIS, PHLEGM, ASTHMA, WHEEZING

Individual Herbal Helpers

See Chapter 3: Anemarrhena, apricot kernel, bamboo sap, bamboo shavings, codonopsis, coltsfoot, ephedra stems, fritillary, gardenia, ginger, jujube dates, lily bulb, pinellia, platycodon, poria cocos, rhubarb, scutellaria, sophora, tangerine peel, trichosanthes

Chinese Patent Formulas

BRONCHITIS PILLS (COMPOUND)   These pills treat acute and chronic bronchitis, chronic asthma, labored breathing from weak lungs and phlegm retention, as well as cough and mucus caused by colds and flu.

Dosage: 2 to 3 capsules, 3 times daily. Available in bottles of 60 capsules.

CHING FEI YI HUO PIAN   This patent formula treats Toxic Heat with thick, sticky, yellow phlegm; painful, swollen throat; fever; dry or raspy coughs; scanty, dark-yellow urine; constipation; mouth or nose sores; bleeding gums; and toothaches.

Dosage: 4 tablets, 2 to 3 times daily. Available in boxes containing 12 vials, each vial holds 8 tablets.

Precautions: Do not take Ching Fei if you are pregnant. Discontinue this patent formula once Heat symptoms subside, or if diarrhea develops.

ERH CHEN WAN   This formula relieves mucus congestion in the stomach, lungs, or face (nose, throat, sinuses), with such symptoms as abdominal distention, chest distention, nausea, dizziness, vertigo, excessive salivation, and hangover resulting from overindulgence in alcohol beverages.

Dosage: 8 pills, 3 times daily. Available in bottles of 200 pills.

HSIAO KEH CHUAN PILLS   This gentle formula is an extremely effective remedy for difficult breathing, asthma, acute or chronic bronchitis, lung congestion, and coughing accompanied by copious, clear- to white-colored mucus.

Dosage: 2 capsules, 3 times daily. Available in bottles of 18 capsules.

HSIAO KEH CHUAN LIQUID (SPECIAL BRONCHITIS MEDICINE)   Similar to the preceding patent except in liquid form. This formula helps build immunity and alleviates frequent, clear urination, as well as lower back pain due to Cold.

Dosage: 1 to 2 tablespoons, 3 times daily. Available in 100-milliliter bottle.

LO HAN KUO INFUSION   This formula soothes the lungs, reduces thirst, resolves phlegm, and relieves itchy throat and chronic coughing (including whooping cough).

Dosage: 1 cube dissolved in 1 cup hot water, 3 to 6 times daily. Available in boxes containing 12 smaller boxes (each containing 2 doses).

NATURAL HERB LOQUAT-FLAVORED SYRUP   This pleasant-tasting syrup relieves acute bronchitis and accompanying sinus congestion, emphysema, acute and chronic coughs from Lung weakness, as well as symptoms of Heat or Dryness accompanied by sticky phlegm.

Dosage: 1 tablespoon, 3 times daily. Available in 5-, 10-, or 25-ounce bottles. Children can take 1 teaspoon, 3 times daily.

PINELLIA EXPECTORANT PILLS (QING QI HUA TAN WAN)   This patent formula relieves bronchial congestion, sinus congestion, and asthma accompanied by excessive, thick, yellow, sticky mucus or nasal discharge.

Dosage: 6 pills, 3 times daily. Available in bottles containing 200 pills.

Precautions: Do not use this formula if chills are present or in case of dry coughing without phlegm.

PULMONARY TONIC PILLS   This formula is used to strengthen the lungs against chronic symptoms of weakness with Heat, such as dry coughing and the expectoration of thick, sticky, yellow phlegm.

Dosage: 5 pills, 3 times daily. Available in bottles containing 60 pills.

Classical Oriental Herbal Prescriptions

MINOR BLUE-DRAGON COMBINATION   This great formula is first mentioned in Chinese medical texts between A.D. 142 and 220. It treats dry coughs, whooping cough, fever, general aching, asthmatic cough, occasional sensation of chills in the back, and conjunctivitis. This formula is not for weak persons or those suffering from night sweats.

Pinellia	6.0 grams *or* approximately 1/6 ounce	
Ephedra Stems	3.0	1/10 ounce
Peony Root (White)	3.0	1/10 ounce
Cinnamon Twigs	3.0	1/10 ounce
Wild Ginger	3.0	1/10 ounce
Ginger	3.0	1/10 ounce
Schisandra	3.0	1/10 ounce
Licorice (Honey-Fried)	3.0	3 to 4 slices

PORIA COCOS (HOELEN) AND SCHISANDRA COMBINATION   This herbal prescription, from the Han dynasty, is suited for persons suffering from bronchial asthma, acute or chronic bronchitis, emphysema, and/or edema who have delicate constitutions, a tendency toward anemia, cold hands and feet, and a feeling of water stagnancy in the stomach.

Poria Cocos	4.0 grams	1/7 ounce
Apricot Seed	4.0	1/7 ounce
Pinellia	4.0	1/7 ounce

Schisandra	3.0	1/10 ounce
Ginger (Dried)	2.0	1/14 ounce
Wild Ginger	2.0	1/14 ounce
Licorice	2.0	3 to 5 slices

EPHEDRA COMBINATION   This formula is for strong persons suffering from a cold or flu with fever, stuffy nose, bronchitis, asthma, rhinitis, general pain, or rheumatoid arthritis. This is another classic from the Han dynasty.

Ephedra	5.0 grams	1/5 ounce
Apricot Seed	5.0	1/5 ounce
Cinnamon Twigs	4.0	1/7 ounce
Licorice	1.5	2 or 3 slices

DIGESTIVE DISORDERS

Individual Herbal Helpers

See Chapter 3: Agastache, atractylodes, cardamom, coix, cyperus, fennel seeds, ginger, hawthorn fruit, kudzu, magnolia bark, peppermint, pinellia, poria cocos, radish seed, tangerine peel

Chinese Patent Formulas

CURING PILL   A gentle, yet extremely effective herbal formula for abdominal upset, Montezuma's revenge (diarrhea), food poisoning, stomach flu accompanied by sudden, violent abdominal cramping, vomiting, headaches, bloating with pain, constipation, nausea, motion sickness, and morning sickness. This patent formula is safe to take during pregnancy and can be given to small children. We never travel outside the United States without a good supply of Curing Pills.

Dosage: 1 to 2 full vials of tiny pills, 2 to 4 times per day, or as needed. Available in boxes, each containing 10 vials filled with pills.

CARMICHAELI TEA PILLS   This formula treats watery diarrhea, poor digestion, nausea, vomiting, pale- to clear-color urine, abdominal fullness, and cold hands and/or feet. This formula contains aconite.

Dosage: 8 to 12 pills, 3 times a day. Available in bottles of 200 pills.

FRUCTUS PERSICA COMPOUND PILLS   This patent herbal prescription treats habitual constipation associated with Dryness or Heat.
Dosage: 4 to 8 pills, 3 times a day. Available in bottles of 200 pills.

GINSENG ROYAL-JELLY VIALS (RENSHENG FENG WANG JIANG)   This formula stimulates appetite and facilitates food absorption. It is particularly helpful following surgery, prolonged illness, childbirth, and in old age.
Dosage: 1 to 2 vials per day. Available in boxes; each contains 10 glass vials holding 10 cc of liquid. The box also contains a glass cutter and 10 small straws to sip the liquid.
Precautions: Do not eat cold foods, citrus, or drink caffeinated beverages while ingesting Ginseng Royal Jelly.

GINSENG STOMACHIC PILLS (REN SHEN JIAN PI WAN)   A great formula to treat low-energy, chronic-digestive problems accompanied by abdominal pain and bloating, diarrhea, poor appetite, and inability to gain or maintain weight.
Dosage: 6 pills, 3 times daily. Available in bottles of 200 pills.
This product also comes without ginseng and is known as Jian Pi Wan.
Precautions: Nursing mothers should avoid this product. Do not consume cold foods while taking Ginseng Stomachic.

LIU JUN ZI TABLETS   This product relieves poor digestion accompanied by reduced appetite, indigestion, acid regurgitation, nausea, and diarrhea.
Dosage: 8 tablets, 3 times daily after meals. Available in bottles containing 96 tablets.
Precautions: Avoid consuming cold foods while taking this formula.

MU XIANG SHUN QI WAN (APLOTAXIS CARMINATIVE PILLS)   This patent treats low stomach acid (hypoacidity). It relieves food congestion accompanied by abdominal distension, poor digestion, foul-smelling belches, bad breath, erratic stools, and constipation.
Dosage: 8 pills, 2 times daily. Available in bottles of 200 pills.
Precautions: Avoid consuming cold foods while taking this formula.

PING WEI PIAN   This formula supports digestion, treats gas, abdominal cramping, bloating, nausea, poor appetite, diarrhea, and pain.
Dosage: 4 tablets, 2 times daily. Available in bottles of 48 tablets.

SAI MEI AN   This formula treats hyperacidity, nonbleeding duodenal and gastric ulcers, stomach irritation and inflammation following meals, and gastritis associated with hyperacidity of the stomach.

Dosage: 3 pills, 3 times daily prior to meals. Available in bottles containing 50 pills.

Note: In case bleeding accompanies the preceding symptoms, combine this patent with Yunnan Paiyao (listed under "Trauma").

Precautions: This patent formula should be discontinued two weeks after the symptoms subside. Long-term use can damage the stomach and digestive process.

SHU KAN WAN   This patent formula reduces Evil Wind or flatulence with abdominal pain, hiccups, belching, poor appetite and digestion, nausea, vomiting, acid regurgitation, cold limbs, and flushed face.

Dosage: 8 pills, 3 times daily. Available in bottles of 120 pills.

Precautions: Do not ingest this product during pregnancy.

WEI TE LING   This product relieves pain and bleeding accompanying gastric and duodenal ulcers, gas, stomach distension, gastritis in conjunction with stomach hyperacidity.

Dosage: 4 to 6 tablets, 3 times daily before meals, or as necessary. Available in bottles of 120 tablets.

Classical Oriental Herbal Prescriptions

PINELLIA-AND-GINGER COMBINATION   This herbal prescription is from the Han dynasty and treats stagnant moisture and food in the stomach, that feeling of everything just sitting there (sometimes, you can actually hear water sloshing around inside). This formula treats gastric distention, sour stomach, diarrhea, nausea, and vomiting.

Pinellia	5.0 grams	*or* approximately 1/6 ounce
Ginseng (Panax)	2.5	1/12 ounce
Scutellaria	2.5	1/12 ounce
Jujube Dates	2.5	1/12 ounce
Licorice	2.5	1/12 ounce
Ginger (Fresh)	2.0	1/14 ounce
Ginger (Dried)	1.5	3 or 4 slices
Coptis	1.0	1/30 ounce

HOELEN FIVE HERB FORMULA   This formula, from the Han dynasty, is particularly helpful for treating the stomach flu with vomiting, fever, diarrhea, and abdominal pain. It can be given to children with the flu as well, but reduce the dosage according to Clark's Rule. (See page 48.) This formula also treats toxemia during pregnancy.

Alisma	6.0 grams	1/5 ounce
Zhu Ling	4.0	1/7 ounce
Poria Cocos	4.0	1/7 ounce
Atractylodes	4.0	1/7 ounce
Cinnamon Twigs	2.0	1/14 ounce

ENERGY TONICS

We experience low energy for a vast number of reasons. It's possible we've been burning the candle on both ends for too long and simply need a vacation. Many personal setbacks also take their toll (such as the death of a loved one, separation or divorce, loss of a job). It's natural to feel drained and fatigued after an emotional trauma. Maybe we're recovering from a chronic illness. Or, quite simply, we're trying to be superhuman. In any case, it's truly important to come to grips with the root cause of our need for more energy. It might be necessary to improve our diet or get our energy moving by taking a 30-minute walk 3 or 4 times a week (it's amazing how energizing a brisk walk in the fresh morning air can be). In any case, before grabbing that next cup of coffee, coke, or ginseng capsule for an energy boost, try to address the real issue at hand. This might mean setting some time aside to be alone so you can truly think things over. Following are some wonderful herbal aids to help you rebuild and rejuvenate on a deeper level.

Before ingesting Qi-Tonifying herbs (such as ginseng), make sure that your Qi is moving in the first place. If you feel tired, lethargic, and are suffering from Stagnant Qi, ingesting Qi-boosting herbs is going to cause only further congestion. Your herbal formula will need herbs to help move or regulate the Qi, such as cyperus or tangerine peel. The same goes for all categories of Tonifying herbs, those that Tonify the Blood, the Yang or the Yin. Oriental herbal formulations are harmonized in this way. Rarely will you find a practitioner of Oriental medicine prescribing one single herb, such as dioscorea or ginseng. Usually, a minimum of three to four herbs are combined to create a balanced formula based on the specific needs of the individual.

Individual Herbal Helpers

See Chapter 3: Astragalus, codonopsis, cuscuta, dang gui, dendrobium, dioscorea, epimedium, eucommia, fenugreek seed, ginseng, glehnia, jujube dates, licorice, lily bulb, longan berries, ophiopogon, peony root (white), polygonum, rehmannia

Chinese Patent Formulas

BU ZHONG YI QI WAN (CENTRAL QI PILLS)   This formula regulates low energy; relieves poor digestion accompanied by gas, pain, bloating and erratic stools; and prevents uterine bleeding, miscarriages, chronic diarrhea, and hypoglycemia. It was originally used for uterine, rectal, colonic, hemorrhoidal, varicose vein, and hernial prolapse.

Dosage: 8 pills, 3 times daily. Available in bottles of 100 pills.

Precautions: Do not ingest cold foods while taking these pills. This patent formula should not be used in the presence of Heat symptoms such as scant, dark-yellow urine, profuse perspiration, aversion to heat, thirst, strong body odor, or yellow-to-red discharges.

EIGHT-TREASURE TEA   This patent is an excellent general tonic, especially for women with the following symptoms: Fatigue, dizziness, palpitations, anemia, pale face, shortness of breath, hypoglycemia, poor appetite, absent or irregular menstruation, or general weakness during pregnancy. This classical formula strengthens energy, nourishes the blood, and speeds recovery after childbirth or chronic illness.

Dosage: 8 pills, 3 times daily. Available in bottles of 200 pills.

GOLDEN BOOK TEA (SEXOTON PILLS)   This formula treats fatigue; low-back and knee pain; poor circulation; clear, frequent urination; edema; infertility; impotence; lowered sex drive; and poor digestion with undigested food particles in the stool.

Dosage: 8 to 10 pills, 3 times daily. Available in bottles of 120 or 200 pills.

Precautions: Not to be taken by persons with Heat symptoms such as aversion to heat, yellow discharges, thirst, facial flushing with fever; or by persons suffering from chronic gastrointestinal weakness. Avoid consuming cold foods when taking this formula.

SHEN QI DA BU WAN   This simple formula is composed only of codonopsis and astragalus root. It is a wonderful tonic for general weakness, fatigue, anemia, and poor digestion due to stomach weakness. This formula helps build the immune response.

Dosage: 8 pills, 3 times daily. Available in bottles of 100 pills.

Six-Flavor Tea (Liu Wei Di Huang Wan) This extraordinary classic formula treats spontaneous sweating and mild night sweats, low energy, sore throats, thirst, dizziness, burning sensations in the soles of the feet or palms of the hands, ringing in the ears (tinnitis), restlessness, insomnia, impotence, nocturnal emission, and urinary incontinence.

Dosage: 8 pills, 3 times daily. Available in bottles of 200 pills.

Yang Rong Wan (Ginseng Tonic Pills) This formula promotes health and longevity. It treats general weakness caused by surgery, trauma, chronic illness, and helps in childbirth.

Dosage: 8 pills, 3 times daily. Available in bottles of 20 pills.

Precautions: Do not take this formula in the presence of Heat symptoms such as yellow or red discharges, thirst, fevers, or aversion to heat. Do not eat cold foods while ingesting these herbs.

Classical Oriental Herbal Prescriptions

So many of the herbs that boost energy are gentle, neutral- to sweet-flavored tonics that can be added to cereals, soups, stews, and desserts. This is one of the best ways to ingest tonifying herbs—as part of a balanced meal. Be sure to see Chapter 5 for some wonderful recipes.

Ginseng and Longan Combination This wonderful formula comes to us from the Sung dynasty. It is specifically for weak persons with a delicate constitution who suffer from such symptoms as anemia, insomnia, palpitations, night sweats, fatigue, gastric ulcer, nervous exhaustion, mild neurosis, genital itching, and/or leukemia.

Ginseng (Panax)	3.0 grams	1/10 ounce
Poria Cocos	3.0	1/10 ounce
Longan Berries	3.0	1/10 ounce
Zizyphus Seeds	3.0	1/10 ounce
Atractylodes	3.0	1/10 ounce
Astragalus	2.0	1/14 ounce
Dang Gui	2.0	1/14 ounce

Polygala	1.0	1/30 ounce
Saussurea	1.0	1/30 ounce
Jujube Dates	1.0	2 fruits
Ginger (Dried)	1.0	3 or 4 pieces
Licorice	1.0	2 or 3 pieces

Note: This formula is available as a Patent Medicine; please see Gui Pi Wan under the section entitled, "Anxiety, Restlessness, and Insomnia."

REHMANNIA SIX FORMULA (LIU WEI DI HUANG WAN) No book on Oriental herbs should be without this extraordinary formula from the Sung dynasty (A.D. 1035–1117). It is available as a Patent medicine; please see the indications for use of this formula listed earlier, entitled, "Six-Flavor Tea." Rehmannia Six is a Kidney Yin tonic that supports an exhausted kidney/adrenal system.

Rehmannia (Cooked)	6.0 grams	1/5 ounce
Alisma	3.0	1/10 ounce
Cornus	3.0	1/10 ounce
Dioscorea	3.0	1/10 ounce
Moutan Peony	3.0	1/10 ounce
Poria Cocos	3.0	1/10 ounce

EYE PROBLEMS

Individual Herbal Helpers

See Chapter 3: Alisma, chrysanthemum, coptis, cornus, dang gui, dendrobium, dioscorea, forsythia, gypsum, lycii fruit, poria cocos, rehmannia (cooked), scutellaria

Chinese Patent Formulas

MING MU DI HUANG WAN This patent is a variation of the classical Liu Wei Di Huang Wan found earlier under "Energy Tonics." It aids vision problems due to Liver Heat and Wind such as red, itchy eyes; dry eyes; photophobia; excessive tearing; glaucoma; and cataract.

Dosage: 10 pills, 3 times daily. Available in bottles of 200 pills.

Ming Mu Shang Ching Pien   This formula treats conjunctivitis; red, itching, tearing eyes; photophobia; vertigo; night blindness; night sweats; scanty, dark-yellow urine; fatigue; fever; and dry mouth and throat.

Dosage: 10 pills, 3 times daily. Available in bottles of 200 pills.

or 4 tablets, 2 times daily. Available in boxes containing 12 vials; each vial holds 8 tablets.

Precautions: Do not use this formula during pregnancy.

Qi Ju Di Huang Wan (Lycii and Chrysanthemum Tea or Lycium-Rehmannia Pills)   Yet another variation of the Kidney Yin-nurturing Liu Wei Di Huang Wan formula, this patent treats poor night vision, blurry vision, dry and painful eyes, intolerance to light, pressure behind the eyes, as well as outbursts of anger, heat in the palms, dizziness, headaches, pain behind the eyes, restlessness, and insomnia.

Dosage: 8 pills, 3 times daily. Available in bottles of 100 pills.

Classical Oriental Herbal Prescriptions

Lycii, Chrysanthemum, and Rehmannia Formula   Here is the prescription for the same excellent formula that precedes, "Qi Ju Di Huang Wan."

Rehmannia (Cooked)	6.0 grams	1/5 ounce
Alisma	3.0	1/10 ounce
Cornus	3.0	1/10 ounce
Dioscorea	3.0	1/10 ounce
Moutan Peony	3.0	1/10 ounce
Poria Cocos	3.0	1/10 ounce
Chrysanthemum	1.0	1/30 ounce
Lycii Fruit	1.0	1/30 ounce

Fatigue

see Energy Tonics

GYNECOLOGICAL DISORDERS

There are hundreds of wonderful herbal prescriptions for women's complaints. Oriental medicine gently treats a great variety of disorders including absent or painful periods, leukorrhea, ovarian cysts, PMS, postpartum depression, hot flashes and other menopausal complaints—the list goes on and on. In fact, in Oriental medicine many disharmonies are often related to gynecological conditions, which in the West we attribute to other causes; examples might include fatigue, headache, shoulder stiffness, dizziness, hysteria, constipation, anemia, abdominal puffiness, high and low blood pressure, shortness of breath, and palpitations. These imbalances take their emotional toll as well, with accompanying feelings of pessimism, anxiety, irritability, insecurity, despair, self-reproach, indecision, and aversion to seeing people.

Help is often as close as a well-balanced herbal formula. I have seen the following herbs and formulas work wonders for hundreds of women (including myself).

Individual Herbal Helpers

See Chapter 3: Atractylodes, bupleurum, cardamom, cinnamon, codonopsis, cohosh, cuscuta, cyperus, dandelion, dang gui, eucommia, gardenia, ginger, jujube dates, licorice, ligusticum, moutan peony, peony, peppermint, polygonum, poria cocos, rehmannia

Chinese Patent Formulas

AN TAI WAN (FOR EMBRYOS) This formula helps prevent miscarriage (accompanied by lower-abdominal pain) during pregnancy. It stops premature uterine contractions and calms a restless fetus.

Dosage: 7 pills, 3 times daily. Available in bottles of 100 pills.

Precautions: During pregnancy, a licensed practitioner of herbal medicine should monitor use of formulas.

BUTIAO TABLETS This formula effectively treats absent or irregular periods, anemia, menstrual pain, and excessive uterine bleeding accompanied by fatigue. I can cite case after case in my practice where this formula brought regularity and relief of menstrual pain to many women.

Dosage: 3 pills, 3 times daily. Available in bottles of 100 pills.

CHIEN CHIN CHIH TAI WAN This formula treats leukorrhea (vaginal discharge), trichomonas, and vaginal infections accompanied by anemia, weakness, low back pain, and abdominal distension and pain. (Also see Yudai Wan listed later.)

Dosage: 10 pills, 2 times daily. Available in bottles of 120 pills.

HSIAO YAO WAN (BUPLEURUM SEDATIVE PILLS)   This formula treats PMS; menstrual complaints including cramps, breast distension, irregular periods, infertility, irritability and depression; headaches; blurred vision; red, painful eyes; and fatigue. It is also used to treat chronic hay fever, food allergies, poor appetite, abdominal fullness and bloating, and hypoglycemia.

Dosage: 8 pills, 3 times daily. Available in bottles of 100 or 200 pills.

PLACENTA COMPOUND RESTORATIVE PILLS (HE CHE DA ZAO WAN) This patent alleviates hot flashes and menopausal night sweats. It is also effective in treating male spermatorrhea. Both male and female conditions may include such symptoms as weak, aching lower back and legs, dizziness, tinnitus, general fatigue, low-grade afternoon fevers, red cheeks, and a hot, flushed face.

Dosage: 8 pills, 3 times daily. Available in bottles of 100 pills.

SHIH SAN TAI PAO WAN   This formula is taken during the first trimester of pregnancy to prevent miscarriage, nausea, anemia, and fatigue.

Dosage: 1 pill, 2 times daily. Available in boxes; each box contains 10 containers (resembling waxed eggs).

Precautions: During pregnancy, a licensed practitioner of herbal medicine should monitor use of formulas.

TANG KWE GIN   This tonic formula treats anemia and fatigue resulting from trauma, surgery, or illness. It treats irregular menses accompanied by pale blood, amenorrhea, postpartum weakness due to loss of blood, palpitations, dizziness, and poor memory.

Dosage: 1 to 2 tablespoons, 2 times daily. Available in bottles of 100 milliliters or 200 cc.

WU CHI PAI FENG WAN (WHITE PHOENIX PILLS)   This formula treats menstrual disorders due to anemia; symptoms include cramps, ovulation pain, prolonged and irregular periods, amenorrhea, headaches, postpartum weakness or bleeding, low back pain, and poor appetite. This formula contains animal products.

Dosage: 5 pills, 3 times daily. Available in bottles of 120 pills

or 1/2 to 1 large chewball pill, 2 times daily. Available in boxes containing 10 large chewballs. This chewball can be cut in pieces, dissolved in water, or dissolved in the mouth.

Yudai Wan   This formula effectively treats acute vaginitis, dark and odorous leukorrhea, and bladder infections due to yeast overgrowth accompanied by low back pain, fatigue, or abdominal distension or pain.
Dosage: 8 pills, 3 times daily. Available in bottles of 100 pills.

Classical Oriental Herbal Prescriptions

BUPLEURUM AND PEONY FORMULA   This excellent formula comes to us from the Sung dynasty (A.D. 1100) and is used to treat menstrual irregularity as well as a host of menopausal complaints (facial flushing, hot flashes, night sweats, depression, anxiety, irritability, insomnia). Other symptoms might include infertility, PMS, constipation, eczema, chronic hepatitis or cirrhosis, dizziness, aching in the arms and legs, earache, and headaches.

Dang gui	3.0 grams	1/10 ounce
Atractylodes	3.0	1/10 ounce
Bupleurum	3.0	1/10 ounce
Peony (White)	3.0	1/10 ounce
Poria Cocos	3.0	1/10 ounce
Moutan Peony	2.0	1/14 ounce
Gardenia	2.0	1/14 ounce
Licorice	2.0	1/14 ounce
Ginger (Dried)	1.0	1/30 ounce
*Peppermint	1.0	1/30 ounce

DANG GUI FORMULA   This wonderful formula from the Han dynasty eases difficult labor, helps prevent spontaneous abortions, and is used to alleviate postpartum problems.

Peony (White)	3.0 grams *or*	1/10 ounce
Ligusticum	3.0	1/10 ounce
Scutellaria	3.0	1/10 ounce
Dang gui	1.5	1/20 ounce
Atractylodes	1.5	1/20 ounce

*Add peppermint after decoction has simmered as directed in Chapter 5, remove the pot from the heat, and let the peppermint steep with the decocted herbs for 20 minutes before straining.

DANG GUI AND PEONY FORMULA   This formula treats both men and women who are constitutionally weak with anemia, fatigue, and pale, with pain in the lower abdomen (patients suffering from nausea, vomiting, or poor appetite should not take this formula). This formula is prescribed for various complaints during pregnancy including abdominal pain, edema, habitual abortion, cystitis, lumbago, and postpartum weakness. It also treats irregular or painful menstruation.

Peony (White)	4.0 grams *or*	1/7 ounce
Alisma	4.0	1/7 ounce
Atractylodes	4.0	1/7 ounce
Poria Cocos	4.0	1/7 ounce
Ligusticum	3.0	1/10 ounce
Dang Gui	3.0	1/10 ounce

PINELLIA AND MAGNOLIA COMBINATION   This formula, from the Han dynasty, treats persons with a somewhat delicate constitution and a tendency toward fatigue who are experiencing gastrointestinal weakness, nausea, vomiting, abdominal fullness or bloating, flaccidity of skin and muscles, insomnia, nervousness or nervous exhaustion, palpitations, edema, fearfulness, esophageal spasm, toxemia during pregnancy, as well as such symptoms as glassy eyes, hoarseness due to the common cold, asthma, whooping cough, and swelling of lymph nodes (particularly in the neck).

Pinellia and Magnolia has truly worked wonders for a number of my patients. I'll never forget Diane's comments after taking it for only a week: "I never thought it was possible to feel so tranquil, centered, and just happy to be alive!" Diane, a small woman measuring in at just over 5 feet tall, had experienced a complete hysterectomy 10 years previously (at only 28 years of age). For 10 years she battled fatigue, nervousness, edema, and many of the symptoms mentioned here.

Pinellia	6.0 grams *or*	1/5 ounce
Poria Cocos	5.0	1/6 ounce
Ginger	4.0	1/7 ounce
Magnolia bark	3.0	1/10 ounce
Perilla Leaves	2.0	1/14 ounce

HEADACHES

Individual Herbal Helpers

Headaches occur for various reasons. In Traditional Oriental Medicine, we treat the root disharmony. For this reason, you are referred to formulas that address main problems responsible for creating the headache. For individual herbal helpers and classical herbal formulations, you can refer back to the sections that follow.

Chinese Patent Formulas

Headache and Fever Due to Cold/Flu: See section titled, "Colds and Flu"—Yin Chiao Tablets or Zhong Gan Ling.

Headache and Chills Due to Cold/Flu: See section titled, "Colds and Flu"—Chuan Xiong Chao Tiao Wan.

Headache and Allergies or Sinusitis: See section titled, "Allergies, Rhinitis, and Sinusitis"—Bi Yan Pian.

Headache and Indigestion: See section titled, "Digestive Disorders"—Curing Pill.

Headache and Muscle Tension or Cramping: See section titled, "Gynecological Disorders"—Hsiao Yao Wan.

Migraine Headache: See section titled, "Pain"—Corydalis Yanhusus Analgesic Tablets.

Migraine Headache and Sensations of Coldness: See section titled, "Arthritis, Rheumatism, Lumbago"—Tian Ma Wan.

HEART DISHARMONIES

Individual Herbal Helpers

See Chapter 3: Achyranthes, bupleurum, cinnamon bark, cyperus, dandelion, dang gui, dragon bone, eucommia, garlic, gastrodia, ginseng, hawthorn, ligusticum, oyster shell, pearl, peony root (red), polygala, rehmannia, safflower, salvia, sophora, zizyphus seed

Chinese Patent Formulas

DANSHEN TABLETCO   This formula treats heart palpitations, chest pains, and angina pectoris with left-arm pain. It reduces blood cholesterol and lipids.

Dosage: 3 pills, 3 times daily. Available in bottles of 50 pills.

Precautions: Any person suffering from the symptoms listed above should immediately consult a licensed healthcare practitioner.

REN SHEN ZAI ZAO WAN (GINSENG RESTORATIVE PILLS)   This herbal patent treats stroke-related symptoms such as facial paralysis (Bell's palsy), speech disturbances, hemiplegia, and spastic, contractive, or flaccid muscle tone in the extremities. This formula contains animal products.

Dosage: 10 pills, once a day. Available in bottles of 50 pills

or 1 large waxed-egg pill, 2 times daily. Available in boxes containing 10 large, chewy pills encased in a waxed, plastic egg-shaped container. This pill can be cut into pieces, dissolved in the mouth, or dissolved in water.

Note: In many cases, heart palpitations can be a symptom of overwork, anxiety, fatigue, anemia, or other disharmonies. Please see other formulas in sections on Chinese Patent Formulas titled, "Anxiety, Restlessness, and Insomnia," and "Gynecological Disorders."

Classical Oriental Herbal Prescriptions

There are innumerable classical formulas that help with disorders of the heart. For example, one known as Poria Cocos, Apricot, and Licorice Combination treats palpitations, chest pain, pain in the back, valvular disease, and bronchial asthma. Another formula called Poria Cocos and Schisandra Combination treats cyanosis, cold extremities, left-sided cardiac weakness, and edema in the lower body. However, before self-prescribing herbs, please see a qualified medical practitioner to determine if your condition is life-threatening. If you wish to pursue treatment with Oriental herbs and dietary modifications, consult a licensed practitioner of Oriental medicine who can guide you with treatment geared for your unique constitution and its imbalances.

HEMORRHOIDS

Individual Herbal Helpers

See Chapter 3: Bupleurum, dang gui, cohosh, ginseng (see pseudoginseng), rhubarb, sanguisorba, scutellaria, sophora

Note: Persons suffering from hemorrhoids should avoid consuming spicy hot, greasy foods and alcohol.

Chinese Patent Formulas

FARGELIN (FOR PILES)   This is an excellent patent formula for acute and chronic hemorrhoids that brings rapid relief (often within 12 to 24 hours) of swelling as well as bleeding, itching, burning, prolapse, and constipation.
Dosage: 3 pills, 3 times daily. Available in bottles of 36 and 60 pills.

Classical Oriental Herbal Prescriptions

COHOSH (CIMICIFUGA) COMBINATION   This formula comes from the Tokugawa era in Japan and was developed by a famous doctor, Hara Nanyou. It is used specifically for hemorrhoids, to treat severe pain, intense itching, bleeding, prolapse of the rectum, and constipation. The rhubarb should be decreased or omitted in cases without constipation.

Dang gui	6.0 grams *or*	1/5 ounce
Bupleurum	5.0	1/6 ounce
Scutellaria	3.0	1/10 ounce
Licorice	2.0	1/14 ounce
Cohosh	1.5	1/20 ounce
Rhubarb	1.0	1/30 ounce

GINSENG AND ASTRAGALUS COMBINATION   This formula, from the Yuan dynasty in China, treats weak patients suffering from severe hemorrhoids accompanied by other symptoms such as fatigue, low-grade fever, headache, night sweats, and lack of appetite.

Astragalus	4.0 grams *or*	1/7 ounce
Ginseng (Panax)	4.0	1/7 ounce
Atractylodes	4.0	1/7 ounce
Dang gui	3.0	1/10 ounce
Citrus Peel	2.0	1/14 ounce
Bupleurum	2.0	1/14 ounce
Ginger	2.0	1/14 ounce

Jujube Dates	2.0	1/14 ounce
Licorice	1.5	1/20 ounce
Cohosh	1.0	1/30 ounce

HYPERTENSION

Individual Herbal Helpers

See Chapter 3: Achyranthes, chrysanthemum, dang gui, eucommia, gambir, gardenia, garlic, gastrodia, poria cocos, scutellaria, sophora

Chinese Patent Formulas

COMPOUND CORTEX EUCOMMIA TABLETS (FU FANG DU ZHONG PIAN)   This formula relieves hypertension with such symptoms as low back pain, fatigue, frequent urination, palpitations, headaches, and a flushed face.
Dosage: 5 pills, 3 times daily. Available in bottles of 100 pills.
Precautions: Do not consume cold foods while taking this formula.

HYPERTENSION-REPRESSING TABLETS (JIANG YA PING PIAN)   This patent treats hypertension accompanied by Heat signs such as scanty, dark-yellow urine; constipation; thirst; yellow phlegm; tinnitus; headaches; dizziness; and a flushed face. This formula is used to lower blood cholesterol and prevent hardening of the arteries. This gentle formula can be ingested for several years without side effects. It contains some animal products.
Dosage: 4 tablets, 3 times daily for six weeks; reevaluate presence of Heat symptoms mentioned above and repeat if needed. Available in boxes with 12 bottles containing 12 pills each.
Precautions: Do not consume hot, spicy, greasy food while taking this formula.
Note: Blood pressure should be monitored on a daily basis, and a licensed health-care practitioner should be consulted if it exceeds the excepted range.

Classical Oriental Herbal Prescriptions

MAJOR BUPLEURUM COMBINATION   This formula comes from the famous Chinese doctor Chang Chung-ching whose herbal prescriptions are recorded in the *Shang han lun*, compiled during the Han dynasty (A.D.

142–220). This formula should be used only by large, robust, strong persons with healthy skin, exhibiting the following symptoms: hypertension, tendency to obesity, chest pain, constipation or diarrhea, irritability, muscle tenseness with such problems as impaired liver function, gallstones, sour stomach, gastric or duodenal ulcers, diabetes, asthma, or impaired hearing.

Bupleurum	6.0 grams *or*	1/5 ounce
Ginger	4.0	1/7 ounce
Scutellaria	3.0	1/10 ounce
Pinellia	3.0	1/10 ounce
Peony (White)	3.0	1/10 ounce
Jujube Dates	3.0	1/10 ounce
*Chih-Shih	2.0	1/14 ounce
Rhubarb	1.0	1/30 ounce

There are innumerable classical formulas that help with hypertension. In the Oriental medical view, however, hypertension is frequently linked to other symptoms that can be quite distinct depending upon the individual and his or her unique body type. For example, one known as Gastrodia and Uncaria Decoction treats essential hypertension, renal hypertension, cerebrovascular disease, epilepsy, and neurosis when accompanied by the following symptoms: headache, ringing in the ears, dizziness, vertigo, blurred vision, insomnia with dream-disturbed sleep, a red tongue, and sensation of heat rushing to the head. Before self-prescribing herbs for this potentially dangerous disharmony, please see a qualified medical practitioner to determine if your condition is life-threatening. If you wish to pursue treatment with Oriental herbs and dietary modifications, consult a licensed practitioner of Oriental medicine who can guide you with treatment geared for your unique constitution and its imbalances.

Insomnia

see section entitled, "Anxiety, Restlessness, and Insomnia"

---

*Chih-Shih is the immature fruit of the bitter orange; like tangerine peel, it regulates Qi. Look for thick, solid dried fruit that is bluish-black in color.

LIVER AND GALLBLADDER DISORDERS

Individual Herbal Helpers

See Chapter 3: Aduki beans, bupleurum, coptis, dandelion, gardenia, garlic, gentian, lonicera, rhubarb, scutellaria

Chinese Patent Formulas

Ji Gu Cao Pills   This excellent herbal patent treats acute or chronic hepatitis with jaundice. For acute hepatitis, combine with Li Gan Pian, which follows. No side effects are noted.
   Dosage: 4 pills, 3 times daily. Available in bottles of 50 pills.

Lidan Tablets   In China, this formula is a specific remedy used to dissolve and remove gallstones. Symptoms include acute or chronic gallstone inflammation and bile-duct inflammation.
   Dosage: 6 pills, 3 times daily. Available in bottles of 120 pills.

Li Gan Pian (Liver-Strengthening Tablets)   This formula can be combined with either of the two preceding formulas. It treats acute or chronic hepatitis, jaundice, and gallstones and decreases liver pain.
   Dosage: 2 to 4 pills, 3 times daily. Available in bottles of 100 pills.

Classical Oriental Herbal Prescriptions

Minor Bupleurum Combination   This extraordinary harmonizing formula was first recorded by the famous Chinese doctor Chang Chung-ching, who lived during the Han dynasty. It is effective for the person of average constitution with such symptoms as pain beneath the ribs when pressure is applied, stomachache, a bitter flavor in the mouth, headaches, neck stiffness, poor appetite, stress, feelings of annoyance or irritability, vertigo, chest pain, white coating on the tongue, and possible recurrent fever and chills. Minor Bupleurum Combo effectively treats a number of disorders such as hepatitis, gallstones, jaundice, stomachache, gastric ulcer, acute and chronic bronchitis, tonsillitis, otitis media, mumps, and impotence in young men. This is a gentle formula that can be given to children exhibiting the preceding symptoms; it improves mental stability and the general physical constitution.

Bupleurum	7.0 grams *or*	1/5 ounce
Pinellia	5.0	1/6 ounce
Ginger	4.0	1/7 ounce
Scutellaria	3.0	1/10 ounce
Ginseng	3.0	1/10 ounce
Jujube Dates	3.0	1/10 ounce
Licorice	2.0	1/14 ounce

BUPLEURUM AND DANG GUI FORMULA   This classical Chinese formula, also known as "Rambling Powder," is reputed to free the spirit, allowing for open-mindedness. Often, the emotional results of congested or constrained liver function are feelings of irritability. We become judgmental and downright grumpy. When Liver Qi is flowing smoothly, our spirit soars or "rambles free" above petty, everyday concerns. Physical symptoms include fatigue, poor appetite, pain or discomfort under the ribs, dry mouth and throat, a bitter taste in the mouth, headache, vertigo, and a pale-red tongue, as well as possible alternating fever and chills. Women may experience irregular periods and painful breasts.

Bupleurum	3.0 grams *or*	1/10 ounce
Dang Gui	3.0	1/10 ounce
Poria Cocos	3.0	1/10 ounce
Peony (White)	3.0	1/10 ounce
Atractylodes	3.0	1/10 ounce
Ginger (Dried)	2.0	1/14 ounce
Licorice (Honey-baked)	1.5	1/25 ounce

Menstrual Irregularities
see Gynecological disorders and Liver and Gallbladder Disorders

Motion Sickness
see Colds and Flu: Chinese Patent Formulas—Huo Hsiang Cheng Chi Pien
Also: Chapter 3—Ginger

PAIN

Individual Herbal Helpers

Pain indicates something is basically wrong in our human garden. Pain, unless due to an injury or accident, never comes alone; it accompanies other symptoms that signal tendencies toward a greater imbalance. Look through the descriptions of the healing qualities of the various herbs and formulas given throughout this book. Once you start treating the root cause of your disharmony, the pain will go away. However, always consult a licensed health-care practitioner in case of severe, unresolved pain. Pain is a messenger and can be indicative of a serious or life-threatening disorder.

Chinese Patent Formulas

CORYDALIS YANHUSUS ANALGESIC TABLETS   This pain-relieving formula is often used in conjunction with other patent formulas that treat the root imbalance. This patent reduces pain due to dysmenorrhea, hepatitis, rheumatism, trauma, gastric- or duodenal-ulcer pain, insomnia due to pain, postpartum pain, stomachaches, abdominal pain, and chest pain. It is also used to treat muscle spasms, seizures, and tremors.

Dosage: 4 to 6 pills, 3 times daily. Available in bottles of 20 pills.

Prostatitis

see Urinary Disorders

Rheumatism

see "Arthritis, Rheumatism, Lumbago"

Rhinitis

see "Allergies, Rhinitis, Sinusitis"

SKIN PROBLEMS

Individual Herbal Helpers

See Chapter 3: Bupleurum, coptis, dandelion, dang gui, forsythia, gardenia, honeysuckle, ligusticum, pearl, peony, phellodendron, rehmannia, rhubarb, schizonepeta, scrophularia, scutellaria, siler, sophora

Chinese Patent Formulas

CHING WAN HUNG   This is an excellent topical ointment that is applied to first-, second-, and third-degree burns and scalds with remarkable results. We always have a tube or jar of Ching Wan Hung in the refrigerator in case of cooking burns. Applied immediately after a burn, blisters rarely appear. This formula reduces pain, swelling, and blistering. It can also be applied topically to acne, bedsores, heat rashes, sunburn, and hemorrhoids.

Dosage: Apply liberally and cover with a bandage; this product will discolor clothes. Clean and change dressing daily. Available in small tubes or larger plastic jars.

LIEN CHIAO PAI TU PIEN   This formula treats acute inflammations and infections such as ulcerated abscesses and carbuncles with pus, as well as itchy skin characterized by redness and rashes.

Dosage: 2 to 4 tablets, 2 times daily. Available in boxes containing 12 vials; each vial holds 8 tablets.

Precautions: Do not take during pregnancy.

MARGARITE ACNE PILLS   Often used to treat adolescent acne, this remedy also relieves itchy skin, rashes, hives, and furuncles. Purchase Plum Flower brand.

Dosage: 6 pills, 2 times daily. Available in bottles containing 30 pills.

Precautions: Reduce dosage if diarrhea develops.

For more skin formulas see section titled, "Sore Throats, Mouth, and Ear Disorders":

Chuan Xin Lian for abscesses and furuncles.

Huang Lien Shang Ching Pien for hives and itching.

Superior Sore-Throat Powder Spray for ulcerative skin lesions.

Also, see the "Coughs, Bronchitis, Phlegm, Asthma, Wheezing" section:

Ching Fei Yi Huo Pian for boils and sores of the nose and mouth.

Classical Oriental Herbal Prescriptions

COPTIS AND SCUTE COMBINATION   From the Chin dynasty, this formula treats strong, robust body types exhibiting Internal Heat symptoms such as severe itching, hives, rashes, hypertension, palpitations, insomnia, vertigo, flushing up, facial reddening, inflammation, nosebleeds, anxiety, and emotional instability.

Scutellaria	3.0 grams *or*	1/10 ounce
Gardenia	2.0	1/20 ounce
Coptis	1.5	1/25 ounce
Phellodendron	1.5	1/25 ounce

DANG GUI AND GARDENIA COMBINATION   This great Chinese formula is a combination of two classical formulas—Dang Gui Four Combination and Coptis and Scutellaria Combination. Best suited for persons with black, brown, or yellowish skin tone, this herbal prescription treats severe itching, dermatitis, eczema, and urticaria. Other symptoms may include ulcers of the mouth, tongue, and checks; hypertension; leukorrhea; peptic and duodenal ulcers; nervous excitement; severe uterine bleeding; and emotional instability.

Dang Gui	4.0 grams	1/7 ounce
Rhemannia	4.0	1/7 ounce
Peony	3.0	1/10 ounce
Ligusticum	3.0	1/10 ounce
Scutellaria	3.0	1/10 ounce
Gardenia	2.0	1/14 ounce
Phellodendron	1.5	1/20 ounce
Coptis	1.5	1/20 ounce

SORE THROATS, MOUTH, AND EAR DISORDERS

Individual Herbal Helpers

See Chapter 3: Anemarrhena, coptis, dandelion, forsythia, gardenia, gypsum, honeysuckle, mint, pearl, platycodon, rhubarb, schizonepeta, scutellaria, siler, sophora, trichosanthes

Chinese Patent Formulas

ANTIPHLOGISTIC PILLS (CHUAN XIN LIAN)   This formula treats fever and swollen glands in acute throat inflammations, including strep. It is used to treat viral infections (including measles, flu, and hepatitis), as well as abscesses, furuncles, and mastitis.

Dosage: 3 pills, 3 times daily. Available in bottles of 60 pills. Take for 1 to 3 days.

HUANG LIEN SHANG CHING PIEN   This formula treats Heat symptoms such as ear infections; sore throats; high fevers; headaches; itching; hives; nosebleeds; toothaches; scanty, dark-yellow urine; red eyes; constipation or diarrhea; and insomnia.

Dosage: 4 tablets, 1 to 2 times daily. Available in boxes containing 12 tubes; each tube holds 8 tablets.

Precautions: This formula should be discontinued once these Heat symptoms have subsided.

LARYNGITIS PILLS   This patent formula treats the following symptoms resulting from Heat: laryngitis, acute tonsillitis, mumps, or sore throats. If a strep infection is present, also take Antiphlogistic Pills listed earlier.

Dosage: 1 pill, 3 times daily—0 to 1 years of age; 2 pills, 3 times daily— 1 to 2 years of age; 3 to 4 pills, 3 times daily—2 to 3 years of age; 5 to 6 pills, 3 times daily—4 to 8 years of age; 8 to 9 pills, 3 times daily—9 to 15 years of age; 10 pills, 3 times daily for adults.

This formula is available in small boxes; each box holds three vials; each vial contains 10 pills.

Precautions: This formula should be taken for short periods of time— one to three days at most. Do not take this formula during pregnancy.

SUPERIOR SORE-THROAT POWDER SPRAY   This is an effective dry powder spray that tastes bad. It is used to eliminate sore throats, mouth ulcers, inflamed sinuses, skin lesions, and middle-ear infections.

Dosage: Spray throat and mouth 3 times daily. Do not inhale through the mouth while you are spraying the powder—hold your breath. For sinusitis, the powder is sprayed in the nose five times daily. Apply the powder to ulcerative skin lesions once daily. Available in bottles containing 2.2 grams.

TSO-TZU OTIC PILLS   This formula treats ringing in the ears (tinnitus), high blood pressure, headaches, insomnia, pressure behind the eyes, eye irritation, and thirst.

Dosage: 8 pills, 3 times daily. Available in bottles of 200 pills.

Note: Please see "Colds and Flu," Ching Fei Yi Huo Pien is an excellent remedy for sore throats.

Classical Oriental Herbal Prescription

PLATYCODON COMBINATION   This simple formula, from the Han dynasty, treats tonsillitis and acute bronchitis with such symptoms as shivering with severe chills, cough with thick phlegm, and dry, swollen, sore throat.

Platycodon	2.0 grams *or*	1/14 ounce
Licorice	3.0	1/10 ounce

Note: Kudzu Combination (also known as Pueraria Combination) treats acute tonsillitis. Please see section titled, "Colds and Flu."

TRAUMA

Individual Herbal Helpers

See Chapter 3: Ginseng "Pseudoginseng"

Chinese Patent Formulas

YUNNAN PAIYAO   This excellent patent formula, comprised primarily of pseudoginseng, treats pain and stops bleeding resulting from cuts and wounds. It also helps reduce excessive menstrual bleeding, serious nosebleeds, and bloody stools and vomit. Yunnan Paiyao reduces swelling from injuries, fractures, muscle and ligament tears, sprains, bone dislocations and breaks, and bruising from falls or blows. This formula is taken internally and can also be applied externally.

Dosage: 1 to 2 capsules, 4 times daily. Available in packets of 20 capsules.

Also available in boxes containing 10 bottles; each bottle holds 4 grams of powder.

For internal use, take .2 to .5 gram powder.

For external use, thoroughly clean the wound first; hold the sides of the cut together and apply the powder directly to the bleeding wound. Hold the wound closed for one to two minutes and then bandage.

Precautions: Not to be taken internally during pregnancy.

Note: In case of serious injury, always see a licensed health professional as quickly as possible.

URINARY DISORDERS

Often, such problems as frequent urination, nighttime urination, urinary incontinence, and lowered sex drive are a signal that our human battery pack (the kidney/adrenal complex in Oriental medicine) is seriously depleted. Golden Book Tea and Six-Flavor Tea, described in the section titled, "Energy Tonics," help address genitourinary problems due to deficient energy.

Individual Herbal Helpers

See Chapter 3: Achyranthes, alisma, astragalus, bupleurum, clematis, codonopsis, coptis, cuscuta, dang gui, du huo, gardenia, gentian, ginseng "pseudoginseng," rehmannia, rhubarb, salvia, scutellaria

Chinese Patent Formulas

KAI KIT WAN   This patent formula is a specific remedy for an enlarged prostate gland accompanied by such symptoms as frequent or nighttime urination, difficult or painful urination, groin pain, and fatigue. This formula is very effective for chronic conditions where swelling is pronounced.
Dosage: 4 to 6 pills, 3 times daily. Available in bottles of 20 pills.

LUNG TAN XIE GAN PILLS   This extremely effective formula treats urinary-tract infections, urethritis, prostatitis, oral and genital herpes, fever blisters in the mouth, headache accompanied by red, burning eyes, ringing in the ears, sore throat, constipation, scant urine, and yellow vaginal discharge (leukorrhea).
Dosage: 6 pills, 2 times daily. Available in bottles of 100 pills.

SPECIFIC DRUG PASSWAN   This formula treats acute or chronic urinary calculi (stones) in the ureters, kidneys, or bladder. It helps dissolve stones and stops pain and bleeding.
Dosage: 6 to 8 capsules, 3 times daily. Available in bottles of 120 capsules.

Classical Oriental Herbal Prescriptions

GARDENIA AND PORIA COCOS (HOELEN) FORMULA   This wonderful formula comes to us from the Sung dynasty. It effectively reduces Internal Heat in the bladder accompanied by acute pain and dark-colored urine. It treats bladder infections, urethritis, and kidney and bladder stones or stones in the ureters, as well as gonorrhea.

Poria Cocos	6.0 grams *or*	1/5 ounce
Dang Gui	3.0	1/10 ounce
Licorice	3.0	1/10 ounce
Peony (White)	2.0	1/14 ounce
Gardenia	2.0	1/14 ounce

Wheezing

see "Coughs, Bronchitis, Phlegm, Asthma, Wheezing"

Chapter 5
Delicious Recipes to Incorporate Healing Herbs and Foods into Your Daily Diet

Healing with Flavor

Over thousands of years of careful observation of patterns in nature and the human garden, our friends in the Orient developed an incredibly sophisticated and effective natural healing system based on 5 Elements, 5 Seasons, 5 Directions, 5 Organ Systems, and 5 Flavors. In this chapter, we revisit the 5 Elements to help each of us determine our unique pathway to balance and health through healing recipes, herbs, foods, and flavors.

Disease does not just drop out of the blue one day. It is preceded by many warning signals. *The Oriental healing system ties psychological or emotional imbalances to physical symptoms.* Most frequently, prevalent or persistent emotional patterns indicate we are headed for a more serious imbalance that will manifest as a physical disharmony. Prevention is the best medicine, and Oriental healing insights into patterns of disease are far more advanced than our own somewhat limited Western preventative measures.

At best, prevention in the West involves trying to eat a more balanced diet, while getting adequate exercise and rest. Too often, we rely simply on popping megadoses of vitamins, minerals, herbs, or prescription drugs, or drinking the newest meal-replacement liquid, thinking these will bring good health and enhanced performance. Unfortunately, we are attracted by the glitz, glitter, and glamour of prefabricated food, trendy diets, or the newest drug, vitamin, mineral, or herb fad with their promises of the perfect body or perfect health.

In contrast, Oriental medical wisdom teaches that we are all unique and each of us, depending upon body type, requires different herbs, amounts of exercise, rest, and diet (this is the key as to why our experts can't seem to agree). All these factors continually vary per individual according to the seasons and the stress levels in our lives.

BALANCING THE "5 FLAVORS"

When we start talking about the "5 Flavors," we are entering the world of our hunting-and-gathering forefathers. Human lives depended upon their ability to distinguish food from poison, healing herbs from potentially dangerous ones. These days we hear a lot of talk about chemicals and more specifically "phyto-chemicals" (or the active ingredients found in our plant allies). Thousands upon thousands of years ago, humankind had already formulated ideas about flavors and their effects on the human body. The flavor of a substance gives us valuable clues about how it can nurture and balance or further imbalance our bodies. Modern research is now confirming what traditional healing systems have long told us, that even our temperaments are greatly affected by everything we ingest. Emotions such as joy, fear, love, or depression are not just attitudes created by our thought processes but are actually produced and reinforced by the biochemical activity of our brain, and those biochemicals come from the foods we eat, as well as the prescription drugs or herbs we ingest.

Unfortunately, our twentieth-century taste buds have been adulterated by two very strong flavors: Sweet and Salty. These are not the naturally occurring sweet and salty flavorings found in whole foods that our ancient ancestors depended upon, but are artificially altered, highly refined foods such as sugary-rich chocolate cake and salted peanuts. On the yin/yang scale, we tend to swing violently back and forth between these extremely strong flavors, first downing a handful of candies or a coke, to be followed by heavily salted food items like potato chips, pretzels, or the like, as we attempt to balance energies in our human garden.

As an aspiring herbalist, it's really important for you to start practicing with flavors in order to get a firsthand experience of how they affect your body, your mind, and your well-being. It would be great for you to clear your palate of strong flavors such as coffee, tobacco, refined sugar, and salt for a few days so that you can really taste the lovely subtlety of the "5 Flavors" used in Oriental healing: *Sour, Bitter, Sweet, Spicy, and Salty.*

THE SOUR FLAVOR   Now, take one raspberry, blackberry, or a few drops of lemon juice and place it on your tongue. Let it sit there for a few minutes as you really taste the *sour flavor*. Sour substances are astringent, detoxifying, and show antibacterial and antiviral activity. The Sour Flavor comes mostly from acids found in herbs or foods (such as lactic, citric, malic, and oxalic acids). These substances have a Cooling and Drying effect on the human body. If we check what's happening flavorwise during springtime (the season associated with the Sour Flavor), in many regions we will find that nature is offering us an abundance of naturally slightly sour herbs and foods that will help clear our liver (the organ associated with the Wood Element and spring-time). All that natural Vitamin C also helps build immunity and protect us against spring colds and flus. Some examples of slightly sour herbs and foods would include lemon, blackberry, quince, raspberry, sour plum, star fruit (carambola), purslane, schisandra, lemon balm, hibiscus, hawthorn berry, and vinegar. (The Sour Flavor is also found in conjunction with the sweet fla-vor in fruits such as cherry, apple, apricot, and so forth.)

I feel that flavor can heal and, in excess, flavor also has the ability to harm. Flavor can be incredibly addictive. Let me tell you about one patient who was addicted to the Sour Flavor. Yes, I said sour! Dana, a wonderful "Wood" lady, came to the clinic complaining of severe muscle cramps, especially around the midriff. Bordering on workaholism, Dana spent 10 to 12 hours a day coordinating the efforts of the camera crew for an adver-tising agency. Loving every minute of the challenge, she never took breaks, rarely had lunch, and pushed herself to the limit. Two to three sessions of acupuncture, herbs, and some dietary changes were not bringing relief and something told me to probe deeper. "Do you like the Sour Flavor?" I asked Dana. "I like it a lot, especially vinegar!" was her reply. Dana reluctantly admitted that she drank one to two cups of apple-cider vinegar daily. Once Dana's habit, "addiction" to vinegar, was addressed, relief was almost immediate.

While an addiction to the Sour Flavor may sound ridiculous to most of us, we think nothing of our own personal taste preference. Which do you prefer?—salty, sweet, spicy, or bitter (such as coffee, dark chocolate, or beer) flavors? Any of these in excess can bring disharmony and disease to our bodies.

THE BITTER FLAVOR The *Nei Ching*, one of the oldest medical texts in Traditional Chinese Medicine, states that the Bitter Flavor Drains and Dries. Bitters aid digestion and have anti-inflammatory, antispasmodic, and antibacterial effects. Major plant constituents imparting the Bitter Flavor are alkaloids, some glycosides, and sesquiterpenes; many are Cooling, while some are Warming.

Remember that the Bitter Flavor is the one associated with the summertime, the Fire Element, and the Heart and Small Intestine and Pericardium and Triple Warmer Meridian Systems. Several important bitter herbal medicines influence the heart. Probably the most well-known is digitalis, which contains digitoxin, a bitter cardiac glycoside. Western herbalists also use bitter herbs to help decongest the lungs. Similarly, according to Oriental medical principles, the Bitter Flavor helps disperse obstruction and increases the flow of oxygen into the lungs.

The Bitter Flavor is relatively unfamiliar in American cuisine. Some examples of herbs and foods that have an abundance of the Bitter Flavor include dandelion root and greens, salad greens, endive, burdock root, borage, honeysuckle, forsythia, gardenia, gentian, goldenseal, plantain, uva ursi, mugwort, echinacea, yellow dock, gotu kola, feverfew, rhubarb root, and yarrow. Persons who lack digestive fire may find that the consumption of raw food results in loose stools filled with undigested food particles. Here, the Bitter Flavor comes to the rescue. Lightly steam and eat plenty of bitter greens such as endive, arugula, or dandelion greens to stimulate digestion. Top them with a touch of lemon, olive oil, and a dash of salt in the fashion of Greek cuisine. Many traditional cultures start their meals with a salad made from bitter greens to aid digestion. Also, it's important to boost your immune system by eating plenty of nature's green antibiotics.

Often, I wonder if our collective "love of coffee" as a nation is not due to an inherent call from nature to add the Bitter Flavor to our diet. Once again, as highly refined sugar and salt do not offer our body the nutrients needed to support health, the Bitter Flavor from coffee diminishes our natural mineral stores. It gives us a false start in the morning and picks us up in the afternoon when our energy begins to sag. Unfortunately, we are drawing on our invaluable Kidney/Adrenal "battery-pack." Let me tell you about Sylvia.

Sylvia is a bright and witty, 52-year-old playwright who spends 12 to 15 hours a day on her computer. She came to the clinic with complaints of insomnia, swollen, arthritic knees and elbows, and bony spurs on the bottoms of her feet. The bony spurs had been surgically removed the previous year but were now growing back. When questioned about drinking coffee, Sylvia said she kept an 18-cup coffee pot beside her computer and drank 15 to 18 cups daily. Scandinavian studies have shown that 435 mg of calcium are excreted in the urine immediately after drinking one cup of coffee (435 mg of calcium is just about our average daily intake). Were Sylvia's bony spurs due to a sedentary lifestyle and excessive consumption of coffee, which resulted in the redistribution of calcium throughout her body? We can't be certain, but she reduced her coffee intake and, after making it through a week or so of severe withdrawal symptoms, felt much better. Needless to say, her insomnia disappeared and the swelling in her elbows and knees went down dramatically.

In order to get a true sense of what is meant by the Bitter Flavor, take a piece of dandelion leaf and slowly chew on it. You might hate this flavor at first, but, interestingly, it grows on you. One day you will actually look forward to eating some of those steamed bitter greens for dinner.

THE SWEET FLAVOR The Full Sweet Flavor associated with the Earth Element, harvesttime or doyo, and the Spleen/Pancreas Meridian System is found in beans, whole grains, root veggies, winter squash, low-fat dairy products, fish, lean meats, and Tonifying herbs. The full Sweet Flavor nourishes and nurtures all body tissues that require protein to rebuild and glucose as their fuel. The energy of these nutrients can range from slightly Cool to Hot. Important immune-enhancing herbs in this category include astragalus, ginseng, codonopsis, dioscorea, licorice, and jujube dates. Most full sweet foods of the Earth Element increase moisture in the human body. If you are experiencing Dryness (dry skin and hair), please remember to balance your constitution by consuming more full sweet foods that moisten. If your human garden is too Damp (bloating or edema), look at the types of sweet foods you are ingesting. Chances are, you are overdoing it on the empty sweet side of the equation (candies, doughnuts, cookies, ice cream).

A 12-ounce can of Coke contains almost 10 teaspoons of sugar; 10 jelly beans contain nearly 7 teaspoons of sugar, and an 8-ounce ice-cream sundae contains 19 teaspoons of sugar. A bowl of Rocky-Road ice cream or a slice of tangy lemon pie might sweeten your existence, but please keep these goodies for special occasions. If you do not have a serious imbalance, once or twice a week you could possibly afford to sit down and indulge, enjoying every last bite of a sugary confection. This can be done in good conscience if you know that the rest of the week you are nourishing your body at a deep, fundamental level with real foods straight from nature. You might be surprised, however, when your sweet cravings start to diminish once your body receives the nutrition it wants and needs. Many of my patients now marvel at how they ever thought the empty Sweet Flavor of white sugar actually tasted good.

It is estimated that every American consumes approximately 135 pounds of sugar per year. This means each person in our country would have to consume about two pounds of sugar per week, amounting to between 500 and 600 empty calories daily. White sugar, in excess, creates congestion and extinguishes digestive fires—it really gums up the works. Sugar causes increased mucus in the body, which results in painful swelling of the joints and extremities. Increased mucus lowers immunity by restricting the ability of our white blood cells to move rapidly to ingest and destroy germ invaders. Sugar bursts into the bloodstream rapidly, giving us a sense of instant energy (usually hyper and scattered) to be followed by a crash, fatigue, depression, and anxiety. If you eliminate sugar products from your diet, you may feel tired, drowsy, and/or depressed for one to five days.

Please remember that sugar cravings can indicate protein deficiency. If you are well-nourished, cravings of all kinds disappear. To experience the full sweetness of the Earth Element, slowly chew on a few grains of cooked brown rice, a bite of sweet potato, a spoonful of butternut squash, or a piece of chicken or halibut—this is the Full Sweet Flavor of nutritious, life-giving, body-building food.

THE SPICY FLAVOR   The flavor associated with autumn, the Metal Element, and Lung/Colon Meridian Systems is described as spicy, acrid, or pungent. The Spicy Flavor is utilized in Traditional Oriental Medicine to Disperse Congestion and Stagnation. It contains essential oils and resins that irritate the mucosa, increasing blood and lymph flow while counteracting mucus production.

During autumn, it is important to increase your immunity by consuming more spicy foods such as onion and garlic. Both of these foods are sources rich in sulfur, a natural antibiotic. And guess what? Nature is looking after us once again! Pungent roots are harvested in late summer and fall, just in time to help us build our immunity to avoid autumn colds and flus. Other spicy foods include leek, scallion, horseradish, radish, ginger, celery and mustard seed, parsnip, black and cayenne pepper, and aromatic spices such as cinnamon, nutmeg, clove, cardamom, thyme, sage, rosemary, fennel, and mint.

The Spicy Flavor can also be quite addictive. Jerry, a 35-year-old counselor and true Fire Type, came to me with an extremely painful case of colitis. He had been undergoing standard medical tests and treatments for about three years, and his doctors had mentioned the possibility of surgery. When Jerry was confronted with this option, he decided to seek alternative therapy. On Jerry's first visit, we spent over an hour talking about his eating habits. The sources of his problem were easy to identify. Usually, he started his day with a couple of glasses of orange juice, followed by another glass or two in the afternoon. Also, Jerry loved corn chips with hot Mexican salsa; in fact, four to five times a week, he downed an 8-ounce jar of his favorite smoking hot salsa with a bag or two of chips. Jerry said that none of his doctors had ever talked to him about diet. I asked him to cut out the acidic orange juice and replace it with unfiltered, naturally sweet organic apple juice. Jerry was to completely refrain from eating all salsa, tomato sauce, and other spices. Jerry was given a gentle Chinese patent medicine call "Curing Pills." Within two days, the bleeding stopped, and after four days he was pain free. It's now five years later and Jerry never has problems with colitis. He occasionally enjoys a spicy Mexican dinner out, but knows not to push his luck anymore with frequent hot salsa fiestas.

THE SALTY FLAVOR   The Salty Flavor is associated with the winter season and Kidney/Urinary Bladder Meridian Systems. In herbalism, when we speak of the Salty Flavor, we are referring to mineral salts that the body requires for optimum functioning. The Salty Flavor and its associated minerals as found in sea veggies is cooling in nature. It nourishes the Kidney/Adrenal complex and softens tissues. In Oriental medicine, kelp is used to dissolve tumors. However, refined salt can have the opposite effect, greatly increasing water retention and heat in the body.

Sources rich in valuable mineral salts include sea veggies such as wakame, kombu, kelp, hijiki, arame, dulse, and nori; seeds such as sesame, pumpkin, and walnuts; and mushrooms such as shiitake, oyster, portabello, chantrell, and reishi. Other sources of the Salty Flavor include miso; liquid amino acids; horsetail rush; nettles; plantain; oyster, clam, and abalone shells; dragon bone; and mineral salts. Parsley and nettles support the Water Element by eliminating Dampness and contributing needed mineral salts to build and maintain a strong skeletal system (remember "Bones" are the body tissue linked to the Kidney System).

Sally, a 38-year-old artist and world traveler came to me a few years ago with two breast lumps, one the size of a chicken egg, the other slightly smaller. She also had many lymph-node swellings in her neck, armpits, and the soles of her feet. Sally told her gynecologist that she wanted to try alternative therapy for a month before taking a biopsy of the lumps. He reluctantly agreed. Sally ate a typical American fast-food diet and suffered from severe salt cravings, downing a can of cashews or peanuts frequently, "just to get at the salt." Sally was one of those incredible model patients; she changed her lifestyle and diet 100 percent during her course of treatment with me. First, and foremost, she consumed only fresh veggies, grains, and beans prepared with lots of seaweed. She was given two Chinese herbal formulas to help dissolve the lumps and lymph-node swellings: Pinellia and Magnolia Formula and Tangkuei (Dang Gui) 16-Herb Combination. By the end of three weeks, the lymph-node swellings were gone, and at the end of six weeks, the breast lumps had disappeared along with her salt cravings. About twice a year Sally sends me a postcard from some exotic location. She says she's feeling great and always mentions that she is still eating seaweed.

Now is the time to start cooking with sea vegetables. The human body is composed of over 70 percent water; the human brain over 90 percent. The chemical composition of the water in our bodies is almost exactly like ocean water, only slightly diluted (like the earth's oceans before the Ice Age). Sea veggies give us valuable mineral salts in the exact proportion our human cells inherently understand because they grow in the oceanic environment where the beginnings of life evolved. Look under "Sea Vegetables" in Chapter 3 to learn important details regarding this important food that has been forgotten in America.

In summation, we can say that the flavor of a substance gives us a good hint as to how it will affect our human garden. *Sour substances are astringent and have a Cooling and Drying effect on the body. The Bitter Flavor Drains, Dries, and aids digestion. The Full Sweet Flavor Builds, Tonifies, and Moistens, while the neutral or bland taste helps remove Dampness, promoting urination. The Spicy Flavor (sometimes described as acrid or pungent) Disperses Congestion and Stagnation. Salty substances generally Purge, Soften, and Cool and can have a Tonifying effect on the Kidney/Adrenal complex.*

In order to enjoy true health, we need to learn how to balance the 5 Healing Flavors in the correct proportion that our unique body requires.

Determining Your Predominant Element

The 5 Element system of thought teaches that while each of us is composed of all 5 Elements (wood, fire, earth, metal, and water), each of us also has a dominant single root Element that is the source of our greatest strengths and weaknesses. Each Element has different characteristics, and one is not better or worse than the other, just different. Ideally, throughout our lifetime, we will learn the lessons of all 5 Elements and be able to draw on each of them at the appropriate time and place. Are you basically a Warrior? a Lover? a Peacemaker? a Sage? or a Philosopher?

The upcoming sections describe a few of the predominate personality characteristics and physical complaints often associated with each of the Five Elemental Types. Try to determine which of the Elements best describes your emotional tendencies and health problems. You're going to have to be honest with yourself. Sometimes that can prove to be a bit of a task, so you might ask a family member or friend to also complete the checklists for you and then compare your answers. Don't be surprised if you check a number of items in both the Excess and Deficiency columns. Since our root Element is the source of our greatest strengths and weaknesses, we may tend to teeter-totter between Excess and Deficiency in this Element. You might be experiencing disharmonies in more than one Element. This is not uncommon since, according to Oriental medical view, each organ system greatly influences the health and well-being of all other organs and tissues in the body. It is also possible that due to stress, overwork, or poor diet you are experiencing an imbalance that does not correspond to your predominant element but one of the other elements (this will be much easier for you to harmonize). Healing herbal recipes follow that can help bring you and your loved ones back into balance. (If you want to delve deeper into Five-Element archetypes, their imbalances and healing methods, please see the Resources Section for books on this subject.)

One note about emotions before we move into the Elements. It is only human, as well as normal, to feel and express grief and depression due to the loss of a loved one, just as it is natural to feel anger, joy, worry, or fear at various times. We should never feel guilty about any emotion we might be experiencing. It's extremely important to recognize, acknowledge, and try to understand our feelings. However, there are also constructive and destructive means of expressing emotions. It is important for each of us to step out of our limited world and recognize how our emotional ups and downs are affecting and perhaps afflicting other persons around us. We might need to seek outside guidance for prolonged emotional problems or look into lifestyle changes for ourselves. Oriental healing teaches that any emotion, in excess, can injure its related organ system just as the health of the organ system can influence our emotions. For example, prolonged grief due to numerous losses over a number of years frequently results in diseases of the Lung/Large Intestine Organ Systems manifesting as frequent colds and flu, bronchitis, or pneumonia. In the same way, if, due to lowered immunity, we experience frequent colds and flu, bronchitis, or pneumonia, the emotional toll is frequently expressed as feelings of depression or grief.

Let's continue our healing adventure and cycle through the seasons once again, but this time we'll be looking at Element Types and the foods and flavors that can help balance and prevent disease. You find a few "Western" herbs in my recipes (most are also used in the Orient). Many of these gentle healing foods (such as dandelion, nettles, burdock, milk thistle, borage, and plantain) grow in our own backyards but have been forgotten and erased from our food lists over the past 50 years. Our ancestors knew about them and used them regularly.

Two simple, ten-question checklists (one for Excess and the other for Deficient disharmonies affecting the five major Organ Systems) precedes healing recipes given for each Element and the Season with which it is associated. In order to help you become more aware of your inclinations toward imbalance, make a check beside each of the Mood Indicators or Body Cues that seems to apply to you on a fairly frequent basis. You will find the checklist for the Wood Element on page 269; Fire Element on page 281; Earth Element on page 289; Metal Element on page 299; and Water Element on page 312.

Once you complete each of the checklists, record the number of ✓'s you made on the following 5-Element Tally Sheet:

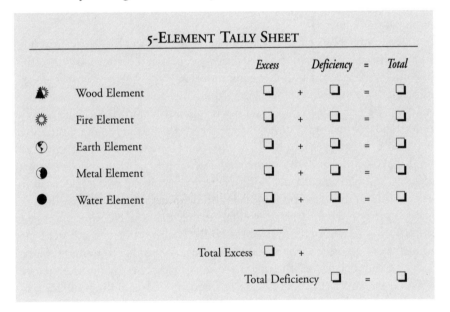

5-ELEMENT TALLY SHEET

		Excess		Deficiency	=	Total
▲	Wood Element	❏	+	❏	=	❏
☀	Fire Element	❏	+	❏	=	❏
☯	Earth Element	❏	+	❏	=	❏
☽	Metal Element	❏	+	❏	=	❏
●	Water Element	❏	+	❏	=	❏

Total Excess ❏ +

Total Deficiency ❏ = ❏

Add the numbers in the Excess column and the Deficiency column and write the results in the blank provided below each column. Work to bring balance to the Element or Elements in which you received the highest scores by gradually introducing more of the healing flavors and foods recommended into your diet. If you have a much higher score in the Excess column than in the Deficiency column, you will need to concentrate on ingesting more cooling, yin-natured foods (fruits and vegetables) and herbs. If your score in the Deficiency column is much greater than the Excess column, then you should consume more warming, yang-natured foods (fish, chicken, miso) and herbs.

Wood Element

Yin Organ: Liver   Yang Organ: Gallbladder

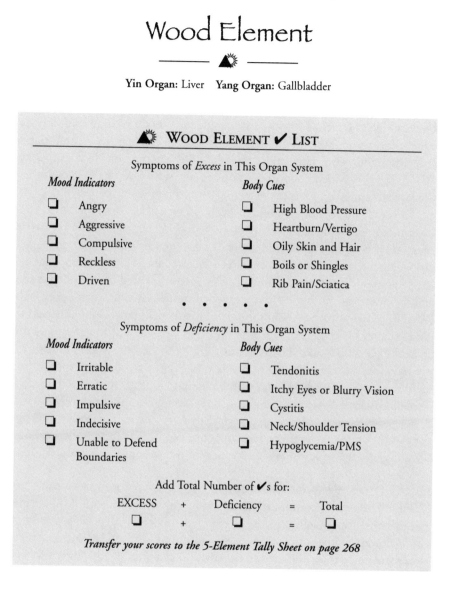

▲ WOOD ELEMENT ✔ LIST

Symptoms of *Excess* in This Organ System

Mood Indicators	*Body Cues*
❏ Angry	❏ High Blood Pressure
❏ Aggressive	❏ Heartburn/Vertigo
❏ Compulsive	❏ Oily Skin and Hair
❏ Reckless	❏ Boils or Shingles
❏ Driven	❏ Rib Pain/Sciatica

• • • • •

Symptoms of *Deficiency* in This Organ System

Mood Indicators	*Body Cues*
❏ Irritable	❏ Tendonitis
❏ Erratic	❏ Itchy Eyes or Blurry Vision
❏ Impulsive	❏ Cystitis
❏ Indecisive	❏ Neck/Shoulder Tension
❏ Unable to Defend Boundaries	❏ Hypoglycemia/PMS

Add Total Number of ✔s for:

EXCESS	+	Deficiency	=	Total
❏	+	❏	=	❏

Transfer your scores to the 5-Element Tally Sheet on page 268

ARE YOU A WOOD TYPE? The Adventurer, pioneer, workaholic, doer and shaker, innovator, achiever—all are adjectives that could apply at times to the character of the true Wood Type. You can find the Warrior blazing new trails across the tundra in Iceland, scaling Mt. Everest, or racing to the finish line—whatever finish line that might be. Warriors are meant to lead, and lead they must; they want to be *the first, the best, and the only* of whatever endeavor sparks their interest. While all of us have a warrior within that we call upon at various times in our lives, the "root" Warrior Type is easily identified. Warriors love action and adventure, skill and speed. They enjoy and work best under pressure since they continually seek challenge. The Warrior, in balance, is confident, bold, courageous, decisive, direct, powerful, and committed to noble causes. One of the greatest challenges for Wood Types is to remain flexible, in body, mind, and spirit. The true lesson in life for Warrior types to learn is when to retreat or yield. Wood types tend to experience vascular headaches, migratory aches and pains, pain under the ribs, and hypertension. In disharmony, Wood Types experience volatile emotions and can find themselves feeling downright cantankerous, intolerant, impatient, judgmental, or peevish.

Even if you are not a Wood type, you can experience emotional and physical symptoms relating to this Element through dietary imbalances and everyday stress. Have you noticed how certain foods affect your moods? Coffee stimulates, giving you a feeling of alertness only to be followed by an energy slump; chocolate soothes, giving you the feeling of being loved, followed by mild depression and the desire for more chocolate; excess red meat fuels your assertiveness, followed by lethargy. Excessive consumption of fatty, rich, processed foods such as pizza, salami, or ice cream, red meat and eggs, alcohol and drugs, coffee and chocolate, or imbalanced hormones can greatly stress our Wood Element or Liver/Gallbladder Organ Systems. If you are a Wood type and are experiencing the disharmonies described here, you will have to work harder to achieve and maintain balance. *Wood types are drawn to the use of stimulants, such as coffee, just to keep up the pace; ultimately, they might have to rely on sedatives to get a decent night's sleep.* If your predominate Element is not Wood, but you are suffering from a Wood disharmony, it will be much easier for you to come back into balance.

HERBS THAT RESTORE HARMONY TO THE WOOD ELEMENT See Chapter 3: Aloe, bupleurum, chrysanthemum, coptis, cyperus, dandelion, dang gui, forsythia fruit, gambir, gardenia, garlic, gastrodia, gentian, ginger, honeysuckle flowers, kudzu, licorice, lycii berries, mung beans, peppermint, peony root, rehmannia, rhubarb, salvia, scutellaria, shiitake mushrooms, turmeric

Also See Chapter 4: Gynecological Disorders and Liver and Gallbladder Complaints for Recommendations on Herbal Formulas that Can Help with Symptoms Related to the Excess or Deficient Conditions Listed earlier

TREATING YOUR WOOD IMBALANCE Dandelion and bupleurum ("Liver Herbs" par excellence) are especially indicated in treating imbalanced Wood conditions. *(Note: If you suffer from migraine headaches, substitute cyperus for bupleurum.)* If, earlier, you checked more items in the Wood

Excess column than you did in the Deficient column, you will need to choose a number of herbs (such as dandelion, bupleurum, or cyperus) that range from neutral to cold in energy to help your body detoxify. If you are plagued with boils or other infections, you will need to add antimicrobial herbs such as coptis, forsythia, honeysuckle, or scutellaria. Cooling, bitter, or spicy herbs such as gardenia, peppermint, lemon balm, and chamomile will help soothe your irritability. Cut out processed meats, fried foods, highly refined fatty foods, coffee, and chocolate. Green tea is an excellent substitute to help you get over your addiction to coffee.

Deficient Wood types often need to increase herbs and foods that are high in mineral salts (such as mushrooms, miso, seaweed, dragon bone, oyster shell, walnuts, or pumpkin seeds), as well as full sweet earth protein foods. An increase in slightly sour fruits and herbs can help improve liver function—lemon, blackberry, strawberry, plum, or vinegar. Warm, sweet, spicy herbs such as dang gui will help build blood and move congestion.

Wood types may want to consider undergoing a one- to three-day "liver-cleansing" fast in the springtime. Excess Wood types would probably do well on a diluted (with spring water) apple-juice fast while Deficient types often benefit from a one-day fast of diluted lemon or lime juice (add a touch each of maple syrup, olive oil, cayenne pepper and garlic). Another alternative is to undertake several half-day fasts with the following Spring Greens Tonic Soup Recipe. Have the soup for breakfast, lunch, and midafternoon snack, then follow up with a light dinner such as the Spring Kicharee or Spring Stir Fry (with tofu or fish) served over kamut (Egyptian wheat) or barley. Plan on taking it easy during the fast—no driving, no work, no marathons. It is best to stay home, rest, take short walks, and drink plenty of water during fasting. You will be amazed at the new energy and mental clarity you feel after giving your body a break from its regular food fare! Be sure to drink plenty of spring water while fasting and *always check with your health practitioner before undertaking a fast.*

One additional note about a Wood Excess condition and Tonifying herbs: You may be attracted to energy enhancing herbs such as ginseng; they are not for you until your Wood Element has come back into balance. Once in balance, you should never take ginseng alone, but always in an energetically balanced formula.

The following recipes are not exclusively for Wood types, but for anyone wishing to enhance the functioning of their Wood Element. Most of us would benefit greatly by clearing our systems with the following healthful spring recipes. Rigorous fasting is not recommended, however, for debilitated persons or vegetarians (if they consume a balanced, healthful diet based on plenty of whole grains, beans, and veggies).

Spring Recipes
Slightly Sour to Lighten and Enliven

SPRING GREENS TONIC SOUP
Basic Recipe for Two Persons:

2 cups water or stock
*3 cups finely chopped greens
(Optional)
squeeze of lemon
fash of Bragg's amino acids
sprinkle of caraway seeds
sprinkle of milk thistle seed gomasio
dash of cayenne pepper
1 to 2 tsp. olive oil
dash of dulse or kelp powder
3 to 6 ounces of soft tofu (required by
    persons with carbohydrate sensitivity)
1 tsp. spirulina (blue-green algae)

• Choose 4 to 5 of the spring greens
  listed—experiment by trying one
  from each elemental category.
• Bring water to a boil.
• Toss in greens and simmer for 5 minutes.
• Puree in blender, adding your choice
  of optional condiments listed at left.
• Drink this liver cleansing tonic for
  breakfast or lunch.

Create your own unique blend!

Suggestions for Supporting Each of the 5 Elements—Wood Element: Celery, Broccoli, Purslane,
Shepherd's Purse, or Bok Choy *Fire Element:* Asparagus, Borage, Dandelion, or Spinach
Earth Element: Carrot, Turnip, or Beet Greens   *Metal Element:* Cabbage, Chinese Cabbage,
Green Onion, or Chives   *Water Element:* Parsley, Collard Greens, Nettles, Watercress

SPRING STIR FRY (APPROX. 20 MINUTES TO PREPARE)
Basic Recipe:

2 leeks
2 cloves garlic
1 to 2 T. olive oil
1/2 cup sliced dandelion roots
3 cups chopped watercress, purslane,
    broccoli, or spinach, bok choy, celery
    kale, collard greens, cabbage, dande-
    lion greens, chard, mung bean sprouts
1/2 cup shiitake mushrooms
1 T. toasted almond slivers
1 T. freshly grated ginger root, squeeze
    of lemon, sea salt, gomasio, or tamari
    to taste

• Saute onion or leeks in oil, add garlic.
• Add desired spices, daikon, and shi-
  itake.
• Cover and simmer 5 minutes in 1/3
  cup water.
• Add remaining veggies, cover, and
  simmer approximately 7 minutes.
• Remove from heat, add tamari,
  gomasio, or sea salt.
• Top with toasted almonds.

Serve over kamut, barley,
quinoa, or rye.

The following recipe for Spring Kicharee is always a phenomenal success with my patients. If you do not have all of the ingredients, don't let that stop you from making it—just improvise. This recipe is particularly great for Wood types. Since carbohydrates ranking low on the glycemic index are used, it is also good for persons who suffer from carbohydrate sensitivity. However, these persons should consume only 1 to 1-1/2 cups of the kicharee along with 3 to 4 blocks of protein (9 to 12 ounces of tofu; 3 to 4 ounces of chicken breast or tuna; 4-1/2 to 6 ounces of fish; or 3/4 to 1 cup of nonfat cottage cheese).

SPRING KICHAREE
Basic Recipe:

10 cups spring water

1 cup pearl barley

1/2 cup quinoa

1/2 cup French green lentils or mung beans

2 to 3 T. canola oil or ghee

1 large onion, minced

5 cloves garlic, minced

1 thinly sliced burdock root

2 parsnips, thinly sliced

2 cups chopped broccoli

1 cup sliced dandelion greens

1 T. dry dandelion root

3 slices fresh ginger (1/2-inch thick)

1/4 cup chopped parsley

1 cup shiitake mushrooms

2 T. chopped cilantro

2 T. nettles

1/3 Arame seaweed

1 tsp. turmeric

2 tsp. mustard seed

1-1/2 tsp. coriander powder

1-1/2 tsp. cumin powder

dash of black or white pepper

dash of cayenne pepper

pinch of asafoetida

sea salt, Bragg's amino acids, or tamari to taste

- Rinse grains well.
- Saute onion, burdock, and garlic in oil.
- Add cumin, coriander, turmeric, asafoetida, and mustard seed—saute until mustard seed starts to pop.
- Add water and grains/beans, ginger, dandelion root, arame.
- Simmer for 50 to 60 minutes on low heat, stirring occasionally.
- Add nettles, mushrooms, parsley, parsnips.
- Simmer another 25 to 30 minutes adding another cup of water if necessary.
- Add chopped broccoli, dandelion greens, cilantro, and pepper.
- Stir, cover, and simmer another 10 to 12 minutes.
- If desired, for a creamier texture, remove 2 cups of the soup and blend.
- Mix blended portion with remaining kicharee.
- Add salty seasoning to taste.

EARTH IN SPRING SOUP
Basic Recipe:

3 cups cubed butternut or kabocha
   squash
4 cups spring water
1 to 2 T. olive oil
1 medium-sized onion
4 cloves minced garlic
1 cup shredded dandelion greens or
   watercress
salty seasoning to taste
chopped parsley

- Simmer squash in 3-1/2 cups water for approximately 30 minutes until tender.
- Saute onions and garlic in oil until opaque.
- Add greens to onion mix with 1/2 cup water and simmer 10 to 15 minutes.
- Puree squash in blender; stir in onion and greens mixture.
- Add salty seasoning to taste.
- Top with a sprinkle of parsley.

Try this recipe with other spring greens.

Note: Since orange-colored veggies rank high on the glycemic index, this yummy recipe (one of my daughter's favorites) is suited only for persons who are not sensitive to carbohydrates.

BARLEY-STUFFED ARTICHOKES
Basic Recipe:

6 artichokes
1 cup pearled barley
3 cups water or stock
1 T. canola oil
1 T. olive oil
1 large onion
4 cloves garlic
3/4 cup shiitake, chantrelle, or portabello
   mushrooms
1/4 cup pine nuts
2 cups shredded arugula, chard, or bok
   choy leaves
1/2 cup grated carrot
dash of black and/or cayenne pepper
1/8 to 1/4 tsp. tarragon
sea salt, tamari, or Bragg's amino acids to
   taste
juice of 1/2 to 1 lemon

- Simmer chokes until done; let cool.
- Meanwhile, simmer barley in liquid for approximately 1 hour until tender.

- Saute onions and garlic in oils until browned.
- Add mushrooms and tarragon; saute 5 min.
- Add green veggies, seeds, carrot, and barley.
- Heat thoroughly until green veggies have wilted but carrots are slightly crunchy.
- Remove from heat, adding pepper, lemon, and salty flavor to taste.
- Cut chokes in half (start cutting at stem).
- Remove thistle down gently with spoon.
- Pile chokes high with grain mix.
- Top with an edible flower or sprig of mint.

Substitute Quinoa for Barley:

1 cup quinoa to 2 cups water

Takes only 15 minutes to cook.

ASPARAGUS AND SPRING GREENS SALAD

Basic Recipe:

1 lb. asparagus, cut diagonally into 1-inch pieces

1/4 cup diced red bell pepper

8 cups favorite spring greens (endive, dandelion, spinach, bok choy, nettles, arugula)

1/2 cup thinly sliced jicama

1/4 cup presoaked lycii berries

sea salt to taste

3 T. toasted pine nuts or almonds

• Separately steam asparagus and greens until tender (careful not to overcook).

• Drain well; add sea salt to taste.

• Artistically arrange veggies: greens on bottom layer, asparagus in center, circled by red pepper and jicama strips.

• Blend listed ingredients for dressing.

Spring Dressing:

1/2 cup raspberries or blackberries

1/3 cup light olive or canola oil

1 tsp. stoneground mustard

1/4 cup lemon juice or rice vinegar

2 T. parsley

1 T. sucanat or maple syrup

1 tsp. stoneground mustard

sea salt and black pepper to taste

• Pulse mustard, oil, and parsley in blender until parsley is chopped.

• Add remaining ingredients and pulse until smooth and creamy but berry flecks are still visible.

• Drizzle dressing over salad.

• Top with toasted nuts and lycii berries.

GET THE HANDLE ON HIGH CHOLESTEROL   High cholesterol is a symptom frequently associated with liver/gallbladder disharmonies. Following is a checklist to help you bring down those numbers. One patient, Ned, adopted the suggestions and dropped 75 points (from a walloping 325 to 250) after only four weeks. By the end of eight weeks, his cholesterol count came in at 190.

Cholesterol Reduction Checklist

• Japanese researchers have found that approximately *3 ounces of shiitake mushrooms* added to the diet on a daily basis lowers serum cholesterol by 12 percent in one week. Even when butter was added to the diet, the shiitake counteracted rises in cholesterol. *Note:* Shiitake mushrooms should always be cooked prior to consumption. Some people have shown allergic reactions to raw shiitake.

• *Garlic* reduces "bad" LDL cholesterol and triglycerides while raising "good" HDL cholesterol. Studies conducted by Dr. Benjamin Lau demonstrated a brief initial rise in LDL when garlic was added to the diet, followed by a considerable drop in serum cholesterol. Thirty-five percent of the persons in this study did not experience a drop in cholesterol; however, they all ate diets extremely high in fat and drank heavily. (Ingest one to two cloves of garlic daily or garlic tablets as directed.)

- Researchers have confirmed that *gugulipid*, an herbal extract, lowers cholesterol 14 to 27 percent and triglycerides 22 to 30 percent in four to twelve weeks. It actually increases the liver's metabolism of LDL cholesterol. (The dosage is approximately 200 mg, four times daily.)
- Several studies have shown that *grapeseed oil* helps lower cholesterol better than other oils according to Elson Haas, M.D., Director of the Preventive Medical Center of Marin in San Rafael, California.
- *Stress* is probably one of the greatest contributors to high cholesterol and heart disease. It's important to check in with your body and mind on a daily basis to identify those stressors that tighten muscles, speed up breathing, and prepare you for the fight-or-flight mode.
- *Exercise* is an essential tool for lowering blood cholesterol and elevating HDL. A simple 30-minute walk, 5 times a week, will do wonders to bring your cholesterol levels back in line.
- Throw out those plastic margarines that stay solid at room temperature and take 30 minutes to prepare your own delicious alternative:

BETTER GHEE (SPECIAL THANKS TO JADE REDMON FOR THE SUGGESTION)

Basic Recipe: Delicious and healthy margarine replacement—spreads nicely.

2 lbs. raw unsalted butter
1-1/2 cup canola or light olive oil

(Optional)
2 cloves minced garlic
1/4 tsp. sea salt
herbs such as 1/4 tsp. tarragon
1/4 tsp. basil
1/2 tsp. chives
Experiment!

- Melt butter in a saucepan over medium heat (watch carefully so it does not burn).
- Let butter come to a slow rolling boil.
- Remove from heat and carefully skim off foam with a spoon.
- Return the pan to the heat and repeat the preceding procedure two more times.
- Let remaining clear liquid (ghee) cool for 30 minutes; then strain through a prewashed piece of muslin cloth.
- Mix in oil and refrigerate mixture; it will melt at room temperature.

Fat Facts

High cholesterol and many other problems related to the functioning of our Liver/Gallbladder System are associated with the types of fat we ingest. Following is a chart of the different types of oils available, along with various fat facts about the properties of each of them.

MONOUNSATURATED FATS				
Lower "bad" LDL cholesterol without lowering "good" HDL.				
Fat	*% Mono*	*% Poly*	*% Sat*	*Description*
Olive Oil	77%	9%	14%	Helps lower cholesterol and may help control diabetes and blood pressure. Buy virgin, expeller-pressed olive oil.
Canola	52%	31%	6%	Canola oil is next best to olive oil and has a very mild flavor. This oil may have the same BP-lowering qualities as fish oil.
Avocado	73%	14%	12%	While excellent for the skin as moisturizers, the strong flavor of these oils makes them unpopular for consumption. Refrigeration is required.
Almond	73%	18%	9%	
Apricot	63%	31%	6%	
Peanut	48%	34%	18%	Though monounsatured, peanut oil appears to promote arteriosclerosis (University of Chicago Pathology Prof. Vasselinovitch). Peanuts, because they grow in damp places, are often contaminated by fungus. These aflatoxins are frequently found in peanuts (and corn) and may cause liver cancer, as well as allergic reactions.
Sesame	42%	43%	15%	A good oil for salad dressings, unrefined sesame oil breaks down easily at high temperatures. Sesame is contraindicated for B blood types.

POLYUNSATURATED FATS

Reduce "bad" LDL cholesterol, as well as "good" HDL.

Fat	% Mono	% Poly	% Sat	Description
Safflower	13%	78%	9%	Safflower and sunflower oil are high in Vitamin E.
Sunflower	20%	69%	11%	
Walnut	24%	66%	10%	Rich in Omega-3 fatty acids and Vitamin E, walnut oil is not good for cooking.
Corn	25%	62%	13%	Possible fungal contamination. Corn oil should be avoided by persons with allergic sensitivities.
Soybean	24%	61%	15%	High Vitamin E content; contains linoleic acid, which is converted to the same fatty acids found in fish oil.
Cottonseed	19%	54%	27%	This oil has the highest content of pesticide residues. It contains cyclopropene fatty acid, which has a toxic effect on the gallbladder and liver. It is commonly used as "vegetable oil" by fast and packaged food manufacturers.

SATURATED FATS

Increase "bad" LDL cholesterol, contributing to heart disease and cancer.

Fat	% Mono	% Poly	% Sat	Description
Coconut	6%	2%	92%	Coconut and palm-kernel oils contain lauric acid, which is linked to arteriosclerosis. Both are frequently used in packaged foods.
Palm Kernel	12%	2%	86%	
Butter	30%	4%	51%	
Palm	39%	10%	51%	

SHIITAKE MUSHROOMS   Don't forget the Japanese studies that have shown that *3 ounces of shiitake mushrooms* added to the diet on a daily basis lowers serum cholesterol by 12 percent in one week. Following are some of my favorite shiitake recipes. *Note:* Shiitake mushrooms should always be cooked prior to consumption. Some people have shown allergic reactions to raw shiitake.

SHIITAKE STOCK
Basic Recipe:

8 cups spring water

2 cups fresh shiitake, sliced, stems removed

2 celery stalks, minced

1 medium onion or 1 large leek

1/2 cup parsley, finely chopped

4 to 6 cloves garlic, minced

3 bay leaves

1 T. ghee or canola oil

1/2 tsp. sage

2 T. nettles

1/4 tsp. tarragon

1/2 tsp. sweet basil

sea salt or tamari to taste

- Saute onion or leek and garlic in oil.
- Combine all ingredients and bring to boil.
- Cover and simmer for 45 minutes.
- Strain the stock; save the mushrooms for other dishes and discard other veggies.
- Continue simmering stock for additional 15 minutes to reduce further and intensify flavor.

Serves as a wonderful base for quick soups—try soba noodles! Stick with barley, oats, or rye or very minor amounts of the other grains if you are carbohydrate sensitive.

SHIITAKE ALMOND PATÉ
Basic Recipe:

3 cups fresh, finely chopped shiitake caps and stems

2 T. ghee

1/2 finely minced onion

2 cloves minced garlic

1/3 cup toasted almonds

3 oz. ricotta cheese, *or*

3 oz. Neufchatel cream cheese *or* 3 oz. Mori-Nu silken tofu (firm)

1/8 tsp. thyme

1/4 tsp. sea salt

1/8 tsp. pepper

1 tsp. nettles

1 tsp. parsley leaves

2 tsp. dry sherry (optional)

- Finely chop shiitakes in blender.
- Saute onion and garlic in ghee; add mushrooms and seasonings.
- Blend above mixture with remaining ingredients (almonds, tofu or cheese, and optional dry sherry) until smooth.
- Spread in serving dish and chill an hour.
- Serve with your favorite crackers or flat bread.

SPRING GREENS SPREAD
Basic Recipe:

1 cup shredded dandelion greens (try other favorites)

1/4 cup nonfat yogurt

1/2 cup nonfat cottage cheese

2 cloves minced garlic

2 tsp. olive oil (optional)

squeeze of lemon

dash of cayenne pepper

sea salt to taste

- Blend all ingredients except greens, salt, and cayenne pepper.
- Add shredded greens to blender and pulse to desired consistency.
- Add seasonings to taste, stirring well.
- Spread in serving dish.
- Let flavors mingle at least an hour before serving.

Deficient Wood types can suffer from anemia. Following is a wonderful recipe to build blood and energy and Tonify our Wood Element.

SPRING CHICKEN HERB SOUP
Basic Recipe:

2 half chicken breast pieces (skinned) cut in strips

9 to 10 cups spring water

1/4 cup arame sea veggie

2 chopped leeks

4 cloves garlic

1 to 2 T. olive oil

3/4 cup pearled barley or rice

1/2 ounce dang gui

1/2 ounce white peony root

2 T. lycii berries

1/2 ounce dioscorea yam

3 slices fresh ginger

1 small American ginseng root

1 cup shiitake mushrooms

2 cups shredded spring greens

1/2 cup chopped celery

2 sliced carrots

3 bay leaves

2 T. nettles

1/4 to 1/2 tsp. thyme

1/2 tsp. basil

sea salt to taste

dash of black pepper

- Brown chicken, leeks, and garlic in oil in a large soup pot.
- Add water, arame, grain, bay, and herbs; bring to boil; simmer 50 minutes over low heat.
- Add remaining ingredients, except spring greens, and simmer 15 minutes.
- Add 2 cups spring greens and simmer 10 minutes.

Fire Element

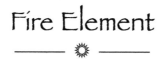

Yin Organs: Heart, Pericardium   **Yang Organs:** Small Intestine, Triple Warmer

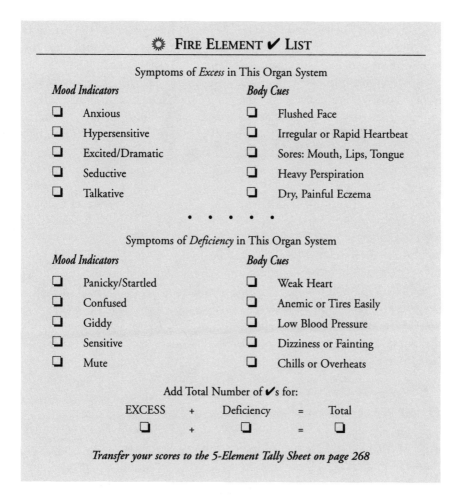

☀ FIRE ELEMENT ✔ LIST

Symptoms of *Excess* in This Organ System

Mood Indicators	*Body Cues*
❏ Anxious	❏ Flushed Face
❏ Hypersensitive	❏ Irregular or Rapid Heartbeat
❏ Excited/Dramatic	❏ Sores: Mouth, Lips, Tongue
❏ Seductive	❏ Heavy Perspiration
❏ Talkative	❏ Dry, Painful Eczema

• • • • •

Symptoms of *Deficiency* in This Organ System

Mood Indicators	*Body Cues*
❏ Panicky/Startled	❏ Weak Heart
❏ Confused	❏ Anemic or Tires Easily
❏ Giddy	❏ Low Blood Pressure
❏ Sensitive	❏ Dizziness or Fainting
❏ Mute	❏ Chills or Overheats

Add Total Number of ✔s for:

EXCESS	+	Deficiency	=	Total
❏	+	❏	=	❏

Transfer your scores to the 5-Element Tally Sheet on page 268

ARE YOU A FIRE TYPE? The optimist, communicator, entertainer, empathizer, lover—all are adjectives that could describe the character of a true Fire Type. Fire Types know how to live in the moment; they love excitement, sensation, intimacy, sentiment, and drama. Frequently, you will find the "Lover" on stage—many artists, actors, dancers, musicians, politicians, and salespeople are Fire Types. If not on stage, they are usually the center of attention at most social gatherings. Keenly intuitive and naturally empathetic, the Fire Type shares your joys and sorrows. Like the bright, hot summer sun, a well-balanced Fire Type spreads joy, light, and laughter. According to 5-Element correspondences, the emotion of joy (or, in its absence, sorrow) and a voice filled with happiness, or the sound of laughter like that of children at play, are associated with the Fire Element. While all of us have a lover within that we call upon to bring fulfillment to our relationships with family and friends, the true "Lover," or Fire Type, is easily identified. In balance, the Lover is optimistic, lively, alert, enthusiastic, tender, devoted, charismatic, and communicative. One of the greatest challenges for true Fire Types is to learn to contain their excitement; to learn to conserve as well as to share their resources. If our Fire Element is in balance, we are able to integrate and express our thoughts, feelings, and sensations and experience love in all its forms. Imbalance in this element can be signaled by such symptoms as palpitations, anorexia, insomnia, chest pain, confusion, anxiety, panic attacks, or ceaseless chatter.

Like all types, Fire Types need to guard against excessive consumption of rich, fatty, highly processed foods. When compared to the four other types, Fire Types can be more inclined to abuse the use of mind-altering substances. *They need to guard against addiction to chocolate, alcohol, and drugs.* If your predominate Element is not Fire, but you are suffering from a Fire disharmony, it will be much easier for you to come back into and maintain balance than it will be for the true Fire Type.

HERBS THAT RESTORE HARMONY TO THE FIRE ELEMENT See Chapter 3: Achyranthes, borage, bupleurum, cinnamon bark, coriander, cyperus, dandelion, dang gui, dragon bone, eucommia, garlic, gastrodia, ginseng, hawthorn, ligusticum, longan, oyster shell, pearl, peony root, polygala, rehmannia, safflower, saffron, salvia, sophora, valerian, zizyphus seeds

Also see Chapter 4: Anxiety, Restlessness, and Insomnia; Energy Tonics; and Heart Disharmonies for Recommendations on Herbal Formulas that Can Help with Symptoms Related to the Excess or Deficient Conditions Listed earlier.

Summer Recipes
Simple, Light, and Fast

MARINATED TOFU
Basic Recipe:

1 pound firm tofu cut into slices

3 T. tamari or soy sauce

2 T. rice wine (Mirin)

1/8 tsp. dry ginger

3 to 4 cloves minced garlic

1/8 tsp. anise

1/2 tsp. parsley

dash of cayenne pepper

1/2 tsp. of any of the following herbs—experiment: basil, oregano, marjoram, oregano, rosemary, thyme

- Preheat oven to 300 degrees.

- Make a marinade with all the ingredients listed below the tofu.

- Place tofu in a saucepan and cover with marinade; add spring water to just cover tofu and simmer 15 to 20 minutes.

- Lightly oil a cookie sheet with canola or olive oil and lay tofu slices on it.

- Bake at 300 degrees for 7 to 10 minutes per side, or until flavor sears in.

JICAMA SUMMER SALAD
Basic Recipe:

1/2 small jicama

1/2 small red bell pepper

1/2 small yellow bell pepper

1 small carrot

1 small zucchini

2 T. extra-virgin cold-pressed olive oil

2 T. lime juice

1 small clove garlic

dash of cayenne pepper

sea salt to taste

- Mince garlic and add olive oil, lime juice, cayenne pepper, and sea salt.

- Wash all veggies, remove skin of jicama and seeds and membranes of bell peppers.

- Cut veggies into long, thin (julienne) strips.

- Toss all ingredients to mix well and let marinate at least 10 minutes before serving.

Seitan Spinach Salad
Basic Recipe:

12 ounce package of seitan

4 T. cold-pressed extra-virgin olive oil

4 to 6 cloves minced garlic

1/3 cup balsamic vinegar

1/2 bag baby spinach greens

1/2 bag mixed baby salad greens

1 cup carrots cut in thin strips

1/4 cup soaked and rinsed arame

1/4 cup gomasio

• Cut seitan into small squares.

• Warm oil in skillet over medium heat. Saute garlic 1 to 2 minutes; add carrots, seitan, and seaweed; continue to heat another 5 to 7 minutes.

• Add vinegar (or your favorite dressing) and continue to warm 2 minutes.

• Pour mixture over greens, then sprinkle with gomasio.

Serve with quinoa, barley, or rice. Try substituting tempeh for seitan.

Sumptuous 5-Flavor Sushi Rolls
(Takes time, but make plenty—the flavor gets even better the next day.)
Basic Recipe:

4 cups cooked brown rice or barley

1 small onion

6 cloves garlic

cold-pressed olive oil

juice of 2 lemons

honey or maple syrup

cayenne pepper

tamari or miso

splash of water

1 grated carrot

1/2 cup parsley

pickled ginger

thin slices of jicama, zucchini, or avocado

nori seaweed sheets for sushi

• Place diced onion and garlic in blender, cover with olive oil, lemon juice, 1 T. sweetener, dash of cayenne, 2 tsp. tamari, 1 T. water, parsley, and blend.

• Taste above mixture and add any of the five flavors to obtain desired result.

• Mix blended ingredients into rice, along with finely grated carrot.

• Roll rice mixture up in nori sheets, including a sliver of ginger and jicama, zucchini, or avocado in the center.

• To boost protein, add 1/2 cup pre-cooked aduki beans to rice.

Be prepared for rave reviews!

Note: If you are on the "Zone" diet, substitute barley for the rice and add appropriate amount of protein to the center of the roll (tofu slices, salmon, halibut, chicken or turkey breast).

SUMMER-GARDEN BURGERS

(TAKES A LITTLE TIME, BUT PREPARE LOTS AND FREEZE.)

Basic Recipe:

8 cups spring water

1 cup small red lentils

2 cups millet

1/2 cup sunflower seeds

1 diced onion

4 cloves garlic, diced

1 sweet red bell pepper

1 grated carrot

1/2 cup diced celery

1/2 cup parsley

1 grated zucchini

1/2 cup finely sliced mushrooms

2 T. canola or olive oil

spice as you like

1/4 cup barley or millet flour

rolled oats as needed

- Wash lentils, millet, and sunflower seeds.

- Cook over medium heat in 8 cups water until water evaporates (+/-30 minutes).

- Meanwhile, saute onion and garlic in oil.

- Add veggies and 2 T. water to onion; cover, allowing to steam for 7 min.

- Stir veggies into millet mixture.

- Stir in 1/4 cup barley or millet flour.

- Let cool, then form burgers—if too moist, add rolled oats to desired consistency.

Serve with rice; or in a sandwich on whole-grain bread; in pita bread with alfalfa sprouts; rolled in a cabbage leaf and gently steamed; rolled in a tortilla; or smothered in mushroom gravy. Yummy!

Now get creative! Substitute other grains for millet (quinoa, amaranth, rice, etc.) and other beans for red lentils (pinto, black, aduki, navy, kidney, mung, garbanzos). Try different combinations of veggies and/or spices. The possibilities are limitless. To increase protein, add a 10 oz. package of silken tofu or nonfat cottage cheese.

Carbohydrate-sensitive individuals should avoid millet, which ranks 103 on the glycemic index. Precook barley and add it to your lentil mixture.

According to Oriental thought, corn is the grain that helps nourish the Fire Element. Following are two great recipes using corn and whole-wheat pastry flour. These are not suitable for carbohydrate-sensitive individuals or for persons suffering from Excess Moisture. They are, however, great recipes for persons suffering from Dryness in their human garden. Kids will love them!

PINE NUT CORN MUFFINS
Basic Recipe:

1-1/4 cups whole-wheat pastry flour

1 cup yellow or blue cornmeal

1 cup coarsely chopped, lightly toasted
   piñon nuts

1/2 cup ghee or canola oil

1-1/4 cup milk, soy milk, or rice dream

2 large eggs

2 tsp. cinnamon

4 tsp. baking powder

1/2 tsp. sea salt

1 tsp. vanilla

1 cup pure maple syrup

- Preheat oven to 400 degrees.
- Thoroughly mix all dry ingredients and pine nuts and set aside.
- Beat eggs well, then add ghee or oil and other wet ingredients.
- Gently combine liquids with dry ingredients. Be careful not to overstir. Stir just enough to produce batter.
- Fill oiled and floured muffin tins 2/3 full.
- Bake for 10 minutes and check.
- Rotate pans so they will brown evenly.
- Bake 4 to 5 more minutes or until golden brown.
- Makes approximately 12 large muffins.

SUMMER SCONES
Basic Recipe:

2 cups whole-wheat pastry flour

1 cup blue or yellow cornmeal

1/3 cup sucanat

3/4 cup ghee or canola oil

1/2 cup soy milk or skim milk

1 T. baking powder

1/2 tsp. baking soda

1/2 tsp. sea salt

2 tsp. cinnamon

1 cup mixture of currants, chopped nuts,
   dried fruits, orange peel, cranberries—your choice!

2 T. lycii berries

- Preheat oven to 425 degrees.
- Thoroughly combine dry ingredients, except nuts and fruits.
- Pour oil or ghee over dry ingredients in a slow, steady stream.
- Gently cut oil in with a fork until mixture resembles small, pea-sized crumbs.
- Gently stir in fruits and nuts and liquid.
- Turn mixture out onto a board sprinkled with 1/2 cup cornmeal.
- Knead lightly and roll out dough to about 1/2" thick.
- Cut dough in desired shapes—squares, triangles, etc., and place on an unoiled cookie sheet.
- Bake 6 minutes—rotate pan to ensure even browning and bake another 5 or 6 minutes.

Serve with your favorite organic fruit-sweetened jam.

FRESH FRUIT PUDDING: SIN FREE!
Basic Recipe:

2 sweet, ripe peaches or 6 apricots or 1 apple

1 cup water

1/2 cup organic apple juice

1 tsp. cinnamon

1/4 tsp. cardamom

1 T. raisins or currants

2 T. sliced almonds, walnuts, or sunflower seeds

1 1/2 cup leftover millet, quinoa, amaranth, rice, or barley

1 heaping T. kudzu dissolved in 2 T. water

2 tsp. vanilla

• Place fruit in bottom of saucepan.
• Then layer with raisins, spices, and nuts.
• Top with leftover grain.
• Gently pour in water and juice without stirring.
• Bring to a boil and simmer approximately 12 minutes—until fruit is soft.
• Stir in kudzu-and-water mixture.
• Remove from heat and add vanilla.
• You can blend, if you want a really creamy texture.

Experiment with other fresh, seasonal fruits: pears, blueberries, black cherries. Try other spices or a dash of lemon peel.

Carbohydrate-sensitive individuals—this recipe is great for you. Stick to oatmeal, barley, or rye flakes. Measure out 3/4 cup of the pudding and add 3/4 cup of nonfat cottage cheese to create a delicious three-block breakfast.

FRESH FRUIT PIE
Basic Recipe:

4 cups fresh, ripe sliced fruit

1 tsp. cinnamon

squeeze of lemon

2 cups organic apple juice

2 T. agar agar flakes

1 T. kudzu dissolved in 1/2 cup water

2 tsp. vanilla

touch of sea salt

• Arrange fruit (blueberries, peaches, apples, apricots, etc.) on precooked pie shell.
• Sprinkle fruit with lemon juice and cinnamon.
• Mix agar agar into apple juice, bring to boil, simmer for 5 minutes.
• Add kudzu-and-water mixture and stir until thick.
• Add vanilla and touch of salt.
• Cool—then pour over fruit.
• Let set in refrigerator before serving.

Carbohydrate-sensitive individuals who are on "The Zone" can blend 2 cups of nonfat cottage cheese and spread on the crust. Arrange the fruit on top of the cottage cheese.

FOOLPROOF PIE CRUST

(JACK BISHOP, NATURAL HEALTH MAGAZINE, 12/95)

Basic Recipe:

1 cup whole-wheat pastry flour

1 cup unbleached all-purpose flour

1/2 tsp. sea salt

2 tsp. Sucanat (optional)

1/2 cup ghee or canola oil

1/4 cup cold milk or soy milk

2 to 3 tsp. cinnamon (optional)

- Mix dry ingredients with fork in large bowl.
- Pour oil over dry ingredients in a slow, steady stream. Mixture should resemble pea-sized crumbs when oil has been added.
- Add soy milk 1 tablespoon at a time until dough comes together.

- Knead together briefly to form large ball; chill in refrigerator for 20 minutes if you have the time (helps roll-out).
- Flatten dough into 5-inch disc and place between 2 large pieces of wax paper.
- Roll into 12-inch circle, starting at center of dough and pushing out toward the edges.
- Remove top sheet of wax paper; invert crust over 9-inch pie pan; carefully remove remaining sheet of wax paper.
- Press dough into edges of pan; trim to 1/4 inch of rim; flute edge.
- If prebaking shell, prick crust with fork, then place in preheated 425° oven for approximately 15 minutes or until golden brown.
- Cool crust before filling.

Remember to steam or simmer foods as quickly as possible to guarantee very little depletion of natural vitamins, minerals, and enzymes. Add spices such as ginger and cayenne to stimulate perspiration—the body's natural mechanism to eliminate stored toxins and summer heat. However, minerals are lost through perspiration, stress, and consumption of refined foods. They need to be replaced by eating the widest variety of produce available; be sure to check your local farmers' market.

Persons with reduced digestive fire may find that the consumption of raw food results in loose stools filled with undigested food particles. Steamed bitter greens such as endive, arugula, or dandelion stimulate digestion. While the Bitter Flavor is relatively unfamiliar in American cuisine, it serves an incredibly important function. Bitters aid digestion as well as having anti-inflammatory, antispasmodic, and antibacterial affects. Many traditional cultures start their meals with a salad made from bitter greens. Get ready for fall and winter by boosting your immune system this summer: Eat plenty of nature's green germ fighters.

Earth Element

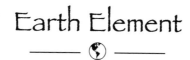

Yin Organ: Spleen/Pancreas   **Yang Organ:** Stomach

🜨 EARTH ELEMENT ✔ LIST

Symptoms of *Excess* in This Organ System

Mood Indicators	*Body Cues*
❑ Worried	❑ Water Retention
❑ Overprotective	❑ Excess Appetite
❑ Meddlesome	❑ Irregular Elimination
❑ Lethargic	❑ Sticky Mucus
❑ Overbearing	❑ PMS and Tender Gums

• • • • •

Symptoms of *Deficiency* in This Organ System

Mood Indicators	*Body Cues*
❑ Wishy-Washy	❑ Difficult Weight Loss
❑ Scattered	❑ Soft Lumps and Swollen Glands
❑ Clinging	❑ Poor Muscle Tone
❑ Submissive	❑ Easy Bruising/Varicose Veins
❑ Spoiling	❑ Slow Healing

Add Total Number of ✔'s for:

EXCESS   +   Deficiency   =   Total

❑   +   ❑   =   ❑

Transfer your scores to the 5-Element Tally Sheet on page 268

Are You An Earth Type?

The peacemaker, nurturer, planner of family and community affairs, Cub or Brownie scout leader—all are roles that the true Earth Type is found playing. Wherever there is need, you will find Earth Types linking, nourishing, and sustaining humanity. Their goal is one involving harmony and togetherness. They love to plan events, be in charge, and then sink into the background, never seeking the limelight. Earth types like to feel involved and needed and sometimes attempt to be all things to all people. Probably the greatest challenge for an Earth Type is to learn how to balance their devotion to nurturing relationships with needed solitude and time to reflect. As well as building community, they need to build self-reliance. The Peacemaker, in balance, is supportive, nurturing, relaxed, considerate, sympathetic, attentive, and agreeable. Some Earth Type problem areas include excessive worry, self-doubt, tendencies to overprotect or meddle, and unrealistic expectations that are followed by disappointments. *More than other types Earth Types are attracted to sugary sweets and carbohydrates*—this can be their undoing. If you are an Earth Type who tends to get caught up on sugar or carbohydrate binges, be sure to look into the diets for carbohydrate-sensitive individuals mentioned in Chapter 1. (A simple carbohydrate-sensitivity quiz follows to help you determine if this might be your problem.) Earth Type physical problems include water retention; difficult weight loss; poor muscle tone; varicose veins; easy bruising; soft lumps and swollen glands; tender, bleeding gums; and lethargy. If your predominate Element is not Earth, but you are simply suffering from an Earth imbalance, it will be much easier for you to come back into balance.

In the same way we plant trees on a hillside to stop erosion (roots sink deeply into the earth to hold it in place), the Wood Element (in the form of the Sour Flavor) helps control the Earth Element in our human garden. Excess Earth conditions can be aided by cutting back on Earth-engendering full sweet foods and increasing the Sour and Spicy Flavors in our diet. Deficient Earth disharmonies often benefit from an increase in full sweet earth foods (usually lean cuts of beef, poultry, and fish) with a corresponding decrease in carbohydrate foods (particularly those high on the glycemic index such as wheat, corn, rice, millet, and potatoes). Also aid digestion by increasing the Bitter Flavor in the form of herbal bitters.

According to Oriental medicine, orange foods such as yam, carrot, winter squash, and millet all help nourish the Earth Element. This is true! If you are an Earth Type and are carbohydrate sensitive, however, these are exactly the foods that you need to avoid (unless you use the following Heller and Heller method.) You will find many wonderful recipes in the following pages containing these Earth-nourishing foods. They are perfect for Metal Types who are experiencing dryness, Excess Wood, Fire, and Water types or anyone who does not suffer from hypoglycemia or carbohydrate sensitivity. Also included in this chapter are two of my recipes for carbohydrate-sensitive individuals who are on "The Zone"—try them out for a few days to see if you do not feel more balanced with fewer sweet cravings. Ultimately, only you can be the judge.

CARBOHYDRATE-SENSITIVITY TEST

(Adapted from The Carbohydrate Addict's Diet *by Rachael F. Heller and Richard F. Heller. Copyright (c) 1991 by Rachael Heller, Ph.D., and Richard Heller, Ph.D. Used by permission of Dutton Signet, a division of Penguin Books USA Inc.)*

Please check ✔ YES or NO to each of the following questions:

Yes   No

❏   ❏   I get tired and/or hungry in the mid-afternoon. (4)

❏   ❏   About an hour or two after eating a full meal that includes dessert, I want more dessert. (5)

❏   ❏   It is harder for me to control my eating for the rest of the day if I have a breakfast containing carbohydrates than it would be if I had only coffee or nothing at all. (3)

❏   ❏   When I want to lose weight, I find it easier not to eat for most of the day than to try to eat several small diet meals. (4)

❏   ❏   Once I start eating sweets, starches, or snack foods, I often have a difficult time stopping. (3)

❏   ❏   I would rather have an ordinary meal that included dessert than a gourmet meal that did not include dessert. (3)

❏   ❏   After finishing a full meal, I sometimes feel as if I could go back and eat the whole meal again. (5)

❏   ❏   A meal of only meat and vegetables leaves me feeling unsatisfied. (3)

❏   ❏   If I'm feeling down, a snack of cake or cookies makes me *feel* better. (3)

❏   ❏   If potatoes, bread, pasta, or dessert are on the table, I will often skip eating vegetables or salad. (3)

❏   ❏   I get a sleepy, almost "drugged" feeling after eating a large meal containing bread or pasta or potatoes and dessert, whereas I feel more energetic after a meal of only meat and salad. (4)

❏   ❏   When I am not eating, the sight of other people eating is sometimes irritating to me. (4)

❏   ❏   I sometimes have a hard time going to sleep without a bedtime snack. (3)

❏   ❏   At times I wake in the middle of the night and can't go back to sleep unless I eat something. (3)

❏   ❏   Before going to dinner at a friend's house, I will sometimes eat something in case dinner is delayed. (5)

❏   ❏   Now and then I think I am a secret eater. (3)

❏   ❏   At a restaurant, I almost always eat too much bread, even before the meal is served. (2)

Total Score: _____

To determine your score, go back over the test, putting the number you find in parenthesis at the end of each question in the blank provided, *ONLY* if you have answered *YES* to the question. For *NO* answers, put a "0" in the space provided, or leave it blank. Tally your total score by adding the numbers. The total possible score is 60, indicating:

(45 to 60) Severe Carbohydrate Addiction
(31 to 44) Moderate Carbohydrate Addiction
(22 to 30) Mild Carbohydrate Addiction
(21 or less) Doubtful Addiction

DOUBTFUL ADDICTION: If you scored 21 or under, you probably are not experiencing problems in controlling your weight or appetite. If you are having such difficulties, the problem is not related to carbohydrate intake.

MILD ADDICTION: A score of 22 to 30 indicates you may have a tendency for carbohydrate addiction, but are frequently able to control your urges. Though you may want to drop a few pounds for health or appearance reasons, weight is not an area of major concern. Sometimes you may eat when stressed, bored, tired, or just out of habit. Sometimes you may eat greater amounts of carbohydrate-rich foods than you intended.

MODERATE ADDICTION: A score from 31 to 44 suggests you may experience bouts of recurring hunger and food cravings that make dieting efforts difficult. Persons with moderate addiction usually have concerns regarding their weight and/or eating patterns. These persons are frequently unhappy or angry with themselves until they understand carbohydrate addiction is a physical disorder.

SEVERE ADDICTION: A score in the 45 to 60 range indicates that weight and/or eating patterns are of great concern. Food cravings and recurring hunger can be overwhelming. Diets are maintained for a while but sooner or later you find yourself eating the very foods you have been trying to avoid. Physical symptoms of severe carbohydrate addiction include mood swings, nervousness, irritability, tiredness, or listlessness. Yo-yo dieting becomes the norm as diet after diet is tried.

Herbs that Restore Harmony to the Earth Element

See Chapter 3: Achyranthes, aconite, agastache, alisma, astragalus, atractylodes, cardamom, cinnamon bark, clematis, codonopsis, coix, cyperus, dang gui, du huo, eucommia, fennel seeds, gastrodia, gentian, ginger, ginseng, hawthorn fruit, kudzu, ligusticum, magnolia bark, peppermint, peony root, pinellia, polygonum, poria cocos, radish seed, rehmannia, safflower flower, salvia, siler, stephania, tangerine peel, zhu ling

Also see Chapter 4: Arthritis, Rheumatism, and Lumbago and Digestive Disorders for Recommendations on Herbal Formulas that Can Help with Symptoms Related to the Earth Element Disharmonies.

Harvest-Time (or Doyo) Taste Treats
Sweet, Centering, Calming, Nurturing

ADUKI SOUP

(GENTLE, NURTURING SOUP THAT HELPS RELIEVE WATER RETENTION)

9 cups spring water

6" strip kombu

1/2 cup aduki beans

1/2 cup coix

1 cup pearl barley

1/2 ounce poria cocos

1 slice astragalus root

1/3 cup chopped parsley

2 stalks celery and leaves

2 scallions

1/2 cup shiitake

2 slices fresh ginger

1 to 2 carrots (optional)

1 T. olive oil

a touch of cayenne pepper

sea salt

• Soak grains and beans overnight with kombu.

• Rinse well, simmer grains, beans, kombu, poria, and astragalus on low heat for 2 hours.

• Add scallions, ginger, celery; simmer 30 minutes; add more water if required.

• Add parsley, shiitake, and optional carrots, simmering 30 more minutes.

• Remove from heat, stir in 1 tablespoon olive oil, dash of cayenne pepper, and sea salt to taste.

• Consume small amounts 3 to 4 times daily.

According to Oriental Medical thought, lean beef nurtures the Spleen/Pancreas Organ system. Add 4 to 8 ounces of lean, organic beef to this recipe to treat fatigue, loose stools, poor appetite, edema, bloating after eating, cold hands and feet. Other vegetables can be added as well.

Soothing Root Stew

6" strip kombu
2 slices astragalus
2 1/2 cups water
1 onion
1 carrot
1 parsnip or turnip
1 stalk celery and leaves
2 cabbage leaves
1 heaping T. kudzu
2 T. cold water
sea salt, tamari, or soy sauce to taste
1/2 tsp. basil or thyme
1/2 cup diced seitan

- Bring kombu and astragalus to boil in water.
- Cover pot and simmer 20 minutes.
- Remove kombu, slice in 1/2" squares, and add back to pot.
- Slice or dice all veggies.
- Add onion, roots, celery, and spices and simmer 15 minutes.
- Add cabbage and seitan, simmering 5 more minutes, or until everything is tender.
- Dissolve kudzu in cold water and stir until stew thickens.
- Add salty flavor as desired.

Carrot/Cashew/Kashi Casserole

(Try saying that rapidly, three times in a row!)

Basic Recipe:

5 medium-sized carrots
2 cups water
1 to 2 cups leftover kashi, millet, or rice
10.5 oz. extra-firm silken tofu
1/4 to 1 cup cashew pieces
1 large onion
6 to 10 garlic cloves
1 to 3 T. canola oil or ghee
1/2 cup finely diced celery
1/4 cup chopped parsley
1 egg (optional)
1/4 cup ketchup or tomato paste (optional)
1/4 to 3/4 cup rolled oats
1 T. sage
sea salt and black pepper to taste

- Simmer carrots in water until soft; discard water and mash carrots.
- Brown onion, garlic, and celery in oil or ghee; stir in sage.
- Mix all ingredients, adding enough rolled oats to create desired consistency.
- Form loaf in lightly oiled casserole dish.
- Cover and bake in preheated 350° oven for 35 minutes.
- Remove cover and brown in oven for 10 to 15 minutes.

For additional crunch, add 1 can water chestnuts when mixing ingredients.

This recipe has always been a favorite!
This recipe is not for persons on "The Zone."

BASIC KICHAREE

(IF YOU ARE NOT CARBOHYDRATE SENSITIVE, THIS IS ONE OF THE MOST NURTURING, HEALING FOODS ON THE PLANET. CARBOHYDRATE-SENSITIVE PEOPLE CAN ENJOY KICHAREE AS WELL; HOWEVER, BEST TO MAKE IT WITH BARLEY. LIMIT YOURSELF TO 3/4 TO 1 CUP AND BALANCE WITH 3 TO 4 BLOCKS OF PROTEIN.)

Basic Recipe:

9 cups spring water

1/2 cup small red lentils or mung beans

1 1/2 cups millet or basmati rice

1 to 3 T. toasted sesame oil or ghee

2 to 6 cloves chopped garlic

1 tsp. black mustard seed

1 1/4 tsp. cumin seed or powder

1 tsp. turmeric powder

1 1/2 tsp. coriander powder

pinch of asafoetida

sea salt or Bragg's amino acids to taste

- Wash lentils, millet, or basmati rice.
- Toast garlic and spices in oil or ghee until mustard seeds start to pop.
- Saute lentils and grains in seed mixture.
- Add water, bring to boil, reduce to simmer for approximately 45 minutes.
- Stir in cilantro and cook 7 to 10 minutes.
- Remove from heat and add sea salt or Bragg's amino acids to taste.
- Add 1 to 2 cups spring water if thinner consistency is desired.

HUMBLE HUMMUS

1 cup garbanzo beans

4 1/4 cups water

2 slices astragalus

2 T. arame sea veggie

2 to 6 cloves garlic

2 to 4 T. toasted sesame seeds

1/4 cup bean cooking liquid

2 T. finely chopped parsley

1 to 2 T. chopped green onion

1 tsp. to 2 T. olive oil (optional)

1 to 2 umeboshi plums

squeeze of lemon juice

- Be sure to sort through beans for rocks.
- Wash and soak beans overnight.
- Rinse beans and simmer in water with sea veggie, astragalus, and garlic for 3 hours.
- Drain beans and reserve cooking liquid.
- Combine ingredients and blend until creamy.
- Freezes wonderfully!

CARROT BUTTER (SPREAD THIS ON YOUR FAVORITE CRACKER!)
Basic Recipe:

6 organic carrots
3/4 cup spring water
1 heaping T. kudzu
2 T. water
1 tsp. ginger or cinnamon
1 to 3 T. ghee or sesame tahini

- Steam sliced carrots in water approximately 20 to 25 minutes until soft.
- Blend water and carrots with spices.
- Dissolve kudzu in water; add to carrot mix; return to low heat and simmer until mixture bubbles.
- Stir in ghee or tahini.

KABOCHA OR BUTTERNUT BUTTER
Basic Recipe:

1 cup precooked kabocha or butternut squash
12 to 25 roasted almonds or 2 to 4 T. sesame seeds
1/4 tsp. cinnamon
pinch of dried ginger (optional)
1 tsp. miso or pinch of sea salt

- Roast sesame seeds (try black for a change) or almonds.
- Blend all ingredients until creamy.
- Substitute almond butter or tahini for sesame seeds if rushed.
- Add water to desired texture.

BAKED FRUIT PIE OR COBBLER (SWEET AND SUGAR-FREE!)
Basic Recipe:

4 cups fresh, ripe, sliced fruit
2 tsp. cinnamon
squeeze of lemon
2 T. kudzu dissolved in 4 T. apple juice
2 tsp. vanilla
3/4 cup unsweetened applesauce
touch of sea salt

- Wash and prepare fruit (blueberries, peaches, apples, apricots, pears, etc.)
- Sprinkle fruit with lemon juice and cinnamon.
- Add kudzu/apple juice mixture to fruit.
- Add vanilla and touch of salt.

- Mix in applesauce to sweeten tart fruits.
- Place mixture in partially prebaked pie shell; topping with remaining 1/2 of uncooked dough.
- For cobbler, simply omit bottom crust and top with crumbled dough (adding coconut flakes, 1/4 cup rolled oats, and 2 to 4 T. maple syrup to mixture).
- Bake in preheated oven (325°) for 40 minutes.
- Raise temperature to 375°, baking pie another 15 to 20 minutes, until brown and fruit is tender (insert toothpick).

See Summer Recipes for a Great Pie Crust!

REVA'S ULTIMATE CARROT CAKE
Basic Recipe:

3/4 cup organic apple juice

1 1/2 cup ghee or canola oil

1 1/2 cup raisins or currants

1/2 cup maple syrup

grated peel of 1 orange

3 medium carrots (grated)

2 to 4 tsp. fresh ginger root (finely grated)

2 to 3 tsp. cinnamon

1/2 tsp. grated nutmeg

1 tsp. nonaluminum baking powder

1 tsp. baking soda

2 cups whole-wheat pastry flour

1/2 tsp. sea salt

1 cup chopped walnuts

- Preheat oven to 350°.
- Blend until smooth: apple juice, 1/2 cup raisins, maple syrup, orange peel, ghee.
- Gently mix in carrots and ginger.
- In a large bowl, mix dry ingredients.
- Fold in apple-juice mixture using as few strokes as possible; it is very important not to overmix the batter.
- Fold in remaining 1 cup raisins or currants and walnuts.
- Pour batter into lightly oiled and floured 8-x-8-inch square or 9-inch round cake pan.
- Bake approximately 35 to 50 minutes until toothpick inserted in middle of cake comes out clean.

OATMEAL BREAKFAST IN THE ZONE
Basic Recipe:

1/2 cup rolled oats (not fast cooking)

1 cup water

1/8 tsp. cinnamon

dash of cardamom

1 fruit from list on the right

3/4 cup nonfat cottage cheese

3 tsp. slivered almonds

The above constitutes 3 blocks. For additional block add (optional) 1/2 cup plain yogurt.

Choose 1 fruit: 1/2 cup blueberries
1 peach
1/2 apple
7 cherries
1/2 cup pineapple
1 cup strawberries
1/3 banana

- Bring oats, water, and spices to a boil. Reduce heat and simmer 5 to 7 minutes.
- Add fruit; remove from heat.
- Stir in cottage cheese, almonds, and optional yogurt.

This is my favorite breakfast. Note to practitioners of Oriental Medicine: In my case, this breakfast has actually reduced dampness. I have no mucus buildup as the result of eating organic, nonfat dairy (which I had avoided for more than 20 years.) I feel genetics has much to do with it.

TOFU, TURKEY, OR TUNA ZONE LOAF

	BLOCKS		
	Protein	*Carbos*	*Fat*
2 cans (6 oz. each) white tuna packed in spring water or 12 oz. ground white turkey breast	12		
32 oz. plain tofu	11		
1 cup chopped onion		1	
2 cups shredded zucchini		2	
1 cup diced bell pepper		1	
1 cup rolled organic oats		4	
1 cup shredded carrots		2	
1 small can Muir organic or V-8 veggie juice		1	
*8 cloves minced garlic			
*3/4 cup minced parsley			
*1/4 cup arame seaweed			
*1+ T Italian seasoning	*4 items above: 1		
Organic cold-pressed olive oil, 1 T. plus 1 tsp.			12
Sea salt and black pepper to taste			

TOTAL: Protein—23 blocks

   Carbos—12

   Fats—12

Mix all of the above together thoroughly and bake for 1-1/2 hours at 375°.

Divide Loaf into 8 equal servings of approximately 3 Blocks of Protein per Serving and 1-1/2 Blocks each of Carbohydrate and Fats. To balance the blocks, have cooked green veggies or salad or 1.5 fruit blocks and 1.5 fat blocks (i.e., 3/4 apple and 3 almonds, *or* 1-1/2 cups steamed broccoli and 3 olives).

Metal Element

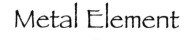

Yin Organ: Lungs   **Yang Organ:** Large Intestine

☽ METAL ELEMENT ✔ LIST

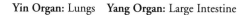

Symptoms of *Excess* in This Organ System

Mood Indicators	*Body Cues*
❏ Dogmatic	❏ Constipation
❏ Self-Righteous	❏ Tight Muscles
❏ Strict/Austere	❏ Dry Skin, Hair, and Mucous Membranes
❏ Perfectionistic	❏ Stiff Posture
❏ Cool or Indifferent	❏ Sinus Headaches

• • • • • •

Symptoms of *Deficiency* in This Organ System

Mood Indicators	*Body Cues*
❏ Petty	❏ Frail Physique
❏ Sloppy	❏ Delicate Skin
❏ Compliant	❏ Moles and Warts
❏ Lacks Conviction	❏ Loss of Body Hair
❏ Numb or Resigned	❏ Clammy Hands and Feet

Add Total Number of ✔s for:

EXCESS	+	Deficiency	=	Total
❏	+	❏	=	❏

Transfer your scores to the 5-Element Tally Sheet on page 268

Are You a Metal Type?

The Sage could be described as the conscience of society. The lawmaker, judge, religious leader—all are roles in which you might find the Sage busily occupied trying to establish order in the midst of chaos. The Sage lives according to reason and principle, respecting discretion, virtue, and authority. The Sage holds him or herself to the highest standards and expects the same of others. Metal types love beauty, refinement, and ceremony and feel most comfortable in a structured, disciplined environment. In balance, the Sage is neat, calm, honorable, reserved, precise, scrupulous, and methodical.

Excess Metal conditions are frequently accompanied by dryness, sinus headaches, and constipation. Antibiotic herbal bitters, such as forsythia fruit, can help eliminate microbes responsible for lung and sinus infections while aloe vera and an increased consumption of healthful oil in the form of pumpkin, sesame or sunflower seeds, almonds, or walnuts, will help relieve constipation and dryness. Once the excess has been eliminated, warming spices and nourishing full sweet foods help combat the cold and dryness afflicting Metal types. Deficient Metal conditions require gentle, warming spices such as ginger, garlic, cinnamon, and fennel as well as an increase in full sweet nurturing foods such as salmon, halibut, cod, chicken or turkey breast, and lean cuts of beef. The climate characteristic of the Fall season is Dryness (to remember, think of the dry leaves and grasses). Metal types suffering from dry skin, hair, and mucus membranes frequently need to increase their consumption of healthful oils such as ghee, canola, or olive. Sesame oil is also good, but should not be consumed by persons with B Blood Type. (*Note:* According to nutritionist Ann Louise Gittleman, persons with Blood Type B should avoid chicken, buckwheat, sesame, and sunflower seeds. These persons have a particular element in their blood that causes blood cells to clump together, or agglutinate, when these foods are eaten.)

Herbs that Restore Balance to the Metal Element

See Chapter 3: Anemarrhena, apricot kernel, bamboo sap, bamboo shavings, bupleurum, chrysanthemum, cocklebur fruit, codonopsis, coltsfoot, coptis, dang gui, dandelion, ephedra stems, forsythia, fritillary, gardenia, ginger, honeysuckle, jujube dates, kudzu, lily bulb, ligusticum, magnolia flower, pearl, peony, peppermint, phellodendron, pinellia, platycodon, poria cocos, rhubarb, schisandra, schizonepeta, scutellaria, siler, sophora, tangerine peel, trichosanthes

Also see Chapter 4: Allergies, Rhinitis, Sinusitis; Colds and Flu; Coughs, Bronchitis, Phlegm, Asthma, Wheezing; Skin Problems; Sore Throats, Mouth, and Ear Disorders

Autumn Recipes
Slightly Spicy to Warm the Spirits

FALL 5-ELEMENT CLEANSE
Basic Recipe:

2 quarts spring water	• Heat 1 quart of water to simmer; add licorice, ginger, and hawthorn berries.
2 lemons or limes	
1-1/2 T. hawthorn berries	
2 slices of licorice root	• Do not boil; cover and simmer 5 to 10 minutes.
7 slices fresh ginger	
(Optional)	• Remove from heat; allow mixture to steep for another 20 minutes.
1 T. maple syrup or honey	
or	• Add second quart of water to cool down mixture.
1/2 cup unfiltered grape juice	
	• Stir in lemon or lime juice and optional sweetener or grape juice.

It is good to give our digestive tract a break once or twice a year. Spring and fall are the best times to undertake fasts. The autumn fast should always be lighter than a spring fast, since we are trying to build Yang energy in the fall to carry us through winter. Undertake fasts only under the guidance of your health practitioner and carry them out over the weekend (when you can stay close to home and rest or take short, quiet walks). Please do not attempt to fast while working or exercising vigorously. First-time fasters might try drinking the preceding 5-element drink throughout the day. Follow it up with a light dinner of steamed veggies, brown rice, and aduki beans. You could follow this procedure for two to three days. More experienced fasters might want to double the recipe and drink it throughout the day (approximately one gallon of liquid). Two to three days will facilitate a good detox. Always follow a fast with two to three days of light meals as already mentioned. No pizza, fried foods, or sweet desserts, please!

Kale, Cauliflower, Cabbage and the Health of Your Colon

In Traditional Oriental Medicine, autumn is the season related to the Metal Element and Lung/Colon acupuncture meridians. Nature, in its elegant simplicity, offers us the exact nourishment we need during the season we need it. Following is a listing of 12 pungent or spicy veggies (the flavor associated with autumn), most of which are readily available in fall. Western medical studies have shown these veggies are high in cancer- and heart-disease fighting phytochemicals such as indoles, glucosinolates, and dithiolthiones.

In botany, flowers having four petals are called cruciferous because of their resemblance to a cross. All members of this botanical family protect against oral esophageal, stomach, and colon cancers. Here are 12 wonderful, life-enhancing cruciferous vegetables that must be added to your shopping list and consumed year-round when available:

Broccoli	Mustard greens
Brussels sprouts	Kohlrabi
Radish	Cabbage
Rutabaga	Cauliflower
Turnip	Horseradish
Watercress	Kale

BROCCOLI: *Lowers risk of colon, lung, esophagus, larynx, stomach, and prostrate cancers.* One study, conducted by Dr. Saxon Graham in Buffalo, New York, showed that persons who consumed more cabbage, broccoli, and Brussels sprouts had a lower incidence of colon and rectal cancer. Another study demonstrated that women who ate more broccoli were less likely to suffer from cancer of the cervix.

BRUSSELS SPROUTS: *Lowers risk of gastrointestinal cancer.* Studies have shown Brussels sprouts have the ability to detoxify aflatoxin (a fungal mold that contaminates corn, peanuts, and rice and is linked to liver cancer). Researchers found that countries where Brussels sprouts are consumed frequently have a lower incidence of stomach and colon cancer.

RADISH: *Aids respiratory infections and colds and flu.* In Traditional Oriental Medicine, radish is used to help dry excess mucus, promote digestion, and soothe headaches.

RUTABAGA: *Clears up mucus; contains anti-cancer phytochemicals; alkalinizes the body.* Rutabaga is a large yellow root and is first cousin to the turnip.

CAULIFLOWER: *Reduces cancer risk, particularly of the stomach, colon, and rectum.* The indoles in cauliflower stimulate the body's natural defense to neutralize carcinogens. It is also high in sulfur compounds (natural antibiotics), potassium, vitamin C, and fiber. Persons with diabetes fare better with cauliflower than with cabbage.

TURNIP: *Reduces mucus, relieves sore throats, asthma, and bronchitis.* This member of the mustard family is high in calcium, iron, and vitamins C and A.

HORSERADISH: *Aids lung disorders such as bronchitis and asthma; stimulates digestion and reduces lymphatic congestion.* This condiment should be used in limited quantities to flavor sauces, meats, and fish.

WATERCRESS: *As a blood purifier, watercress helps relieve liver and pancreatic imbalances, arthritis and gout, as well as symptoms of colds and flu.* Watercress is an incredible power food too frequently absent from the American diet. It is rich in iron (helping to relieve anemia), potassium, sulfur, calcium, and vitamin A. It is excellent served fresh in salads.

KALE: *A high source of calcium and carotenoids, kale is probably one of the best cancer-fighting veggies on earth.* The calcium in kale is easily assimilated, making it an ideal food for people suffering from arthritis and osteoporosis. It is also rich in iron, magnesium, potassium, sulfur, and vitamins A and C.

MUSTARD GREENS: *Superior to spinach because they do not have the high oxalic acid content; mustard greens are high in calcium, iron, and vitamin A.*

KOHLRABI: *A great digestive aid, kohlrabi helps with diabetes, jaundice, alcoholism, and lymphatic cleansing.*

CABBAGE: *Prevents cancer (particularly colon), heals ulcers, stimulates immunity, and kills bacteria.*
According to one study, eating cabbage at least once a week could reduce your risk of getting colon cancer by 60 percent. Another study, conducted in Japan in 1986, showed that persons who ate the most cabbage experienced the lowest death rate from *all* cancers. Bok Choy and Chinese cabbage also belong to the cruciferous family and contain the same anti-cancer phytochemicals.

Upon changing their diet for the better, many people complain of increased flatulence or gas (Evil Wind in Chinese medicine). Most health practitioners (Chinese or Western) will agree that ill health or disease comes from hyperacidity. Unfortunately, the average American diet supports exactly this condition. Highly refined convenience foods coat the intestinal lining, creating an acidic environment that kills off our friendly bacteria. What happens when you mix white flour with water? You get glue, and this is exactly what happens inside the human body. Autopsies show that the average American is carrying around 12 pounds of fecal matter encrusted on the walls of his or her intestines.

But, back to the question of gas. As you change your diet for the better, unfriendly bacteria, living in the highly acidic environment promoted by convenience foods, start to die off. This is one of the major reasons you experience gas—the death of many unwanted micro-organisms creates that Evil Wind. As your system becomes more alkaline (a process supported by the consumption of fresh, nonacidic fruits and veggies), healthy bacteria that aid digestion will begin to proliferate. Eat one to two tablespoons of yogurt daily to increase the number of friendly bacteria in your intestinal tract. (If you cannot consume milk products, it is important to support the growth of favorable bacteria by taking acidophilus and bifidus supplements). Beano is a product (available at many stores) that is reputed to help those stubborn cases of excess Evil Wind.

Autumn Kicharee
Basic Recipe:

10 cups spring water	1 cup shiitake mushrooms
1 cup brown rice	2 T. chopped cilantro
1/2 cup brown basmati	2 T. nettles
1/2 cup red or brown lentils	1/3 Arame seaweed
2 to 3 T. canola or olive oil	1 tsp. turmeric
1 large onion, minced	2 tsp. mustard seed
7 cloves garlic, minced	1-1/2 tsp. coriander powder
1 thinly sliced burdock root	1-1/2 tsp. cumin powder
2 parsnips, thinly sliced	dash of black or white pepper
1-1/2 cups chopped apple	dash of cayenne pepper
1 cup kale or turnip greens	pinch of asafoetida
2 slices astragalus	sea salt, Bragg's amino acids, or tamari to taste
5 slices fresh ginger (1/2 inch thick)	
1/4 cup chopped parsley	

Basic Recipe (continued):

- Rinse grains well.
- Saute onion, burdock, and garlic in oil.
- Add cumin, coriander, turmeric, asafoetida, and mustard seed; saute until mustard seed starts to pop.
- Add water and grains and beans, ginger, burdock root, arame, astragalus.
- Simmer for 50 to 60 minutes on low heat, stirring occasionally.
- Add nettles, mushrooms, parsley, parsnips.
- Simmer another 25 to 30 minutes adding another cup of water if necessary.
- Add chopped apple, greens, cilantro, and pepper.
- Stir, cover, and simmer another 10 to 12 minutes.
- If desired, for a creamier texture, remove 2 cups of the soup and blend.
- Mix blended portion with remaining kicharee.
- Add salty seasoning to taste.

When shopping, look for young delicate turnips. Always peel them before blanching for one minute in boiling water. This removes any bitterness (discard blanching water).

TUMMY-TINGLING TURNIP SOUP
Basic Recipe:

6 to 8 small turnips (2" diameter)

6 cups water

1/3 cup ghee or canola oil

1/2 cup water

1/4 tsp. thyme

1 large onion or 2 leeks

5 cloves garlic

1/2 cup shiitake, chantrelle, or button mushrooms

4 cups 1% milk

dash of black and/or cayenne pepper

2 cups chopped turnip greens

1/2 cup grated and chopped carrot

1 T. ghee or oil

sea salt to taste

1 T. chopped parsley

- Peel turnips and slice into rounds.
- Bring 6 cups water and 2 tsp. sea salt to boil; add turnips and cook 1 minute.
- Drain turnips and discard water.
- Saute onion, garlic, mushrooms, and thyme in ghee.
- Add 1/2 cup water, turnips, and cook 5 minutes.
- Add milk and heat slowly; *do not allow* to boil.
- Cook on *low* until turnips are tender; stir occasionally.
- Cool soup slightly, then blend with sea salt and pepper to taste.
- Saute carrots and chopped greens in ghee until tender (5 to 7 minutes).
- Add to carrots and greens to soup.
- Garnish with chopped parsley and serve.

You can substitute water for milk, if desired, and blend with 10-ounce pack of silken tofu to create creamy consistency.

MASHED TURNIPS
Basic Recipe:

10 to 12 small turnips

1 to 2 T. ghee

6 cups water for blanching

3 cups water for simmering

1/8 tsp. nutmeg

sea salt to taste

- Peel, cut, and blanch turnips as indicated; discard blanching water.
- Add 3 cups fresh water and simmer until soft.
- Add ghee, nutmeg, and sea salt; mash or puree in blender.
- Add a small amount of liquid (milk or water) if needed.

Get creative! Experiment with other autumn root veggies such as rutabaga (they're delicious) or parsnips. Omit nutmeg and use black pepper or other spices such as cinnamon. Remember, you can always increase protein by blending in 4 to 8 ounces of silken tofu. Tofu is versatile and does not add any flavor to a dish you are cooking—instead, it absorbs the flavors available.

GOMASIO: SESAME-SEED SALT
Basic Recipe:

14 T. sesame seeds

1 T. sea salt

If the gomasio becomes bitter, DO NOT use it.

Bitterness indicates the oil in the seeds has become rancid.

- Wash seeds thoroughly by swirling them in at least 2 cups water.
- Drain well in a fine-mesh strainer.
- Evenly disperse seeds on bottom of a thick cast-iron pot or skillet.
- A spread of seeds about 1 inch thick helps prevent them from popping out of the pan.
- Roast seeds, *stirring constantly*, over high heat until they become fragrant. Be careful not to scorch any of the seeds.
- Grind seeds in grinder or with mortar and pestle. Add salt and continue to grind for 10 more minutes.
- Store in airtight jar in refrigerator.

For a healthful change of pace, and to enhance Liver function, make Milk-Thistle Seed Gomasio following these instructions. Milk thistle seeds are available at most health-food stores that carry bulk herbs.

ROASTED EGGPLANT DIP
Basic Recipe:

3 medium eggplants

1 head minced garlic

1/3 cup olive oil

1 large minced onion

2 T. balsamic vinegar

(optional) 8 oz. tofu (Mori-Nu silken tofu (firm)

1/8 tsp. thyme

1/4 tsp. oregano

1/8 tsp. pepper

1/4 tsp. sea salt

3 T. parsley leaves

- Poke holes in eggplants with fork.
- Barbecue eggplant over coals or in oven at 325° until soft.
- Remove eggplant skin and seeds.
- Blend all ingredients.
- Spread in dish and chill at least an hour. It's even better the next day.
- Serve with your favorite crackers or flat bread.

AUTUMN VEGGIE SPREAD
Basic Recipe:

1/2 cup shredded red cabbage

1/2 cup shredded green cabbage

1/4 cup nonfat yogurt

1/2 cup nonfat cottage cheese

3 cloves minced garlic

2 tsp. olive oil

squeeze of lemon

dash of cayenne pepper

sea salt to taste

- Blend all ingredients except cabbage, salt, and cayenne pepper.
- Add shredded cabbage to blender and pulse to desired consistency.
- Add seasonings to taste; stirring well.
- Spread in serving dish.
- Let flavors mingle at least an hour before serving.

AUTUMN HALIBUT STEW (THIS IS A FAVORITE OF MY WORKSHOP PARTICIPANTS!)
Basic Recipe:

1-1/2 pounds halibut or cod (skinned) cut in 1" cubes

3 cups spring water

1/4 cup arame sea veggie

4 chopped leeks or 2 onions

6 to 8 cloves minced garlic

2 to 3 T. olive oil

4 small cans Muir Glen organic veggie juice or V-8 tomato juice

1 small butternut squash

3 medium-sized potatoes, cubed

1/2 cup chopped celery

Basic Recipe (continued):

1/3 cup minced parsley

1" by 3" strip of orange peel

2 bay leaves

1/2 tsp. saffron threads

1/2 tsp. ground fennel seed

dash of ground clove

1 T. fresh lemon juice

sea salt to taste

dash of black pepper

- Slowly cook leeks or onion and garlic in oil with dash of salt until opaque.
- Add clove and fennel and cook for one minute before stirring in saffron, bay leaf, orange peel.
- Add water and veggie juice, celery, arame squash, potatoes. Cook partially covered over medium heat for approximately 20 minutes until veggies are tender.
- Add the fish and cook only 5 to 7 more minutes, just until it is done.
- Remove from heat. Remove bay leaves and orange peel.
- Squeeze with lemon juice, sea salt, and pepper to taste.
- Garnish with parsley.

Carbohydrate-sensitive individuals who are on "The Zone" should omit the potatoes and serve with barley or minor amounts of brown and/or wild rice or quinoa.

AUTUMN STIR-FRY (APPROXIMATELY 30 MINUTES TO PREPARE)
Basic Recipe:

1 onion or 2 leeks

4 cloves garlic

1 to 2 T. olive oil

1 cup sliced parsnips

3 cups chopped watercress, broccoli, or spinach bok choy, celery, kale, collard greens, cabbage

1/2 cup shiitake mushrooms

1/4 cup toasted almond slivers or 1 T. freshly grated ginger root

dash of cayenne, sea salt, sesame gomasio, black pepper, or tamari to taste

- Saute onion or leeks in oil, add garlic.
- Add desired spices, parsnips, and shiitake.
- Cover and simmer 5 minutes in 1/3 cup water.
- Add remaining veggies, cover, and simmer approximately 7 minutes.
- Remove from heat, add tamari, gomasio, or sea salt.
- Top with toasted almonds or cashew bits.

Serve over brown rice, barley, quinoa, or rye.
Add slices of prebaked tofu or tempeh to increase protein.

Thrice-Spiced Braised Tempeh

(Tempeh is a great source of vegetable protein made from soybeans and quite easy to digest.)

Basic Recipe:

16 ounces tempeh, cut into 12 to 16 strips
1 large onion, diced
1/2 cup ghee or canola oil
4 cloves minced garlic
1 T. olive oil
1 tsp. basil
1/4 tsp. oregano
1/2 tsp. thyme
1/2 tsp. ground cumin
1/2 tsp. ground coriander
1/4 tsp. ground fennel
1 bay leaf
1 clove garlic
1 clove (spice)
1 cup dry red cooking wine
1 T. soy sauce or tamari
1" × 3" strip of lemon peel
2 tsp. Dijon mustard
spring water, as required

- Lightly brown tempeh in ghee.
- Remove tempeh from frying pan, place on absorbent paper, and set aside.

- Add 1 T. olive oil to frying pan.
- Saute onion and garlic until brown (medium heat approx. 10 min.).
- Add the herbs and spices in *italics* and continue to saute, stirring constantly, for approximately 45 seconds to one minute; stick clove spice into garlic.
- Add wine, lemon peel, garlic with clove, soy sauce, tempeh, and enough water to cover ingredients.
- Bring liquid to boil, then lower heat to simmer for 30 minutes; turn tempeh over once.
- Add water, if needed, to maintain the original amount of liquid.
- Toss out garlic clove, lemon peel, and bay leaf.
- Remove tempeh from sauce and arrange on serving platter.
- Stir mustard into reserved cooking liquid to create a sauce and spoon over tempeh.
- Serve with steamed veggies over your favorite grain.

You can substitute firm tofu, seitan, or chicken breast for the tempeh.

Wild Rice for Fall

Basic Recipe

1 cup wild rice
2 tsp. olive oil
2 cups spring water
10 to 12 baby pearl onions
2 T. rinsed arame seaweed
2 cloves minced garlic
1 tsp. rosemary
2 T. soy sauce or tamari
1 bunch fresh-chopped chives

- Rinse and drain wild rice, then toast in dry skillet, stirring constantly over low to medium-low heat until most of the grains pop (approx. 10 minutes).
- Add oil, garlic, seaweed, and rosemary, stirring gently to coat rice with oil.
- Add water and soy sauce; cover and simmer 45 to 50 minutes (do not stir) until rice is tender. Garnish with chives.

QUINOA SESAME PILAF
Basic Recipe:

1 cup quinoa

1 minced leek or onion

2 cloves garlic

3 cups spring water

1 to 2 T. ghee or olive oil

2 T. sesame or poppy seeds

1 grated carrot or parsnip

1 small grated zucchini

3 T. chopped parsley

sea salt to taste

dash of black pepper

- Slowly cook leeks or onion and garlic in oil with dash of salt until opaque.
- Add water, and just before it boils, add quinoa, sesame or poppy seeds, and black pepper.
- Lower heat to medium-low, cover, and simmer for 20 minutes.
- Remove from heat; gently toss or fluff in carrots, zucchini, and parsley.
- Cover and let set 5 minutes for flavors to mingle.

CREAMY AUTUMN ALMOND GREEN BEANS
Basic Recipe:

1 pound fresh green beans

4 cloves minced garlic

1 to 2 T. olive oil

1 medium chopped onion

1 T. kudzu dissolved in 1/3 cup spring water

1/4 cup slivered almonds

1/2 cup plain yogurt or blended Mori-Nu silken tofu (soft)

dash of cayenne, sea salt, and black pepper

- Put fresh, cleaned green beans in a saucepan with just enough water to cover.
- Add salt and simmer for 15 to 20 minutes.
- Saute onion in oil; add garlic and 1/2 of almonds.
- Stir kudzu and spring water into onion mixture, then add yogurt or blended tofu.
- Once sauce thickens, remove it from heat, add sea salt, cayenne, or black pepper.
- Drain green beans and top with sauce and remaining almond slivers.

CAULIFLOWER OR BROCCOLI CASSEROLE
Basic Recipe:

1 cup cooked brown rice or barley

4 cloves minced garlic

1 to 2 T. olive oil

1 medium chopped onion

1/2 cup chopped bell pepper

3 cups broccoli or cauliflower florets

1/4 cup slivered almonds

2 cups mashed tofu or low-fat cottage cheese

1 cup grated low-fat cheese

dash of nutmeg or black pepper

sea salt to taste

- Saute onion in oil; add garlic.
- In casserole dish, mix all ingredients including onion and garlic.
- Top with grated cheese and almonds; cover casserole.
- Bake in preheated oven set at 350° for 30 to 45 minutes.
- Remove cover last 5 to 7 minutes to slightly brown almond slivers.

SPICY YAM BISCUITS
Basic Recipe:

1 cup mashed garnet yams

1/4 cup maple syrup

1/2 cup ghee or canola oil

2 cups whole-wheat pastry flour

1 to 2 T. ghee or olive oil

2 tsp. Rumford's aluminum-free baking powder

1 to 2 tsp. ginger powder

2 tsp. cinnamon

dash of nutmeg

dash of sea salt

3/4 cup plain yogurt

- Preheat oven to 400°.
- In a large bowl, mash prebaked yams and mix in maple syrup and oil.
- Sift dry ingredients together in a separate bowl and mix thoroughly.
- Add dry ingredients and yogurt to yam mixture; mix gently by hand until soft dough forms. *Do not overmix!*
- Place dough on floured board and roll out to 1/2" thick; cut into desired shapes and place on ungreased cookie sheet.
- Bake 18 to 20 minutes until lightly browned.

Water Element

———— ● ————

Yin Organ: Kidney/Adrenals   **Yang Organ:** Urinary Bladder

● WATER ELEMENT ✔ LIST

Symptoms of *Excess* in This Organ System

Mood Indicators	*Body Cues*
❑ Cynical or Blunt	❑ High Blood Pressure
❑ Covetous	❑ Headaches Above Eyes
❑ Demanding	❑ Hardening of Arteries
❑ Suspicious	❑ Kidney Stones
❑ Withdrawn or Detached	❑ Bony Tumors

• • • • •

Symptoms of *Deficiency* in This Organ System

Mood Indicators	*Body Cues*
❑ Sarcastic or Critical	❑ Ringing in Ears
❑ Phobic	❑ Weak, Stiff Spine and Joints
❑ Miserly	❑ Infertility
❑ Fussy	❑ Frequent Urination
❑ Alienated	❑ Cold Buttocks, Legs, and Feet

Add Total Number of ✔s for:

EXCESS	+	Deficiency	=	Total
❑	+	❑	=	❑

Transfer your scores to the 5-Element Tally Sheet on page 268

Are You a Water Type?

In their ceaseless search for truth and meaning, the philosopher will leave no stone unturned. While the Wood Warrior Type will scale the highest mountain peaks just for the challenge, the true Water Type digs into the deepest recesses of the mind to uncover life's mysteries. The research scientist, the poet, the intellectual—you might find them poring over texts in the library or simply sitting, thinking, while their minds plumb the depths of the universe. The world of ideas belongs to the philosopher. Often possessing a quiet, serious demeanor, the Water Type is loyal and committed, refusing to sacrifice personal principles for peace or pleasure. The philosopher can be tough, self-reliant, and unconventional, preferring to remain hidden and anonymous in social gatherings. In balance, the Water Type is gentle, modest, thoughtful, ingenious, and original. In disharmony, the philosopher can become lonely and isolated, tactless, unforgiving, and suspicious.

Even if you are not a Water Type, you can experience emotional and physical symptoms related to this Element due to dietary imbalances and everyday stress. Ice-cold food and drink as well as excessive raw food stresses our Water type, as does excessive sugar and refined salt. The Water Type is associated with the Salty Flavor (mineral salts) and the Kidney/Adrenal and Urinary Bladder Organ Systems. Water can be controlled by the Earth type. Just imagine building dikes of earth to direct the flow of waterways the way our ancestors did in ages past. In much the same manner, full sweet moistening Earth-type foods will control an Excess Water condition characterized by high blood pressure; scanty, dark urine; headaches above the eyes; and low back pain. In this case we may wish to minimize foods containing animal protein (to ease stress on the Kidneys) and concentrate on nourishing whole grains, beans, tofu, and veggies (particularly sweet orange ones such as yams, sweet potatoes, winter squash, and carrots) unless carbohydrate sensitivity is an issue. Sour herbs such as cornus or schisandra may be called for while other herbal helpers could include eucommia, rhemannia, codonopsis, and astragalus.

Deficient Water-type symptoms (including frequent, pale urine, cold extremities; weak knees; ringing in the ears; and low sexual energy) benefit from increased Salty Flavor in the form of mineral-rich sea veggies, miso, mushrooms, pumpkin and sunflower seeds, dragon bone, and nettles. Coldness is the climate associated with Water, and Deficient Water types can use wonderful warming spices such as ginger, garlic, cinnamon, cloves, cardamom, and nutmeg to stoke the fires. Fennel, baked licorice root, rehmannia, cuscuta, and ginseng could also be indicated. According to Oriental Medical thought, a light, lean pork stew with lots of veggies will help strengthen the Kidney/Adrenal complex.

Warming Winter Recipes
Delicious, Nutritious, and Building

DRAGON'S NEST SOUP
Basic Recipe:

7 cups water or stock
1/2 cup sliced burdock
1/2 cup rinsed arame
1 medium sized onion
4 to 6 cloves garlic
1/2 cup water chestnuts
*1 cup preferred veggie
1 to 2 T. oil (canola, ghee, or olive)
1/2 cup mushrooms
mello white or barley miso to taste
1 T. freshly grated ginger root
1 to 2 T. kudzu
1/4 cup cold water
1 egg (optional)

- Bring 7 cups water or stock to boil with arame seaweed.
- Saute diced onion, garlic, burdock, and mushrooms in oil.
- Add preferred veggie-and-onion mixture to boiling liquid with ginger and any additional herbs or spices.
- Simmer for 20 minutes.
- Dissolve kudzu root in cold water and stir into soup to thicken slightly.
- Move arame and veggies to one side of the pot; drop optional egg into the liquid while gently stirring.
- Remove from heat and add miso.
- Sprinkle with parsley and enjoy!

Suggestions—Fire Element: Mung Bean Sprouts, Borage, or Spinach *Earth Element:* Butternut Squash or Carrot *Metal Element:* Daikon Radish, Chinese Cabbage, or Tofu *Water Element:* Aduki Beans, Collard Greens, Nettles, or Lotus Root *Wood Element:* Celery, Broccoli, or Bok Choy

WINTER STIR FRY (APPROXIMATELY 30 MINUTES TO PREPARE)
Basic Recipe:

1 large onion or 2 leeks
4 cloves garlic
2 to 3 T. olive oil
2 carrots or parsnips; or 1 turnip, yam, or burdock root
2 cups broccoli, or spinach, bok choy, lotus root, collard greens, cabbage, snow peas, chard—you name it!
1/2 cup shiitake mushrooms
1/4 cup toasted almond or walnut bits
1 T. freshly grated ginger root
sea salt, gomasio, or tamari to taste
Non-vegetarians: Saute 1/2 cup thinly sliced meat strips with onions and garlic.

- Saute onion or leeks in oil, add garlic.
- Add desired spices and sliced root vegetable.
- Cover and simmer 5 minutes in 1/3 cup water.
- Add remaining veggies, cover and simmer approximately 7 minutes.
- Remove from heat, add tamari, gomasio, or sea salt.
- Top with toasted almonds or cashew bits.

Serve over brown rice, barley, millet, quinoa, or kashi.

Barley Pilaf
Basic Recipe:

1 cup pearled barley

3 cups water or stock

1 T. canola oil

1 T. olive oil

1 large onion

4 cloves garlic

3/4 cup shiitake, portabello, or brown
   mushrooms

3/4 cup button mushrooms

2 cups loosely packed spinach, chard, or
   bok choy leaves

1/2 cup grated carrot

dash of black pepper

dash of cayenne pepper

2 T. pine nuts or sesame or sunflower seeds

sea salt, tamari, or Bragg's amino acids to
   taste

- Simmer barley in liquid for approximately 1 hour until tender.
- Saute onions and garlic in oils until brown.
- Add mushrooms; saute 5 more minutes.
- Add green veggie, seeds, carrot, and barley.
- Heat thoroughly until green veggie has wilted, but carrots are slightly crunchy.
- Remove from heat; add pepper and salty flavor to taste.

For a nice change of pace, add 1 T. grated organic orange peel after removing from heat.

Buckwheat Burgers
Basic Recipe:

1 cup cooked buckwheat

1-1/2 cups cooked garbanzos

1 medium-sized red onion, minced

1/2 cup finely minced celery

1/2 cup finely grated carrots

3 T. finely minced parsley

3+ cloves of garlic

1 T. ghee or canola oil

1/2 cup pumpkin or sunflower seeds

1/2 tsp. basil

1/2 tsp. thyme

1/2 tsp. marjoram

1/2 cup sourdough bread crumbs

1 to 2 tsp. Bragg's or tamari

1/4 tsp. cayenne pepper or black pepper
   to taste

1/3 cup water (approximately)

- Saute onion and garlic in oil.
- Add celery, carrots, and spices, continuing to braise for another 5 minutes.
- Mash garbanzos until smooth.
- Add all ingredients and mix with just enough water to moisten so that mixture is not sticky but rather stiff.
- Shape into patties.
- Place on oiled cookie sheet and bake in preheated oven at 375° until the top is slightly crisp.

Serve in pita bread with sprouts or smothered in shiitake-mushroom gravy.

YAMMY CABBAGE/APPLE SALAD
Basic Salad:

5 medium yams cut into 1"-circles
2 thinly sliced Red Delicious, Gala, or Granny Smith apples
1/2 cup shredded green cabbage
1/2 cup shredded red cabbage
2 thinly sliced scallions
1/4 cup thinly sliced celery
1/2 cup tamari toasted pumpkin or sunflower seeds

- Bring yams to boil in large saucepan over medium heat until tender (approx. 15 minutes).
- Drain yams and rinse under cold water; remove skin.
- Combine salad ingredients in serving bowl.

Dressing:

1/3 cup cranberries
1/2 cup canola oil
1/4 cup balsamic, red wine, or rice vinegar
2 T. parsley
2 T. lime or lemon juice
2 tsp. mustard
1 T. sucanat or maple syrup
sea salt and black pepper to taste

- Pulse cranberries and parsley in blender until chopped.
- Add remaining ingredients and pulse until smooth and creamy, but red cranberry flecks are still visible.
- Drizzle desired amount of dressing over salad.
- Top with toasted seeds.

BROTHER EARL'S HONEY-NUT GINGERBREAD
Basic Recipe:

1 cup organic apple juice
1/2 cup honey or maple syrup
2 whole fresh eggs, well beaten
1/3 cup canola oil or ghee
2 cups whole-wheat pastry flour
2 tsp. baking powder
1/2 tsp. baking soda
1 to 3 tsp. ginger powder
2 tsp. ground cinnamon
1/2 tsp. sea salt
1 cup chopped walnuts or pecans
3/4 cup presoaked raisins

- Preheat oven to 350°.
- Thoroughly cream oil and sweetener together.
- Gradually add apple juice.
- Mix all dry ingredients and sift over nuts and raisins.
- Add (thoroughly mixed) dry ingredients to liquid.
- Blend together, then pour batter into a square (oiled and floured) baking dish.
- Bake until firm in center (approx. 45 minutes).

Yummy—Serve warm!

YAM SPREAD
Basic Recipe:

3 to 4 medium-sized yams

2 T. almond or sesame butter

1 tsp. ground cinnamon

1/4 tsp. ground clove

1/4 tsp. nutmeg

dash of ground ginger

- Bake or steam yams.
- Remove skin.
- Mix in blender with other ingredients until creamy.
- Top with toasted almonds or sesame seeds.

KEFFI'S PATÉ
(SPECIAL THANKS TO THE OWNER OF THE FORMER KEFFI'S RESTAURANT FOR THIS RECIPE.) START THIS RECIPE THE NIGHT BEFORE YOU WISH TO SERVE IT.

Basic Recipe:

1 cup raw sunflower seeds

1 cup raw pumpkin seeds

4 cups spring water

squeeze of lemon juice

1/2 cup red onion

1 T. basil

2 T. Bragg's liquid amino acids, tamari, or soy sauce

freshly ground black pepper to taste

- Rinse seeds well, then place in quart jar with 4 cups spring water.
- Soak at least 12 hours.
- Discard water and rinse well.
- Blend all ingredients in food processor.

This will become a favorite! Serve with your favorite crackers or flatbread.

TIERRA'S MINERAL-RICH SEASONING SALT
Basic Recipe:

1 tsp. each of the following herbs: garlic powder, parsley, basil, thyme, oregano, marjoram, kelp or dulse powder, nettle, rosehips, capsicum, 1/4 tsp. dandelion root powder and burdock root powder

Experiment and invent your own!

MOCHI (A TRADITIONAL JAPANESE NEW YEAR'S TREAT)
Basic Recipe:

2 cups sweet brown mochi rice

4 cups water

pinch sea salt

(Optional flavorings)

1 T. vanilla, or

1 T. cinnamon, or

3 T. chopped, roasted almonds

Toppings:

raisins

pumpkin or sesame seeds

cinnamon

- Wash and drain rice.
- Add water, bring to boil.
- Reduce heat and let simmer until done; add flavorings.
- Gather friends or family around table and take turns pounding mochi with a mortar and pestle.
- The consistency becomes sticky and taffy-like (the smoother the better).
- Form cookie-sized shapes and press them on a well-oiled cookie pan.
- Decorate with pumpkin seeds, raisins, sesame seeds, etc.
- Bake in preheated oven at 400° for approximately 20 minutes or until they have puffed up and are crispy on top.

Mochi is a wonderful winter treat eaten by the Japanese to warm the body and increase stamina. Japanese monks could work all day, experiencing no fatigue, by eating one small piece of mochi in the morning. If you elected to make the preceding recipe, it is possible to dry part of the mixture on a cookie sheet, then store it in the refrigerator for later use; it will look and feel like cardboard, but not to worry—once heated up, it regains its moist, chewy texture.

If you weren't adventurous, however, Mochi is available in most health-food stores and comes in a variety of flavors including mugwort, garlic, plain, and cinnamon-raisin. It can be baked, then split open and filled with your favorite spread (try sesame tahini mixed with barley miso; or a date stuffed with a walnut and miso). A piece of mochi can be placed in a heated waffle iron to create a mochi waffle. Or small pieces of mochi can be added to soups to create "dumplings."

Mochi has a warming yang energy that is especially helpful for vegetarians, persons with sensitive digestive systems, or those who are overly tired and weak. Mochi is contraindicated for persons who are carbohydrate sensitive, unless consumed with sufficient protein and fat to counteract its insulin-inducing qualities (it falls around 100 on the glycemic index).

WINTER KICHAREE
Basic Recipe:

10 cups spring water	• Rinse grains well.
1/2 cup red lentils or masoori dahl	• Saute onion, burdock, and garlic in ghee.
1 cup millet or brown rice	
1/2 cup basmati rice	• Add cumin, coriander, turmeric, asafoetida, and mustard seed; saute for 2 to 3 more minutes.
2 T. ghee or canola oil	
1 large onion, minced	
8 to 10 garlic cloves, minced	• Add water and grains, astragalus, ginger, saffron, nettles, arame.
1 burdock root, thinly sliced	
2 pieces of astragalus root	• Simmer for 45 to 60 minutes on low heat.
2 carrots, sliced	
2 cups butternut or kabocha squash (leave the skin on the kabocha)	• Add carrots, squash, parsley, and black and cayenne pepper.
5 slices of fresh ginger (1/2 inch thick)	• Check if kicharee needs more water, if so, add a cup.
4 T. parsley, minced	
2 T. fresh cilantro, minced	• Simmer another 30 minutes or until veggies are tender.
2 T. nettles	
2 tsp. mustard seed	• Remove from heat and add fresh cilantro and salt.
1 tsp. turmeric	
1/3 cup Arame seaweed	
1-1/2 tsp. coriander powder	
1-1/4 tsp. cumin powder	
1/4 tsp. saffron	
1/4 tsp. black pepper	
1/4 tsp. cayenne pepper	
pinch of asafoetida	
sea salt, Bragg's or tamari to taste	

Wonderful warming winter food that nourishes to the core—great for strengthening our Earth and Water Elements.

TIERRA'S DATE DELICACY (A RELATIVELY HARMLESS HOLIDAY TREAT!)
Basic Recipe:

12 to 24 madjool dates	• Rinse dates and walnuts; dry them well.
12 to 24 walnut halves	
aged barley miso	• Remove pit from dates and spread a small amount of miso inside the date—anywhere from 1/4 to 1/2 tsp. each (to taste).
	• Split the walnut half down the middle and arrange the pieces longitudinally in the center of the date.

WHOLE-GRAIN COOKING CHART

One Cup Dry Grain	Water	Cooking Time	Yield
Amaranth	3 cups	30 minutes	2 1/2 cups
Barley	3 cups	1 1/4 hour	3 1/2 cups
Brown rice	2 cups	1 hour	3 cups
Buckwheat	2 cups	15 minutes	2 1/2 cups
Bulgur wheat	2 cups	15–20 minutes	2 1/2 cups
Millet	3 cups	45 minutes	2 1/3 cups
Polenta	4 cups	25 minutes	3 1/2 cups
Wild rice	3 cups	1 hour	4 cups
Wheat berries	3 cups	2 hours	2 2/3 cups
Quinoa	2 cups	15 minutes	2 1/2 cups

WHOLE-BEAN COOKING CHART

One Cup Dry Beans	Water	Cooking Time	Yield
Aduki	3 cups	45 minutes	3 cups
Black beans	4 cups	1 1/2 hour	2 cups
Black-eyed peas	3 cups	1 hour	2 cups
Garbanzos	4 cups	3 hours	2 cups
Kidney beans	3 cups	1 1/2 hours	2 cups
Lentils and split peas	3 cups	45 minutes	2 1/4 cups
Baby lima beans	2 cups	1 1/2 hours	1 3/4 cups
Pinto beans	3 cups	2 1/2 hours	2 cups
Red beans	3 cups	3 hours	2 cups
Small white beans	3 cups	2 1/2 hours	2 cups
Soybeans	4 cups	3 hours	2 cups

ROAD TO RECOVERY SHOPPING LIST

Whole Grains
- ❏ Millet
- ❏ Brown Rice
- ❏ Basmati Rice
- ❏ Kamut
- ❏ Spelt
- ❏ Barley
- ❏ Corn
- ❏ Oatmeal
- ❏ Buckwheat
- ❏ Amaranth
- ❏ Quinoa
- ❏ Kashi (Mixed grains)
- ❏ Brown Sweet Rice
- ❏ White Basmati
- ❏ Seitan (Wheat Meat)

Beans
- ❏ Aduki
- ❏ Red Lentil
- ❏ Red Dahl
- ❏ Mung
- ❏ Red Kidney
- ❏ Anasazi
- ❏ Pinto
- ❏ Green/Brown Lentils
- ❏ Garbanzo
- ❏ White Navy
- ❏ Lima
- ❏ Peas
- ❏ Black Beans
- ❏ Tofu
- ❏ Tempeh

Sea Veggies
- ❏ Arame
- ❏ Dulse
- ❏ Nori
- ❏ Kombu
- ❏ Hiziki
- ❏ Nori
- ❏ Wakame
- ❏ Kelp
- ❏ Sea Palm
- ❏ Agar Agar

Other Items
- ❏ Umeboshi Plums
- ❏ Kuzu Root Powder
- ❏ Bancha (Twig) Tea
- ❏ Ginger Root

Root Veggies and Winter Squash
- ❏ Burdock
- ❏ Carrot
- ❏ Parsnip
- ❏ Onion
- ❏ Garlic
- ❏ Scallion
- ❏ Leek
- ❏ Turnip
- ❏ Rutabaga
- ❏ Yam
- ❏ Radish
- ❏ Butternut
- ❏ Acorn
- ❏ Kabocha
- ❏ Delicata
- ❏ Spaghetti
- ❏ Hubbard
- ❏ Pumpkin
- ❏ Beet
- ❏ Daikon Radish
- ❏ Lotus Root
- ❏ Jerusalem Artichoke

Leafy Greens and Veggies
- ❏ Broccoli
- ❏ Parsley
- ❏ Nettles
- ❏ Cauliflower
- ❏ Cabbage
- ❏ Watercress
- ❏ Cilantro
- ❏ Celery
- ❏ Zucchini
- ❏ Arugula
- ❏ Kale
- ❏ Dandelion
- ❏ Mustard
- ❏ Bok Choy
- ❏ Artichoke
- ❏ Asparagus
- ❏ Chard
- ❏ Purslane
- ❏ Spinach

Local Fruits and Nuts/Seeds
- ❏ Apple
- ❏ Pear
- ❏ Peach
- ❏ Cherry
- ❏ Berries
- ❏ Grapes
- ❏ Kiwi
- ❏ Lime
- ❏ Orange
- ❏ Grapefruit
- ❏ Lemon
- ❏ Almond
- ❏ Walnut
- ❏ Pistachio
- ❏ Pine Nut
- ❏ Chestnut
- ❏ Sunflower
- ❏ Pumpkin
- ❏ Sesame
- ❏ Peanuts

Nightshades
- ❏ Chile Peppers
- ❏ Tomatoes
- ❏ Potatoes
- ❏ Bell Peppers

Dairy
- ❏ Hard Cheese
- ❏ Feta
- ❏ Yogurt
- ❏ Cottage Cheese
- ❏ Soft Cheese
- ❏ Goat Cheese
- ❏ Milk

Animal Products
- ❏ Eggs
- ❏ Beef
- ❏ Turkey
- ❏ Fish
- ❏ Lamb
- ❏ Pork
- ❏ Chicken
- ❏ Shellfish

Sweeteners (Use sparingly)
- ❏ Rice Syrup
- ❏ Barley Malt
- ❏ Maple Syrup
- ❏ Molasses
- ❏ Honey
- ❏ Sucanat
- ❏ Fructose

Oils
- ❏ Olive
- ❏ Canola
- ❏ Sesame
- ❏ Ghee
- ❏ Safflower
- ❏ Sunflower
- ❏ Flax
- ❏ Soybean

Tropical Fruits
- ❏ Mango
- ❏ Papaya
- ❏ Passion Fruit
- ❏ Banana
- ❏ Coconut

Chapter 6

Simple Ways to Understand the Nature of Your Disease

Before we talk about the nature of disease, herbs, and food, we need to distinguish two different ways of treating disease—*symptomatically* in the West versus *energetically* in traditional Oriental healing arts. Then you'll get to meet two of my patients; both suffer from the same chronic disharmony. Next you'll be given a few basic rules—the one plus one of Traditional Oriental Medical diagnoses, which gives you three different ways to understand the nature of your unique body type and its tendencies toward imbalance or disease:

1. The adventure starts with *qi! What is qi* and why is it that sometimes only one lemon in a bag full of lemons becomes covered with greenish-white mold?

2. You'll take a simple quiz to interpret the yin/yang balance of your individual constitutional type; then we'll discuss

3. The yin/yang energies of the herbs and foods that can help you restore balance.

WINNING STRATEGY: TREATING ENERGIES VERSUS SYMPTOMS OF DISEASE

Traditional Oriental Medicine is based on the concept of matching exactly the right energy of the treatment or herb to the constitution and disease of the person afflicted.

While most "herbal cures" are not always miraculous, well-directed herbal treatment based on energetics can produce some dramatic results. One recent case immediately comes to mind. Helen, a 49-year-old biologist, came to me in February 1997, seeking help for what she termed "lifelong" chronic sinusitus. She had exhausted the plethora of Western treatments including pharmaceutical drugs, allergy tests, and shots. She also complained of low energy, frequent headaches, sore throats, low immunity, bloating, and difficulty in breathing through blocked nasal passages that were constantly dry, raw, and encrusted. Herbal treatment was geared to correct her energetic imbalances. After one month of weekly visits, Helen mentioned a walnut-sized cyst on the back of her head for the first time; it had been her companion for more than 25 years. She was amazed that the cyst had reduced in size by at least 60 percent over the past four weeks of acupuncture and herbal treatment. Also, for the first time in years, her nasal passages were no longer raw and encrusted. While we had not addressed the issue of the cyst directly, in treating the overall energetic imbalances, Helen's body was able to rally and start healing the underlying problem that was responsible for creating the cyst and all her other symptoms. It is amazing what the human body can do for itself once it receives the proper nutrients in the form of special herbs and foods.

Like me, most practitioners of Traditional Oriental Medicine treat energetically. What exactly does this mean?

First, let's talk about treating something simple like a headache symptomatically. We often take an aspirin or other pain relievers simply to get rid of the pain, which is a valid intervention. No one likes pain. If we happen to be a Western herbalist, we might take willow bark, meadowsweet, or perhaps rosemary, in one form or another (all are sources of salicin, which converts to salicylic acid in the stomach—the pain-relieving component found in aspirin). In either case, pharmaceutical or herbal, we are treating the headache symptomatically. We give the same herb or drug to every person regardless of the person's age, state of health, or unique genetic characteristics.

CREATING FAIR WEATHER IN OUR HUMAN GARDEN

In the West, pain is viewed as the enemy. We take pharmaceuticals to relieve the discomfort and help us forget it was there in the first place. To the contrary, in traditional healing systems we view pain as an important messenger. It is trying to tell us something about our bodies. Serious illness does not just come to us one day out of the blue. The first signs that a storm is brewing in our human garden include such symptoms as minor aches, pains, and headaches as well as fatigue, indigestion, feeling chilled or flushed, nervousness, irritability, depression, listlessness, frustration, or forgetfulness. We can take pain relievers to ease the discomfort, but we also need to address the imbalance responsible for creating the problem. If not, we are setting the stage for more serious symptoms (the equivalent of torrential rains) to set in, such as insomnia, sinusitis, allergies, frequent colds and flu, chronic aches and pains, PMS, skin eruptions, high blood pressure, high cholesterol, and mood swings with emotional outbursts, to mention a few. Unfortunately, too many of us get caught up in the turmoil of just trying to make ends meet—we put off that badly needed vacation and paint our house instead. Sound familiar? After trying for years to warn us that something is not right, our body finally succumbs to the hurricane—a serious illness in the form of diabetes, arthritis, cancer, heart disease, . . . the list goes on.

To the contrary, in the Orient, a headache is not just a headache. Where the pain is located (temples, forehead, behind the eyes, top of the head, or occipital region) gives an indication of the organ system responsible for the discomfort. For example, headaches in the forehead region could indicate an imbalance in the Stomach Organ System. A dull pain in the forehead points to Stomach Deficiency, while a sharp pain can mean Stomach Heat. Sharp, throbbing pain above the ears and in the temples is referred to as Liver-Fire, Liver-Yang, or Liver-Wind Rising. This area corresponds to the Gall Bladder acupuncture meridian. Chronic headaches in the occiput, or back of the head, is often due to Kidney Deficiency. A headache that occurs only on the top of the head is often due to Deficient Liver-Blood. In Oriental herbology we might give dandelion or cyperus to someone with sharp throbbing pain in the temples to help decongest the liver; cinnamon to eliminate weakness associated with the Kidney-Deficiency headache, or a simple digestive aid such as ginger for the dull Stomach headache.

TWO WONDERFUL WOMEN— ONE CHRONIC DISEASE

Let me tell you about the lives of two wonderful people, patients who came to me for herbal and acupuncture treatment for rheumatoid arthritis. Because treatment for Barbara and Gloria was tailored for their unique body types, they received very different herbal formulas and dietary recommendations.

Western Medical Approach

Since we live in the West, let's first take a look at this crippling illness from the Western medical perspective. Rheumatoid arthritis is a chronic systemic disease that is characterized by joint inflammation resulting in crippling deformities. Causes offered by researchers include possible viral or bacterial origins or an auto-immune-system failure related to an antigen-antibody reaction. *Taber's Cyclopedic Medical Dictionary* states, "there is no specific therapy" for rheumatoid arthritis. Salicylates, such as aspirin, are the drugs most commonly used. Other drugs that are prescribed include anti-inflammatory agents such as Ibuprofen, corticosteroids, and gold compounds. Acute inflammation of synovial tissue of one or two joints may be treated by intra-articular injection of corticosteriods. Such local injections are usually effective for up to 21 days. The basic disease process is not halted by the local or systemic use of corticosteroids. The *American Medical Association Family Medical Guide* advises a patient, "The best thing you can do is to come to terms with what may be a permanent condition."

Because of their many side effects, including gastric ulcer, adrenal suppression and osteoporosis, corticosteroids should be prescribed with caution. The "natural, expected and unavoidable drug actions" of Prednisone, a potent drug of the cortisone class frequently used for major rheumatic disorders, include increased appetite, weight gain, retention or salt and water, and increased susceptibility to infection. While mild adverse effects can include skin rash, headache, insomnia, muscle cramping, and excessive growth of facial hair, serious adverse effects include, but are not limited to, mental and emotional disturbances of serious magnitude, increased blood pressure, development of peptic ulcer, pulmonary embolism, and the list goes on. Possible effects of long-term use include diabetes, thinning and fragility of the skin, osteoporosis, cataracts, increased fat deposits on the trunk of the body, and so on. Prednisone is also habit forming.

Oriental Healing Approach

Traditional Oriental healing systems offer many herbal formulations for the treatment of rheumatoid arthritis. Formulations are modified based on the practitioner's observation of the patient's unique constitutional characteristics. Since no two people are exactly alike, it follows that their illnesses are different, and therefore, treatments should reflect these differences. Let me tell you about just one basic herbal formulation known by the Chinese as I-Yi-Jen-Tang, or Coix Combination.

Coix Combination comes to us from the Tang dynasty, A.D. 618 to 906; it has been used for more than 13 centuries in the treatment of rheumatoid arthritis. This formulation is without side effects. Almost 33 percent of the formula consists of Coicis Lachryma-jobi seeds, known in English as Coix, or Job's Tears. In Traditional Oriental Medicine, the properties of Coix are considered to be sweet, bland, and cool. It is a grain and was eaten as a dietary staple in ages past, much as rice is eaten today. Medicinally, Coix is used for reducing edema, for increasing joint mobility, and for clearing "damp heat," and it is also indicated in the treatment of some digestive problems. Coix is but one of any number of safe, gentle herbs that are selectively prescribed based upon how the illness manifests itself in the individual.

Acupuncture, involving the insertion of thin stainless-steel needles into specific points on the body, as dictated by the patient's condition, can provide symptomatic pain relief and stimulate the body's natural healing forces. Many patients find the treatments incredibly relaxing, and, once again, there are no side effects.

Oriental medicine places much emphasis on prevention of disease, and the practitioner will recommend dietary changes and exercises to the patient. The mind/body complex is viewed as a whole in the Orient, an inseparable unity. Whatever affects the body will affect the mind, and anything affecting the mind will also affect the body. Therefore, patients are normally encouraged to ask questions or to express any concerns regarding treatment. They are also encouraged to discuss any personal problems that are creating stress in their lives. Healing is viewed as a partnership, and the patient is encouraged to actively participate in the treatment process.

Case History No. 1: Gloria

Gloria, a 23-year-old woman in her second year at a community college, first came to me in July 1991 requesting treatment for chronic rheumatoid arthritis. Gloria had been treated by a local rheumatologist for more than a year and was taking regular dosages of Prednisone, Plaquenil, and Motrin for symptomatic relief of the disease. Gloria's condition was diagnosed as Stage III, severe rheumatoid arthritis—all joints in her feet, hands, wrists, ankles, knees, elbows, neck, and right shoulder were affected. X-ray films showed evidence of cartilage and bone destruction, and a few soft-tissue nodules were evident in her fingers. Because Gloria's condition was not improving, her rheumatologist recommended the administration of gold therapy. When he described the side effects to Gloria (which included severe liver damage), she refused treatment and told him she wished to try some alternatives, perhaps herbal therapy. Gloria's rheumatologist said he would not work with her if she chose to undergo any alternative treatment.

Gloria came to me in this way, abandoned by her doctor and addicted to the Prednisone she had been taking for more than a year. She had gained 54 pounds as a result of the drug treatment. All her joints were badly swollen, with severe melanosis (blue discoloration) apparent in the joints of her hands, elbows, and knees. Melanosis is a side effect of Plaquenil.

As a result of her Mexican heritage, Gloria readily identified with herbal therapy and the traditional hot/cold classifications of disease and food. We agreed that Gloria would slowly reduce her Western meds over a ten-week period. In addition, she would make some dietary changes, adding seaweed, astragalus, coix, and aduki beans into the pinto beans her Mom served on a daily basis. She was to avoid all saturated fats and eliminate animal products from her diet. Gloria was given Du Huo Jisheng Wan (you can find this formula in Chapter 4) and instructed to take it at least two hours after taking her Western meds to avoid any drug and herbal interactions (though I have never seen any interactions, it is always better to be safe). She agreed to make the dietary changes and to increase her daily exercise.

In subsequent visits, we discussed Gloria's life prior to the onset of rheumatoid arthritis. Two years earlier, immediately after a disastrous earthquake in the area where Gloria lived, she experienced a severe case of conjunctivitis that went untreated for a prolonged period. We discussed other traumatic events in her life in great detail and how stress could be related to her disease.

Gloria followed advice on diet, exercise, and herbs to the letter. What a joy to watch the changes! At the end of ten weeks and after ten visits, Gloria had been off her Western meds for a week. She lost approximately ten pounds with joint swelling and melanosis improving significantly. At this point, she wrote the following note:

> I feel overjoyed at this stage in my life! The treatment plan I've followed—acupuncture, herbs, changing my diet and getting off Prednisone and Plaquenil has been a great success. My rheumatoid arthritis is now under control, and I am pain free.

I told Gloria she had graduated. Up to this point many hours were spent discussing how she could help herself, and now Gloria was capable of making the correct dietary and herbal decisions. She was given stronger herbal preparations with antibiotic effects, since the herbs would no longer be competing with the Western pharmaceuticals. She was told to call with any questions and make appointments on an as-needed basis. For the next year, Gloria chose to come in for follow-up every two to three weeks.

Twelve months after our first consultation all melanosis was gone, with only slight swelling remaining in some of Gloria's fingers and left ankle. Her weight had stabilized at its pre-Prednisone level (she had lost a total of 54 pounds). At this point in time, Gloria was a vibrant young lady who was able to go dancing just like any other 24 year old. She was participating in regular aerobics and yoga classes at the community college. Gloria brought her fiancé to a treatment session so we could meet. They were married in June 1992. In May 1993 she gave birth to a healthy nine-pound baby boy—no complications.

Case History No. 2: Barbara

Barbara, a 34-year-old Caucasian woman, hard-working mother of three young children, came to me in January 1993, suffering from an acute attack of rheumatoid arthritis—all joints in the neck, shoulders, arms, hands, hips, knees, and feet were badly swollen. Even though she was taking Vicodin and Voltaren to suppress pain, Barbara described the discomfort as "excruciating" and being unable to move any of her joints freely. Barbara had suffered from a similar acute attack approximately seven years previously. In addition to the Vicodin and Voltaren, Barbara's family doctor prescribed Plaquenil, which she took for a few days prior to seeking me out. Her doctor indicated he would be happy to work with an alternative health practitioner and forwarded all Barbara's health records to me immediately. Barbara's medical history indicated she had suffered from numerous strep infections the previous year.

Barbara's body is, constitutionally, quite different from the body of Gloria. In Traditional Oriental Medicine, Barbara is considered a Full Earth type, while Gloria is a Deficient Water/Fire type. Although Barbara and Gloria had been diagnosed as having the same disease, rheumatoid arthritis, the treatment would be quite distinct for both.

When we discussed diet, Barbara indicated she had been overindulging in fried fast foods, ice cream, sweets, and so on. Sweet foods tend to be the undoing of Earth types. I knew we had some work to do. (In my experience, many Americans do not take as easily to hot/cold designations of food and disease; it is not part of their culture. Americans have grown up with the body as machine metaphor, and they often hope to be "fixed" by the health practitioner.) The first two weeks were rough for both of us. We spent a couple of hours on the phone over weekends to answer questions, dispel fears, and help her pull through the crisis. The time was well spent.

To improve liver function, Barbara needed to detox quickly. I recommended one-day lemon-juice fasts followed by three days of unlimited quantities of whole grains, including coix, legumes, and homemade vegetable soups (which included seaweed) for the first three weeks. Barbara was to refrain from eating all saturated fats and animal products including eggs, milk, and cheese. Herbal formulas used were those aimed at purifying the blood (Planetary River of Life formula), and colon cleansing (an East Indian Ayurvedic formula known as Triphala); also included were natural antibiotics such as honeysuckle and forsythia; and Coix Combination (previously mentioned). Pueraria Combination was added at the end of the detox period.

Barbara discontinued Western pharmaceuticals at the end of the first week with her doctor's approval. She received acupuncture treatments twice weekly for the first three weeks, at the end of which time most of the pain had subsided and the swelling was greatly reduced.

Over the next five months, while eating abundantly of a healthy vegetarian diet, Barbara lost 30 pounds that had troubled her for a number of years. She came to truly enjoy the diet and was happy with the weight loss. All symptoms of rheumatoid arthritis were gone.

QI–YOUR BODY'S VITAL ENERGY

At the heart of Oriental healing systems you will find ideas regarding *qi* (pronounced "chee"). Qi forms the foundation of all Oriental thought and in its simplicity might be the hardest concept for Western minds to grasp. It's really not difficult once we understand why our thinking process fails to recognize its existence. Don't worry, this is really easy. In the West, our thinking is always in terms of either/or—*either* spiritual *or* physical—there is no continuum between these two realms. To the contrary, the Eastern mind sees a continuous, flowing spectrum from the invisible, or spiritual part of our universe to the concrete, or material world. There is no split.

Many modern chemists and physicists have actually bridged the spirit/matter chasm in Western thinking and see this remarkable universe as one gigantic energy field, somewhat as ancient Oriental philosophers did. So, we might say that qi is energy. Modern Big Bang theory explains the birth of our universe from a scientific perspective. We are told that the Universe burst into being approximately 15 billion years ago from a point 1/10th the size of a pin head. This infinitely dense and hot point in space exploded in the "Big Bang" and is responsible for creating our visible universe and reality as we know it today. Physicists tell us that all energy and matter were concentrated in that rapidly expanding primordial fireball, which doubled its size every second. All the stuff that stars are made of actually came into being as the universe began to cool down and condense into gaseous matter that later formed the heavier elements that became solid matter . . . and much, much later became your dog, your car, your kids, and you.

We could say that qi is matter taking shape and that matter is frozen or congealed qi. In the Orient, there is a tendency to view material manifestations and their transformations in this unitary way. Qi is the foundation of structure and, simultaneously, is also the catalyst for its transformation and movement. Qi governs the shape and activity of all animate and inanimate objects; in Oriental thought there is no differentiation between the two. In the same way qi governs the forming, organizing, and reshaping of earth, it envelops and permeates all of nature—a grain of sand, a lovely rose, an elephant, or the human body.

It's time to see how qi is actually defined in the Orient. According to Huang Ch'ao-Ch'uan, in his book called *K'an-yu ao pi* (or *Secrets of Siting*), "In the cosmos there is only a single Ch'i (qi). Light pure ch'i ascends and constitutes the sun, moon, planets, stars, winds, clouds, thunder and rain. Heavy, turbid ch'i descends and constitutes mountains, rivers, land and rock formations, lakes, seas and the Chiang and Ho [or the Yangtze and Yellow Rivers]. There is no moment at which the ch'i of the sky does not move downward to contact that of the earth, and no moment at which that of the earth does not rise up." All life between heaven and earth, as we know it, is dependent upon this interaction of heavenly and earthly qi.

Lemons, Qi, and You

So, now, let's get basic. What in the world does qi have to do with a lemon? And for that matter, what does it have to do with you?.

Have you ever had 6 to 12 lemons piled together in a bag or bowl, then, when you pick up a few to make a pitcher of lemonade notice that one of them is totally covered in greenish-white mold? You examine all the lemons and notice that, for some reason, only one of them is moldy. Why didn't more of the other lemons that were directly in contact with the fuzzy monster also succumb to the mold? Oriental medicine can explain this neatly. The life energy, or Defensive Qi of the moldy lemon was not strong enough to fight off the green invader. If you suffer from frequent colds, flus, or fatigue, you are suffering from Deficient Protective Qi in Oriental thought. Just like that poor moldy lemon, your body's qi is not strong enough to fight off unwanted visitors.

As we have delved into Oriental healing with herbs, you have seen the word *qi* a lot, along with the words *yin* and *yang* (pronounced yong as in *song*). It does not do justice to these three words even to try to translate them into a word in English. Now let's get a better idea of the yin and yang of things and what that means in your life.

YIN/YANG BALANCE
YOUR KEY TO PERFECT HEALTH

It's time to play pretend. This yin/yang stuff is really not as foreign as it sounds and is actually pretty practical. By the end of the chapter you will begin to understand why it is the key to perfect health. Let's take ourselves back in time some 10,000 years ago: We're Chinese rice farmers living on the eastern-facing slopes of a low mountain range; if you listen carefully you can hear the sounds of the wide river that cuts through our lush green valley below. We have chosen to build our hut on the eastern slope of the mountain in order to catch the first warming rays of the sun as it peeks up over the horizon at dawn. With the sun comes warmth, light, and the day's activities. In Chinese characters, *Yang* corresponds to the sunny side of our mountain as well as to light, sun, brightness, heat, dryness, activity, and heaven.

Evening approaches and our day's activities come to a halt as the sun slowly sinks into the mountain range behind us. First we experience cooling shade, twilight, and then absolute darkness—the incredible stillness of the night. It's time to rest as the moon and stars move across the vault of the midnight sky and a mysterious mist rises from the river below. *Yin,* in Chinese characters, corresponds to the shady side of our mountain, darkness, moon, coolness, moisture, rest, and earth.

From observing nature's two opposite stages in time—day and night—we form the foundation of how we see the world. Every phenomenon in our universe is perceived in this way—two opposing, yet interdependent and complementary pairs of opposites. Without day we could not have night; without light we could not have darkness; without rest we cannot have activity. The very nature of our universe is determined by the interaction of these two forces. Yin and yang are constantly interacting, re-forming each other, in a never-ending cosmic dance. Mountains (yang), coupled with waters (yin) form a single unit—completeness. Balance or harmony, in Oriental thought, means the proportions of the yin principle (represented by water, cold, dark, passive, receptive, female) and the yang principle (mountains, high, light, active, aggressive, male) are relatively balanced; disharmony indicates the proportions are unequal. However, the balance is dynamic and constantly changing, like our cyclical universe, from day to night, from winter to spring, from summer to fall.

Qualities of Yin and Yang

Yin	Yang
Cold	Hot
Moist	Dry
Night	Day
Dark	Bright
Female	Male
Receptive	Active
Soft	Hard
Water	Fire
Inactive	Active
Matter	Energy
Space	Time
Earth	Heaven

It's important not to confuse Chinese yin/yang concepts with our Western black/white, good/bad bipolar thought of oppositions. There is little room for "black and white" in the Oriental view—yin simply could not and would not exist if it were not for yang. In Western thought, light is often considered superior to darkness. In Oriental thought, however, Yang is not inherently better than Yin because it is associated with light. Yin and Yang are equal and complementary to each other, like two sides of the same coin. Following is the ancient yin/yang symbol called the "Supreme Ultimate." Note how there is a black circle in the white half of the symbol, indicating the seed of darkness in light and vice versa. There's a white circle in the black, yin half, indicating the seed of yang or light resides in yin.

If you would spin this ancient black and white yin/yang symbol like a top, then the true picture would emerge. As the symbol spins, in the cyclical fashion characteristic of Oriental thought, black and white blend in to ever-changing shades of gray.

At a recent workshop one participant questioned, "If the sun represents yang energy, then what yin characteristics could possibly be attributed to it?" This was a great question. The sun is composed of gaseous matter. Though the sun is infinitely hot and light, it still has some substance; that substance is its yin nature. Everything is composed of a combination of yin and yang characteristics. And everything is yin or yang relative to what it is being compared to. A rather calm, quiet, withdrawn man might be considered relatively "yin" when compared to a more "yang" assertive, talkative woman. There are four principles that explain the dynamic, ever-changing relationship between Yin and Yang: (1) All phenomena contain two innate opposing aspects; (2) Yin and Yang are co-dependent; (3) Yin and Yang nurture each other; and (4) Between Yin and Yang there exists a transformative potential.

We are about ready to move on to the fun stuff, discovering the yin and yang of you, of your disease, and of the herbs that can help. However, no book on Oriental herbalism would be complete without the following Laws and Theorems of Yin and Yang. Don't let the words "laws" or "theorems" intimidate you. You might want to read them over a couple of times; it's amazing how much the theorems sound like principles from a beginning chemistry class (simply substitute "positive charge" for yang and "negative charge" for yin).

Laws Governing Yin and Yang

1. All things are the differentiated apparatus of One infinity.

   (A much easier way to say this might be: "All of creation comes from One Source.")

2. Everything changes.

3. All antagonisms are complementary.

4. No two things are identical.

5. Every condition has its opposite.

6. Extremes always produce their opposite.

7. Whatever begins has an end.

Theorems of Yin and Yang

1. Infinity divides itself into Yin and Yang.
2. Yin and Yang result from the infinite movement of the universe.
3. Yin is centripetal (spirals inward) and Yang is centrifugal (spirals outward); together they produce all energy and phenomena.
4. Yin attracts Yang and Yang attracts Yin.
5. Yin repels Yin and Yang repels Yang.
6. The force of attraction and repulsion between any two phenomena is proportional to the difference between their Yin/Yang constitution.
7. All things are ephemeral and changing their Yin/Yang constitution.
8. Nothing is neutral; either Yin or Yang is dominant.
9. Nothing is solely Yin or Yang; everything involves polarity.
10. Yin and Yang are relative; large Yin attracts small Yin, and large Yang attracts small Yang.
11. At the extremes of manifestation, Yin produces Yang and Yang produces Yin.
12. All physical forms are Yin at the center and Yang on the surface.

In the human body, the preceding list translates into the following: The head is yang relative to the feet, which are considered yin; your fingers are yang in relation to the palm of your hand; the front of your body is considered yin while your backside is yang; your internal organs are yin when compared to your skin, which is considered more yang. If we examine a piece of fruit (which is normally considered a yin food), the peach skin is considered yang in comparison to the peach flesh and pit, which are considered more yin. If we compare that peach to a watermelon, the watermelon is more yin than the peach because of its extremely watery nature.

Yin and Yang of You

Let's get down to figuring out the yin and yang of you and your loved ones. This is important because, energetically speaking, we don't want to treat your disease with yang (hot or warm) herbs if you are basically a yang individual with a yang disharmony (acute, feverish condition). We need to cool you down. However, watch out, because cold herbs could be too extreme for your system. Likewise, if you are constitutionally a more yin person with a chronic, cold condition (such as frequent colds with chills), then we do not want to give you cooling herbs. Something of a warm nature would be more appropriate.

HOT AND COLD CLASSIFICATION OF DISEASES   We need to stop and talk a bit about Western misconceptions regarding the "Hot" and "Cold" classification of diseases used in many traditional healing systems. Just as simple rules regarding addition, subtraction, multiplication, and division form the basis for advanced scientific calculations, in the same way, concepts regarding Hot/Cold, Dry/Damp, Yin/Yang are simple metaphors used as a foundation for a complex and sophisticated healing system that is well over 23 centuries (written history) old.

In comparison, according to Western biomedicine's viewpoint, nature, and therefore human beings, are machines that are governed by mechanical laws. The human body is a machine whose parts can be removed, repaired, or replaced. This line of thinking reduces the human body to structural parts that the mechanic/doctor is able to remove or fix in isolation from other tissues or organs.

Traditional Oriental Medicine views the human body as a living, dynamic ecological system. Disease is described in terms of climates and weather conditions. A fever might be viewed as a "Heat" imbalance while chills could indicate a "Cold" imbalance. Puffiness or edema is considered a condition related to excess "Damp," while cracking of the skin and lips could be a sign of "Dryness." To take the symbolism a little deeper, let's reconsider the disease previously discussed. Rheumatoid arthritis, in many cases, would be described as "Damp Heat Obstructing the Joints." This description is really not so far from the Western conception if you remember that "Heat" for the practitioner of Oriental treatment principles refers to inflammation, and "Dampness" refers to fluid accumulation or retention. To translate the Traditional Chinese Medical (TCM) diagnosis to Western terms based on treatment principles, it could be said that rheumatoid arthritis is viewed as a weakening of the autoimmune system, which was (in many cases) precursed by a severe and lingering infection leading to inflammation and swelling of the joints.

It's time for you to become acquainted with some of this language and how it relates to you and your loved ones. Following is a simple test for you to take in order to determine your basic yin/yang constitutional type. Circle the description that best describes your natural tendencies; then write the corresponding number that appears in the column above your selection (0, 25, 50, 75, or 100) on the blank line provided to the right. Total your score. Just to double-check, review your answers with a friend or family member. Frequently, we do not realize if we have a faint or a loud voice.

THE YIN AND YANG OF YOU!

	YIN			YANG		
	●	◐	🌍	🔥	☀	*Record*
	Cold	Cool	Neutral	Warm	Hot	
Possible						
Score	*0*	*25*	*50*	*75*	*100*	*TOTAL*
Character	Withdrawn	Quiet	Somewhere in-between	Assertive	Aggressive	____
Build	Emaciated or heavy and Flabby	Thin	Average	Muscular	Large and Robust or Thin and Wiry	____
Activity	Lethargic	Little Movement	Normally Active	Animated	Hyperactive	____
Posture	Limp	Hunched Over	Relaxed	Erect	Rigid	____
Voice	Whisper	Faint	Moderate	Strong	Loud	____
Body Odors	Extremely Faint	Faint	Mild	Strong	Very Strong	____
Breathing	Soft Sighs	Light and Shallow	Normal	Stretching and Loud Sighing	Heavy and Loud	____
Mucus	Clear and Copious	Thin and Clear or White	White, Slight,	Thick White, Yellow, or Green	Thick Dark Yellow or Red	____
*Urine Color	Clear	Very Pale Yellow	Golden	Dark Yellow	Very Dark Orange or Red	____
Stool	Light Colored, Very Loose	Light and Slightly Formed	Medium	Firm and Slightly Dark	Dark and Hard	____
				Add to Determine TOTAL SCORE:		____

0 to 199:   Yipes, you're ready to go into hibernation! Concentrate on neutral to warm foods and herbs. Gradually introduce those of a "Hot" nature—they could present a shock to your constitution.

200 to 349:   You are definitely running a little cool. Concentrate on neutral to hot herbs and foods to bring yourself into balance.

350 to 649:   You are basically in balance and can choose herbs and foods ranging from "Cold" to 'Hot' depending upon the current condition.

650 to 799:   You are definitely running on the warm side. Concentrate on neutral-to-cold herbs and foods to bring yourself back into balance.

800 to 1000:   Hot chile peppers! A two-week vacation in the Antarctic might be in order! Concentrate on neutral-to-cool foods and herbs, gradually introducing those of a "Cold" nature. They could present a shock to your constitution.

B Vitamins Color Your Urine Yellow—Discontinue Them for a Few Days to Verify the True Color.

YIN AND YANG OF HERBS AND FOODS

Now that you've arrived at your yin/yang balance in the ever-changing dance of life, you need to know how to arrive at correct decisions as to which herbs and foods will help bring you back to balance.

Yin foods usually include those that grow and mature quickly such as zucchini, watermelon, or peaches. They tend to be large, soft, or leafy vegetables, leaves, flowers, and fruits or fast-growing roots such as carrot, turnip, or sweet potato. An herb or food that is considered "yin" cools and moistens the body. *Most yin herbs and foods have a tranquilizing or relaxing effect. Yang foods and herbs, on the other hand, are warming, energizing, and increase circulation.* Most herbs in the "yang" category grow more slowly than their yin counterparts. They are smaller, more hard, and compact. Yang herbs are frequently slow-growing roots such as ginseng, root bark, or tree bark like cinnamon. Yang foods include most of the acid-forming foods such as meat and dairy products, grains (with the exception of millet), and eggs.

Often, herbs found growing in warm climates (like the tropics and subtropics) are flowers and fruits that tend to be more yin or cooling and eliminating in nature. Nature provides what the human body requires for the climate in which it lives. People living in warmer climates need cooling nutrients to help cool the body down. In contrast, people living in cold climates require warming nutrients, and this is exactly where you find compact, warming yang roots and herbs such as ginseng (in Siberia) or heat-producing, nutrient-dense foods such as elk and caribou in Alaska.

In Chapter 3, you found 108 herbs with recommendations for herbal treatment based on symptoms, as well as herbal treatment based on herbal energetics. I urge you to take a little time to play with the idea of herbal energetics. While treating with herbs symptomatically can produce some really great results, the treatment is bound to be much more profound, with lasting effects, if you treat the whole person versus treating the condition.

Chapter 7

EASY WAYS TO DECIDE WHICH HERBS/FOODS WILL HEAL YOU AND YOUR FAMILY

Experiencing stormy weather in your human garden? Sunny skies might be just as close as a warm cup of ginger or peppermint tea. As an aspiring herbalist, in this chapter you are going to begin mastering some basic principles of herbalism. You already learned some of the most fundamental rules in preceding chapters, and now we gradually build on that foundation. The description accompanying each of the herbs in Chapter 3 talks about the herb's usage to relieve symptoms as well as the herb's energetics. If you decide to go no further and simply want to try to match the herb with the symptom, you will have some success. In Chapter 6, however, you learned the "one plus one" of treating energetically with herbs. This involves determining the yin/yang balance of your constitution, your discomfort, and then selecting the herbs that might help.

In this chapter, we expand the yin (cold)/yang (hot) principles in order to (1) Classify nutrients according to their 4 Natures. Then on to (2) "4 Directions" in Treating Acute versus Chronic Discomforts, where you will learn how to direct herbs and foods to the parts of the body in need of healing energy. If you decide to stop there, you will have gained an invaluable foundation for helping yourself and your family with well-targeted, gentle herbal healers. If you would like to get into the "multiplication and division" of herbalism, however, you'll want to (3) Enter the world of the master herbalist who knows How to Direct Healing Herbs to the "Organ and Meridian Systems Affected." The last section in this chapter, (4) Quick Reference Guide to the 18 Categories of Herbs in Traditional Oriental Herbalism, is a bridge between two different worlds. The poetic Oriental "body as garden" view of disease is translated into our Western symptomatic language. It's not difficult and really starts to make lots of sense once you begin to view your body as an ecological system versus viewing it as a machine.

UNDERSTANDING THE "FOUR NATURES" OF NUTRIENTS

Ancient healing systems such as Traditional Oriental Medicine and East Indian Ayurveda classify foods and herbs according to their nature or effect on the human body. Traditionally, the "Four Natures" of nutrients are (1) Cold, (2) Cool, (3) Warm, and (4) Hot. Yin-natured nutrients are cold or cool foods and herbs; and Yang nutrients are considered hot or warm in nature. In actuality, a number of herbs and foods are only very slightly cooling or warming. They are considered mild or neutral in nature and can be used to treat either hot or cold diseases. If this sounds familiar—it is! You got the basis for this in Chapter 6, and now we're just going to build on it. In Chapter 3, all herbs were coded with the following five symbols to indicate their nature:

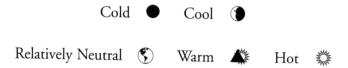

Cold ●   Cool ◐

Relatively Neutral 🜨   Warm 🔺   Hot ☀

Always treat substances at the extremes of hot and cold with great respect. These nutrients usually have strong medicinal qualities and are not meant for long-term, everyday ingestion except in herbal formulas that are energetically balanced. Even then, most herbalists recommend that you take long-term herbal formulas six days a week and rest the seventh; others recommend that you take them only five days a week and rest two. Formulas for chronic conditions may be taken three months at a time, rest two weeks, and repeat if indicated. More often, however, it is appropriate to change formulas on a seasonal basis to make up for the changing weather conditions. Always discontinue Tonifying herbs and formulas if you come down with an acute condition such as a cold or flu, sore throat, and so forth.

"FOUR DIRECTIONS" IN TREATING ACUTE VERSUS CHRONIC DISCOMFORTS

Have you ever taken a bite of hot Chinese mustard while enjoying a delicious Oriental dinner? Did you notice how all of the energy seemed to go directly to your head? Your nasal passages cleared immediately, your eyes started tearing, and quite possibly your ears turned red and felt fiery hot. All substances that we ingest affect us in one way or another, but less dramatically. "Hot" or "warm" Yang foods and herbs (like that Chinese mustard) have a tendency to move upward in the body while "cold" or "cool" yin substances move downward.

Remember the energies of the Five Seasons? As the creative energy of springtime surges upward, the sap rises in the trees. For this reason, the *ascending direction* is associated with yang energy and springtime. Summer is the most yang, or full yang time of year, where the ascending energy of springtime has reached its maximum potential—the sap can't rise any higher! Shortly, the cycle must change—energy, or the sap, is just kind of floating at the top, waiting for the seasonal transition. Therefore, *floating is the direction* assigned to summer. Lighter herbs, such as flowers and leaves (so abundant in spring and summer) are used to treat many yang diseases. These substances are useful for treating more acute disharmonies such as everyday colds, flus, and inflammations. For example, in Oriental herbalism, honeysuckle flowers and forsythia fruit, both herbal antibiotics, are often used to treat acute yang infections and inflammations such as sore throats, minor infections, and inflammations.

In autumn (the cool, yin, time of year) the sap begins to descend once again; the *direction associated with fall is descending.* The most yin time of year, however, is the cold winter season; the sap has sunk. Therefore, the *direction associated with winter is sinking.* Roots and barks (heavier substances) have the tendency to carry energies deeper. The descending and sinking energies of these substances are more useful in treating chronic diseases.

The chart on the following page is intended as a general guideline into the yin/yang, cooling and warming energies of herbs and foods. Remember that in the yin/yang continuum there are no hard and fast rules—everything is relative to what it is being compared to. That is why it is of great benefit to also take into consideration the inherent energy and flavor of an herb to determine its primary action, which takes us even deeper into herbal energetics as we learn to balance the "5 Flavors" and direct their healing energies to the affected organ systems.

ENERGETICS OF HERBS AND FOODS

	YIN *Chronic*			YANG *Acute*	
Cold	Cool	Neutral	Warm	Hot
Winter	Fall	Doyo	Spring	Summer
Sinking	Descending	Center	Ascending	Floating

Fruits/Flowers/Leaves/Fast Growing Roots/Seeds/Twigs/Barks/Slow Growing Roots

mineral salts   bitter   sour   bland   full sweet   hot spicy or pungent

fruit/leafy veggies/root veggies/seaweed/beans/grains/milk products/fish/fowl/red meat

HOW TO DIRECT HEALING HERBS TO THE "ORGAN AND MERIDIAN SYSTEMS AFFECTED"

Traditional Chinese Medicine connects foods and herbs to specific organic effects and classifies them according to the acupuncture organ systems and meridian pathways they influence. In Oriental thought, the organ systems are connected, interdependent, and constantly influencing each other. This is different from our Western view that separates, analyzes, and defines the specialized functions of each organ, such as the heart, kidney, or liver, apart from the rest of the body/machine.

Let's take a look at the Wood Element that governs the *Liver (yin organ)* and *Gallbladder (yang organ)* acupuncture pathways. Remember that the green of young plants in springtime is the color associated with Wood, as is the sour flavor. Most green, leafy foods and herbs that promote the release of bile and help calm hypertension are believed to influence the Liver/Gallbladder Organ System and acupuncture pathways.

Spring is followed by the heat of summer, which is associated with the red color, bitter flavor, and the *Heart (yin)/Small Intestine (yang)* and *Pericardium (yin)/Triple Warmer (yang) Organ Systems* and acupuncture meridians. Most herbs that are bitter, red, and help clear cholesterol from the arteries and veins affect the Fire Element organs and acupuncture pathways. The Small Intestine (where much of our digestion and assimilation of food actually occurs) is the yang organ that counterbalances the yin Heart. Bitter herbs that aid digestion and halt disharmonies that may produce blood in the urine fall within this category as well.

Our Earth Element, which is associated with the full sweet flavor and orange/yellow color, rules digestion and assimilation of nutrients. The *Spleen/Pancreas (yin organs)* are counterbalanced by the *Stomach (yang organ)*. Nutritive, tonic, neutral, and warming herbs and foods influence the Spleen/Pancreas while more carminative herbs that aid digestion are associated with the Stomach Organ System.

The seasons cycle on into fall and the Metal Element, which is associated with the spicy or pungent flavor, the white color, and the *Lung (yin organ)* and *Colon (yang organ)* acupuncture meridians. In Oriental thought, the Lungs are associated with mucus production and rule the skin (our outer lung that helps remove body toxins through perspiration). Often, white, mucilaginous herbs are used to Tonify and Moisten the Lungs. Pungent or spicy herbs that are diaphoretic, or promote perspiration, are often given during the initial stages of colds and flus since these diseases are considered superficial. These herbs also help clear skin blemishes.

Winter invariably follows autumn and is associated with our Water Element and the *Kidney/Adrenal (yin)* and *Urinary Bladder (yang)* Organ Systems. Herbs that are heavy and dark in color influence these organs and corresponding acupuncture pathways. Those with nourishing, tonic, or aphrodisiac qualities are associated with the Kidney/Adrenals while lighter herbs with diuretic actions are used to influence the Urinary Bladder.

In Chapter 3, you will notice that each herb has a section titled "Healing Qualities of (the Herb's name)." In this section, the healing energies of each herb are listed according to traditional Oriental herbalism. First, the predominate flavors (sour, bitter, sweet, spicy, or salty) of the herb are listed; second comes the herb's nature (cold, cool, neutral, warm, or hot); third, you find the Element and Organ or Meridian System this herb affects; and, fourth you are given the healing category of the herb, which naturally leads us into our next topic: The "18 Categories of Herbs in Oriental Herbalism." This section is meant to be a quick reference guide as you begin to experiment with healing herbs. Don't get overwhelmed and don't expect to remember all the categories. You can't become a master herbalist in a day. That needn't stop you, however, from harnessing the healing power of some gentle herbal helpers; you'll find plenty of recipes and formulas in the preceding chapters. At first you might want to start by concentrating on those herbal categories that best seem to describe your own particular disharmonies.

QUICK REFERENCE GUIDE
TO THE EIGHTEEN CATEGORIES OF HERBS
IN TRADITIONAL ORIENTAL HERBALISM

1. Herbs that Release the Exterior

You know that "kinda-achy-all-over" before-the-flu-or-a-cold-sets-in feeling? When germs first make their appearance in our human garden, Oriental medicine says that the disease is at the first layer—the layer of the skin—and sweating will bring it out. The skin is considered the exterior of the body, so we turn to "Herbs that Release the Exterior" to promote sweating. Symptoms associated with exterior conditions are chills, fevers, general muscle aches, headache, or perhaps a stiff neck (called Wind-Cold, Wind-Heat, Wind-Dampness, or Summerheat in Oriental medicine).

When we are losing the battle and the invader penetrates a little deeper, the disease is said to be lodged in the muscles. Symptoms at this stage include general body aches, fevers, and profuse sweating. If the patient has perspired without any relief in his or her condition, it is important to turn to another group of herbs in this category that release the muscles. Cinnamon twigs is probably the most well-known herb used for this purpose.

Herbs that Release the Exterior are also used to stop coughing and wheezing, to control spasms and pain, and to help bring rashes (such as measles and other similar diseases) to the surface.

Herbs that Release the Exterior are divided into two types: (1) Warm and Acrid (Spicy) and (2) Cool and Acrid Herbs.

WARM, ACRID HERBS THAT RELEASE THE EXTERIOR   Ever had shivers associated with the chills? Those shivers are the Oriental equivalent of wind shaking the branches and leaves in our human garden. Warm, spicy herbs help eliminate Wind-Cold conditions such as mild fevers with severe chills, headache, body and neck pains, and absence of thirst.

See Chapter 3: Herbs in This Category include Cinnamon Twigs, Ephedra, Ginger (Fresh), Magnolia Flower, Schizonepeta, Siler

COOL, ACRID HERBS THAT RELEASE THE EXTERIOR   Cool, spicy herbs help eliminate Wind-Heat conditions in our human garden. Symptoms include mild chills with a severe fever and sore throat. Some of these herbs are also used to bring rashes to the surface (in order to move them from the interior to the exterior, or out of the body.) or in treating eye problems (such as red, itchy eyes associated with allergies).

For herbs in this category, see Chapter 3: Bupleurum, Chrysanthemum Flower, Cohosh, Kudzu, Peppermint

2. Herbs that Clear Heat

Herbs that Clear Heat, from a biomedical view, are anti-inflammatory, antimicrobial, and antipyretic (reduce fevers). Most of these herbs, divided into the following four distinct categories, are Cold in nature. In Traditional Oriental Medicine, Heat not only refers to febrile diseases but to any condition that shows Heat signs such as a dry throat, red eyes, yellow tongue coating, red face, dry stool, rapid pulse, or a sensation of heat in the palms of the hand, soles of the feet, or sternum (known as the "Five Centers"). Exterior Heat conditions refer to symptoms such as fever, chills, thirst, and moderate sweating, while Interior Heat conditions include thirst, dry mouth, scanty and dark urine, fever without chills, yellow tongue coating, abdominal distention, and diarrhea or constipation.

HERBS THAT QUELL FIRE   Herbs that Quell Fire are some of the coldest substances used in Oriental herbalism and are used for treating high fevers, delirium associated with febrile diseases, irritability, and thirst.

For herbs in this category, see Chapter 3: Anemarrhena, Gardenia

HERBS THAT COOL THE BLOOD   In Oriental Herbal Medicine, herbs that Cool the Blood are used for the most serious stage of an infectious disease, which should always be treated by a qualified health-care professional. At this stage, internal organs become inflamed and congested; common symptoms include nosebleed and spitting up blood. These herbs reduce fevers and promote coagulation of blood.

Herbs that Cool the Blood are also used for treating Heat symptoms that come as a result of deficiency; symptoms include low fevers in the afternoon or evening, night sweats, reddish or purple tongue, and dry throat.

For herbs in this category, see Chapter 3: Lycii Root Cortex, Moutan Cortex, Rehmannia (Raw), Scrophularia

HERBS THAT CLEAR HEAT AND DRY DAMP   Herbs from this group are used to clear Damp Heat. Imagine the steaming, murky waters in a jungle swamp, the perfect breeding ground for unfriendly microbes. Most herbs that help Clear the Heat and Dry the Dampness have cold, bitter properties and are anti-inflammatory, antimicrobial, and reduce fevers. This class of herbs is used for dysentery, furuncles, high fevers accompanied by sores and swellings with thick yellow pus, and painful urinary infections.

For herbs in this category, see Chapter 3: Coptis, Gentian, Phellodendron, Scutellaria

HERBS THAT CLEAR HEAT AND RELIEVE TOXICITY   This group of herbs is often used to treat hot, toxic swellings such as mastitis, appendicitis, pulmonary and breast abscesses, and certain viral infections such as mumps. You know that a swelling is Hot if it is painful. These herbs have antimicrobial and antiviral effects, reduce inflammation, and also have diuretic qualities.

For herbs in this category, see Chapter 3: Dandelion Root, Forsythia Fruit, Honeysuckle Flower

HERBS THAT CLEAR AND RELIEVE SUMMER HEAT   Summerheat is a condition that occurs primarily in the hot summer months and is associated with fever, diarrhea, sweating, thirst, and irritability. The herbs in this group reduce fevers, eliminate thirst, and produce fluids.

For herbs in this category, see Chapter 3: Mung Bean, Watermelon

3. Downward-Draining Herbs

Downward-Draining Herbs are those that (in Western terms) help unclog the drains—by moving retained stool through the intestines, relieving constipation. These herbs are divided into three groups whose therapeutic actions are quite different.

PURGATIVES   Most Purgatives are cold and bitter in nature and help relieve constipation due to Interior Heat and Interior Cold conditions. Interior Heat is usually the result of a febrile disease that depletes body fluids and causes constipation. Interior Cold is usually the result of weak intestinal function or lack of peristalsis to move the stool out of the body. In case of Interior Cold, it is extremely important to add herbs that warm Interior Cold to the herbal formula.

For herbs in this category, see Chapter 3: Aloe, Rhubarb Rhizome

MOIST LAXATIVES   Moist Laxatives are mild substances, usually seeds or nuts, that help move stool by lubricating the intestines. This type of laxative is appropriate for weak or elderly persons and for new moms, to aid elimination after childbirth.

For the herb in this category, see Chapter 3: Prune Seeds

HARSH EXPELLANTS   These strong laxative herbs are used only in severe cases of constipation. The violent effect of these strong substances induces diarrhea. They have diuretic properties and are used in the treatment of ascites and pleurisy.

Herbs in this category include pharbitis, euphorbia, and daphnes. They are not included in this text because of their toxic properties and should be administered only for a brief time by a qualified, licensed professional.

4. Herbs that Drain Dampness

In Traditional Oriental Medicine, Dampness refers to (1) edema and congested fluids that have accumulated in the body, particularly below the waist and in the legs and feet and (2) Damp-Heat with signs of Heat and Stagnation (dark or yellow secretions, fever, and burning sensations). In case of the second category, herbs that Drain Dampness are normally combined with herbs that Clear Heat and Dry Damp.

Since Draining Damp is a matter of increasing urination to relieve the accumulation of fluids in the body, many of these herbs are diuretics. It is extremely important that herbs in this group not be given to persons with depleted body fluids or Yin Deficiency.

For herbs in this category, see Chapter 3: Aduki Bean, Alisma, Coix, Poria Cocos, Stephania, Zhu Ling

5. Herbs that Dispel Wind-Dampness

In Traditional Oriental Medicine, joint and muscle pain and numbness is caused by Wind, Dampness, Cold, and Heat. The four types are distinguished as follows:

When the pain is caused mostly by Wind, the pain is migratory or moves from joint to joint. The image in Oriental thought might be of wind moving across the countryside, jostling branches and leaves.

If the pain is due to Cold, think of the contractive quality of ice—pain here is severe, fixed, aggravated by exposure to cold, and results in reduced joint mobility.

When there is Dampness in the body, the pain is fixed in location and results in numbing of the muscles and skin and swelling of the extremities.

The fourth type of disharmony is described as a Hot Painful Obstruction and results from an acute disorder. Symptoms include pain, heat and swelling of the joints, fever, thirst, and a yellow tongue coating.

Herbs in this group have analgesic properties, are anti-inflammatory, antipyretic, and promote circulation. Herbs are selected based on the location of the pain, the type of disorder (Wind, Cold, Damp, or Heat), the stage of the disease (acute or chronic), and the strength and age of the patient.

The application of herbal plasters and liniments, acupuncture, and massage therapy are all helpful tools in treating these conditions.

For herbs in this category, see Chapter 3: Clematis, Cocklebur Fruit, Du Huo

6. Herbs that Transform Phlegm and Stop Coughing

When we hear the word *phlegm* in the West, we think of the thick fluid that collects in our throat and lungs. In Oriental thought, however, phlegm accumulation is responsible for a number of disorders including epilepsy, simple goiter, chronic skin problems, chronic lymphadenitis, convulsions, and scrofula.

HERBS THAT COOL AND TRANSFORM PHLEGM-HEAT   This group of herbs is cold in nature and is used to treat Phlegm-Heat and Dry-Phlegm conditions including coughs, scrofula, goiter, and convulsions (due to Phlegm-Heat). Included in this group are anti-inflammatory, expectorant herbs that relieve coughs and have sedative qualities.

For herbs in this category, see Chapter 3: Bamboo Sap and Shavings, Fritillary, Kelp (see Seaweed), Trichosanthes

WARM HERBS THAT TRANSFORM PHLEGM-COLD   These warming herbs treat Phlegm-Dampness and Phlegm-Cold conditions such as nodules in the neck, lymphadenitis, and chronic coughs that produce mucus.

For herbs in this category, see Chapter 3: Pinellia, Platycodon

HERBS THAT RELIEVE COUGHING AND WHEEZING   These herbs treat the "symptom" by stopping coughing and wheezing. It is important, however, to use them in conjunction with herbs that address the "root" problem. If the cough is due to an external factor, they should be combined with herbs that Release the Exterior; if the cough is due to internal weakness or injury, they are combined with Tonifying herbs; if the cough is Cold (producing clear or white mucus), they are combined with Warming herbs; if the cough is Hot (producing thick, yellow mucus), they are combined with herbs that Clear Heat.

For herbs in this category, see Chapter 3: Apricot Kernel, Coltsfoot, Mulberry Root Bark

7. Aromatic Herbs that Transform Dampness

Herbs in this category are warm, spicy, fragrant substances that Dry Dampness in the Middle Burner (or Stomach and Spleen area). This type of Dampness is frequently the result of food poisoning or an acute case of gastroenteritis. Symptoms of this type of disorder include feelings of fullness in the abdomen, loss of appetite, nausea, vomiting of sour fluids, diarrhea, and headache or body aches. If you suspect food poisoning, please consult a qualified health-care practitioner immediately.

For herbs in this category, see Chapter 3: Agastache, Cardamom Seed, Magnolia Bark

8. Herbs that Relieve Food Stagnation

Herbs in this category aid digestion by stimulating gastrointestinal secretions. Food Stagnation is generally classified as either Hot or Cold. The Cold type of Stagnation can result from consuming too much cold, congesting food or because of Spleen/Stomach weakness or Deficiency. Symptoms of the Cold type would include nausea, abdominal distention, spitting up of clear liquids, a white, greasy tongue coating, and preference for hot foods and drinks. To treat this type of disorder, herbs that Warm the Interior are added to the formula.

The Hot type of Food Stagnation is accompanied by extremely bad breath, abdominal distention, a yellow, greasy tongue coating, and aversion to hot food and drinks with a preference for those that are cold. These symptoms are often due to externally contracted microbes, and herbs that Clear Heat are added to the formula.

For herbs in this category, see Chapter 3: Hawthorn Fruit, Radish Seed

9. Herbs that Regulate the Qi

There are basically two Qi disharmonies: Qi Stagnation or Congestion and Qi Deficiency. Herbs that treat Qi Deficiency are those that Tonify or strengthen Qi and can be found under Herbal Category number 12, Tonifying Herbs.

When our energy gets stuck, we experience pain due to Blockage of our Qi (energy) along acupuncture channels. This usually occurs in the head or extremities, but it can actually appear anywhere in the body. Usually, herbs that Expel Wind-Dampness in the channels are effective for treating this type of stagnation; they were discussed under Herbal Category number 5, Herbs that Dispel Wind-Dampness.

Herbs in the Regulate-Qi-healing category are aimed at breaking up Qi Congestion affecting the Organ Systems. Symptoms usually involve pain in the abdomen or chest. For example, Stagnant Stomach and Spleen Qi manifest as belching, gas, acid regurgitation, epigastric and abdominal pain, nausea, vomiting, and loose stool or constipation. Congested Liver Qi includes such symptoms as irritability, pain in the flanks, loss of appetite, and a stifling feeling in the chest. Stagnant Lung Qi is characterized by a stifling feeling in the chest that is accompanied by coughing and wheezing.

From a Western medical standpoint, it could be said that herbs in this category are aimed at correcting a gastrointestinal dysfunction responsible for creating pain.

These herbs are aromatic and Dry in nature and should be used cautiously by persons with Yin or Qi Deficiency. Simmer Qi-Regulating herbs for no more than 15 minutes, since therapeutic volatile oils will be lost if they are cooked longer.

For herbs in this category, see Chapter 3: Cyperus, Persimmon Calyx, Tangerine Peel

10. Herbs that Regulate the Blood

There are three categories of Blood-Regulating herbs: (1) those that Stop Bleeding; (2) those that Invigorate or move the Blood; and (3) Blood Tonifiers. The first two groups of herbs are covered here. Please see Herbal Category number 12 for herbs that Tonify the Blood.

HERBS THAT STOP BLEEDING   It is extremely important to remember that herbs in this category should never be used alone, but in conjunction with herbs that treat the root of the problem. If bleeding is due to Hot Blood, then herbs that Cool the Blood should be added to the herbal formula; if bleeding is due to Deficient Spleen Qi, then herbal Spleen Tonifiers are indicated. If Blood Stasis is the cause of imbalance, then herbs that Invigorate the Blood would be added to the herbal prescription. Always consult a qualified medical professional in case of severe bleeding.

For herbs in this category, see Chapter 3: Agrimony, Mugwort, Pseudoginseng (see Ginseng), Sanguisorba, Sophora

HERBS THAT INVIGORATE THE BLOOD   In Traditional Oriental Medicine, if pain is not caused by infection or injury, it is thought to be the result of Congestion or Stagnation of Blood and Qi. Just imagine a clogged irrigation ditch in your garden; debris accumulates and life-giving water and nutrients do not reach the plants. The same is true in our human garden. Due to lack of exercise and many hours driving to work and then sitting at our desks, our blood, lymph, and energy do not flow as they should. Our cells are denied oxygen and food; toxins are not carried away. The result is often localized pain that is deep, sharp, and colicky in nature. This type of pain is most often associated with lower abdominal pain; difficult, painful, or absent menstrual cycles (dysmenorrhea or amenorrhea); low back and knee pain; chest pain; or lingering pain caused by an old accident.

For herbs in this category, see Chapter 3: Achyranthes, Ligusticum, Peony Root (Red), Safflower Flower, Salvia, Turmeric

11. Herbs that Warm the Interior and Expel Cold

When deep Cold enters the body, symptoms include cold hands and feet, a pale complexion, fear of the cold, loose stools, a white tongue coating, lack of thirst, but possible desire to drink hot liquids. Serious cases would include profuse sweating and ice-cold extremities (often seen when someone is in shock). When the Cold invades the Spleen or Stomach Organ Systems, symptoms might include cold, painful sensations in the abdomen or chest, nausea, vomiting, belching, and diarrhea (often seen in cases of acute gastroenteritis or gastritis).

Most herbs in this healing category are spicy, Warm, and Drying and should be used with caution during pregnancy or in cases with Heat symptoms or Yin Deficiency.

For herbs in this category, see Chapter 3: Aconite, Fennel Seeds, Ginger (Dried)

12. Tonifying Herbs

Remember that poor moldy lemon in Chapter 6? The lemon suffered from lack of Protective or Defensive Qi. While Tonifying herbs can't help the lemon, they are an important key in strengthening our human body's defenses against invaders. These herbal friends are great for boosting our health and can aid in the recovery of persons with chronic of degenerative diseases by strengthening Deficiencies in Blood, Qi, Yang, or Yin. Please remember, however, that herbs are only one piece of the healing puzzle; of equal important is attention to a nourishing diet and physical and breathing exercises. Also, Tonic herbs should be discontinued if you are suffering from an acute illness, such as a cold, sore throat, or flu.

A few people have great difficulty absorbing rich, Tonifying herbs. Basically there are two distinct patterns that can be recognized. The first type has a weak digestive system that can't absorb the herbs; symptoms can include bloating, loss of appetite, and/or nausea. In the second type, Heat symptoms due to Deficiency appear; these include insomnia, irritability, dry mouth and lips, and indigestion. Watch for any of these signs and discontinue Tonifying herbs in tea form until the person is sufficiently strengthened by eating a balanced, nourishing diet. (*Note:* It is possible the person could ingest small quantities of Tonifying herbs by adding them to a favorite soup or stew. You'll find some tasty recipes in Chapter 5.)

HERBS THAT TONIFY THE QI Herbs that Tonify Qi are commonly used in treating weakness of the Spleen or Lung Organ Systems. Think of it this way: The Spleen is responsible for extracting Qi from food while our Lungs are responsible for extracting Qi from the air. If we lack Qi, then one of these systems is probably not functioning up to par. Symptoms of Deficient Spleen Qi include lack of appetite, loose stools or diarrhea, a feeling of heaviness in the arms and legs, and tiredness. Lung Qi Deficiency is signaled by a pale complexion, weak voice, shallow breathing, shortness of breath, and spontaneous sweating.

Qi-Tonifying herbs are usually rich and sweet in nature, so it's important to combine them with small quantities of herbs that Move and Regulate the Qi as well.

For herbs in this category, see Chapter 3: Astragalus, Atractylodes, Codonopsis, Dioscorea, Ginseng, Jujube Date Fruit, Licorice

HERBS THAT TONIFY THE BLOOD In Traditional Oriental Medicine it is said that the Liver System stores the Blood while the Heart System directs it (through veins and arteries). Symptoms of Deficient Blood include a pale complexion and lips, restless fatigue, dry skin, dizziness, vertigo, diminished vision, palpitations, a pale tongue, and menstrual irregularities. Not all symptoms of Blood Deficiency are associated with anemia, but can be the result of a variety of other problems such as chronic hepatitis or heart failure. Most of the herbs in this category strengthen the body through nutrition, increasing the number of circulating blood cells.

These herbs are rarely, if ever, taken alone. They are often given with Yin-Tonifying herbs to increase their actions. Frequently, Blood and Qi Deficiency occur simultaneously, so Qi-Tonifying herbs are added to the herbal formula. Overuse of Blood Tonifiers can cause indigestion; for this reason, stomach-strengthening herbs often make their way into the prescription as well.

For herbs in this category, see Chapter 3: Dang Gui, Longan Berries, Lycii Fruit, Peony Root (White), Polygonum, Rehmannia (Cooked)

HERBS THAT TONIFY THE YANG When Kidney Yang is Deficient, our whole system is in a state of exhaustion. Since the Kidney System is considered the root of our body's yang energy, herbs in this category Tonify Kidney Yang, as well as Deficient Spleen and Heart Yang. While in the West we associate kidney function with managing our body fluids, Oriental thought regards the Kidney System as the storehouse of our body's "essence." The adrenal glands are small organs that sit on top of our kidneys and produce important hormones that regulate body functions. The adrenal glands, as well as our reproductive glands, are part of the Kidney System in Oriental thought. Symptoms of Kidney Yang Deficiency include frequent urination, cold extremities, fear of the cold, pale tongue, weak and sore lower back and extremities, infertility, impotence, watery vaginal discharge, spermatorrhea, diarrhea early in the morning, wheezing, and feelings of despair or paranoia.

Most herbs that Tonify Kidney Yang are drying and warm in nature and should not be used by persons who suffer from Heat symptoms due to Yin Deficiency.

For herbs in this category, see Chapter 3: Cuscuta, Epimedium, Eucommia, Fenugreek Seed

HERBS THAT TONIFY THE YIN   Yin-Tonifying herbs cool, nourish, and moisten. Herbs in this category are used primarily to tonify the Yin of the Liver, Stomach, Lungs, and Kidneys. You will find herbs that nurture Heart Yin under Herbal Healing Category number 14.

There are two major patterns of Liver Yin Deficiency. The first pattern is similar to Deficient Liver Blood except the patient feels a sensation of low-grade heat plus the Blood Deficiency symptoms of dizziness; ringing in the ears; dry nails; night blindness; dry, dull eyes; and poor eyesight. In this case, herbs that nourish the blood should be added to a Liver Yin-tonifying formula. The second pattern of Deficient Liver Yin includes symptoms of Liver Yang Rising such as insomnia, a red tongue, ringing in the ears, vertigo, and a dry mouth and throat.

Deficient Stomach Yin is a lack of fluids in the stomach. This type of condition is seen after a severe disease with high fevers. Symptoms include constipation, lack of appetite, thirst, a dry mouth, and irritability.

Deficient Lung Yin is characterized by a dry cough and throat, dry skin, thirst, loss of voice and, occasionally, spitting up of thick phlegm. If the disharmony is not addressed, it becomes lung consumption with a chronic cough (sometimes with blood in the phlegm), night sweats, and low-grade afternoon fevers.

Kidney Yin Deficiency can be found at the root of many chronic diseases. General symptoms include weakness of the lower back and knees; dizziness; ringing in the ears; warm palms of the hands and soles of the feet; dark, scanty urine; a red and dry tongue; and a low-grade fever in the afternoons.

Yin Tonic herbs are usually quite sweet, cold, and rich in nature. They are extremely difficult for persons with Spleen or Stomach Deficiency to digest. Their energy, unless drastically altered by the inclusion of other warming, carminative herbs in the formula, is not appropriate for persons suffering from Dampness or Phlegm, diarrhea, or abdominal distention.

For herbs in this category, see Chapter 3: American Ginseng Root (see Ginseng), Dendrobium, Glehnia, Lily Bulb, Ophiopogon

13. Herbs that Stabilize and Bind

Herbs that Stabilize and Bind are astringent or sour substances that halt excessive bodily discharges such as excessive urination or sweating and diarrhea. They also treat conditions where structures in the body are slipping away from their correct positions, such as prolapse of the rectum or uterus. Most of these slipping-away conditions are due to old age or chronic disease that has caused extreme weakness in the elasticity of the smooth muscle tissue.

While herbs from this category treat the symptom, they should be combined with herbs that treat the root of the problem. Often, the root is Deficiency in one form or another. These herbs should not be used by people who are experiencing Dampness in the form of Stagnation or Congestion, or by people with symptoms of Constrained Heat. Conditions related to Damp or Heat Congestion should be addressed and eliminated prior to the use of Herbs that Stabilize and Bind.

For herbs in this category, see Chapter 3: Cornus, Ginkgo, Pomegranate Husk, Schisandra

14. Substances that Calm the Spirit

When someone is experiencing symptoms such as insomnia, irritability, palpitations accompanied by anxiety, or forms of mental instability, these substances are used to Calm the Spirit. In Oriental thought, the spirit resides in the Heart while the soul resides in the Liver. Disorders of both organ systems manifest with similar symptoms.

SUBSTANCES THAT ANCHOR, SETTLE, AND CALM THE SPIRIT Heavy, dense shells or minerals that "weigh" down the Heart Calm the Spirit by eliminating insomnia and palpitations with feelings of anxiety. They also hold down or anchor Liver Yang energy that rises up and creates dizziness, a bad temper, flushed face, or headaches. In the case of excessive belching, vomiting, or hiccoughs, they settle the Stomach and direct that Rebellious Qi downwards. These substances have tranquilizing and sedative properties, from a Western biomedical point of view.

For herbs in this category, see Chapter 3: Dragon Bone, Oyster Shell, Pearl

HERBS THAT NOURISH THE HEART AND CALM THE SPIRIT   Most herbs that Nourish the Heart and Calm the Spirit are gentle substances. They are used primarily to relieve palpitations with anxiety and insomnia.

For herbs in this category, see Chapter 3: Biota, Polygala, Zizyphus Seed

15. Aromatic Substances that Open the Orifices

Since these substances are used in severe cases of delirium or disease in Traditional Oriental Medicine, always consult a licensed medical practitioner to treat the disorders listed in this section.

When a person experiences a stroke, coma, or seizures, aromatic substances that open the orifices are used in the Orient. Remember that the Heart governs the Spirit in Oriental thought, and when someone suffers from a seizure, or coma, their Spirit is "Locked Up." Aromatic substances release the person's Spirit by opening up the Sensory Orifices.

There are basically two categories of disharmonies treated by these substances: (1) Cold Closed Disorder and (2) Hot Closed Disorder. You're becoming familiar with Cold symptoms by now, aren't you? Symptoms of a Cold Closed Disorder include a cold body, white tongue coating, and a bluish or ashen face coloring. These symptoms often accompany a coma following a stroke or poisonings. The person might collapse or foam at the mouth. The Hot Closed Disorder occurs in cases of diseases such as encephalitis, meningitis, severe pneumonia, severe infections, heat stroke, or the last stage in liver disease. Symptoms include delirium, yellow tongue coating, red face, convulsions, heavy breathing, and a high fever.

From a Western view, these substances revive someone from a coma by stimulating the central nervous system. At the same time, they have tranquilizing effects that make them useful in stopping spasms and relieving irritability.

For the herb in this category, see Chapter 3: Acorus Rhizome

16. Substances that Extinguish Wind and Stop Tremors

Substances in this category are used to treat Internal Wind, usually due to imbalances in the Liver or Kidney Organ Systems. Yin Deficiency of the Kidney and Liver or Liver Yang Rising include such symptoms as headache, blurred vision, dizziness, and ringing in the ears. Severe cases might include palpitations with feelings of anxiety, irritability, muscle twitches, and vomiting. From a Western biomedical viewpoint, the person is suffering from atherosclerosis or hypertension.

Internal Wind can also be the result of Deficient Blood signaled by dizziness, ringing in the ears, blurred vision, and numbing of the extremities. The person could be suffering from a serious illness and in severe cases can lose consciousness or go into convulsions. It is very important to see a qualified medical practitioner in such cases.

Extremely high fevers can also cause convulsions. Please contact a qualified medical practitioner immediately.

Most of the herbs and other substances used to treat Internal Wind are mild sedatives and antihypertensives.

For herbs in this category, see Chapter 3: Gambir, Gastrodia

17. Herbs that Expel Parasites

Persons with unwanted visitors such as roundworms, hookworms, and tapeworms might experience symptoms such as vomiting, a change in appetite, or itching of the nose, ears, or rectum. If the condition goes untreated, they can experience fatigue and emaciated bodies with distended abdomens. Sometimes, however, parasites can be detected only by stool examination.

The herbs in this category are usually more gentle than antiparasitic drugs but should still always be used with caution. Herbs that Expel Parasites are to be used with caution during pregnancy and should be avoided in case of severe stomach pain or fever.

For herbs in this category, see Chapter 3: Garlic, Pumpkin Seeds and Husks

18. Substances for External Application

Oriental medicine has a wonderful array of healing powders, ointments, and salves. Some practitioners of Oriental herbal medicine have dedicated their whole lives to perfecting such formulas.

Almost all herbs or substances in this particular category, if taken internally, have side effects. Therefore, the prescription of such agents is monitored carefully and they are not included in this book. However, healing herbs in other categories can often be applied externally. Where appropriate, in the description of individual herbs throughout Chapter 3, I have indicated means of applying healing herbs externally. Also, in Chapter 2, you will find simple recipes for external applications in the form of herbal compresses, baths, gargles, liniments, oils, and salves.

Resource Guide

Books

BLOOD TYPES AND DIETARY REQUIREMENTS

D'Adamo, Peter J., *Eat Right for Your Type*. New York, New York: G.P. Putnam's Sons, 1996.

Gittleman, Ann Louise, M.S. *Your Body Knows Best*. New York: Simon & Schuster, Inc., 1996.

CARBOHYDRATE SENSITIVITY AND WEIGHT LOSS

Heller, Rachael F., Ph.D., and Richard F. Heller, Ph.D. *The Carbohydrate Addict's Diet*. New York: Penguin Books, 1993.

Sears, Barry, Ph.D. *Enter the Zone*. New York: HarperCollins Publishers, 1995.

___. *Mastering the Zone*. New York: HarperCollins Publishers, 1997.

FATS IN OUR DIET

Erasmus, Udo. *Fats that Heal—Fats that Kill*. Burnaby, BC, Canada: Alive Books, 1986.

5 ELEMENT ARCHETYPES AND CHINESE MEDICINE

Beinfield, Harriet, L.Ac., and Efrem Korngold, L.Ac., O.M.D. *Between Heaven and Earth—A Guide to Chinese Medicine*. New York: Ballantine Books, 1991. This is an extraordinary introduction to Chinese medicine.

FOOD THERAPY (CHINESE)

Note: Carbohydrate-sensitive individuals can take advantage of the use of medicinal herbal soups and porridges given in *The Book of Jook;* however, substitute pearl barley, coix, or oatmeal for rice (which is high on the glycemic index). Consume your porridge with the appropriate amount of protein and fat as recommended by Sears in *The Zone*. If you follow the Heller and Heller method, consume a medicinal rice porridge during your daily "one-hour Reward Meal."

Flaws, Bob. *The Book of Jook—Chinese Medicinal Porridges*. Boulder, CO: Blue Poppy Press, 1995.

Flaws, Bob, and Honora Wolfe. *Prince Wen Hui's Cook—Chinese Dietary Therapy.* Brookline, MA: Paradigm Publications, 1983.

Lu, Henry C. *Chinese System of Food Cures—Prevention and Remedies.* New York: Sterling Publishing Company, 1986.

___. *Chinese Foods for Longevity.* New York: Sterling Publishing Company, 1986.

HERBALS

Bensky, Dan, and Andrew Gamble (translators). *Chinese Herbal Medicine Materia Medica.* Seattle, WA: Eastland Press, 1993.

Fratkin, Jake. *Chinese Herbal Patent Formulas—A Practical Guide.* Boulder, CO: SHYA Publications, 1993.

Hobbs, Christopher. *The Ginsengs—A User's Guide.* Santa Cruz, CA: Botanica Press, 1996.

Tierra, Lesley, L.Ac. *The Herbs of Life—Health and Healing Using Western and Chinese Techniques.* Freedom, CA: The Crossing Press, 1992.

Tierra, Michael, L.Ac., O.M.D. *Planetary Herbology.* Santa Fe, NM: Lotus Press, 1988.

HERBAL ORGANIZATIONS

American Botanical Council
P.O. Box 201660W
Austin, TX 78720
Tel: (512) 331-8868

American Herbalists Guild
P.O. Box 746555
Arvada, CO 8006-6555
Tel: (303) 423-8800
Fax: (303) 428-8828

The "AHG" is a professional body of herbalists dedicated to promoting and maintaining criteria for the practice of professional herbalism in America.

Herb Research Foundation
1007 Pearl Street, Suite 200F
Boulder, CO 80302

American Herbalists Association
P.O. Box 1673
Nevada City, CA 95959

International Herb Growers and Marketers Association
Box 77123
Baton Rouge, LA 70879

HERBAL STUDIES
East West Herbal Correspondence School
by Michael and Lesley Tierra
P.O. Box 712, Santa Cruz, CA 95061

Chinese Herbs

The following companies sell Chinese herbs by mail order in the United States:

Spring Wind Herb Company
2325 Fourth Street Suite 6
Berkeley, CA 94710
Tel: (510) 849-1820
Fax: (510) 849-4886

Mayway Trading Corporation
1338 Mandela Parkway
Oakland, CA 94607
Tel: (510) 208-3123; 1 (800) 262-9929

Nuherbs Company
3820 Penniman Avenue
Oakland, CA 94619
Tel: (415) 534-4372; 1 (800) 233-4307

East West Herb Products
317 West 100th Street
New York, NY 10025
In New York: (212) 864-5508
Outside New York: 1 (800) 542-6544

China Herb Company
6333 Wayne Avenue
Philadelphia, PA 19144
Tel: (215) 843-5864; 1 (800) 221-4372
Fax: (215) 849-3338

Persons living in the United Kingdom can order most of the medicinals in this book from:

Acumedic Ltd.
101–105 Camden High Street
London NW1 7JN
Tel: 071-388-6704/5783
Fax: 071-387-5766

Harmony Acupuncture Supplies Center
629 High Road Leytonstone
London E11 4PA
Tel: 081-518-7337
Fax: 081-518-7338

Mayway Herbal Emporium
40 Sapcote Trading Estate, Dudden Hill Lane
London NW10 2DJ
Tel: 081-459-1812
Fax: 081-459-1727

Persons living in Europe can order most of the medicinals in this book from:

Tai Yang Chinese Herb Store
Elverdignsestr, 90A
8900 Ieper, Belgium
Tel: 057-21-86-69
Fax: 057-21-97-78

Apotheek Gouka
Goenelaan 111
3114 CE Schiedam, Netherlands
Tel: 010-426-46-33
Fax: 010-473-08-45

Persons living in Australia can order most of the medicinals in this book from:

Chinaherb
29A Albion Street
Surry Hills, NSW 2010
Tel: 02-281-2122

LIVE HERBS AND SEEDS
Shephards Garden Seeds
6116 Highway 9
Felton, CA 95018

Taylor's Garden, Inc.
1535 Lone Oak Road
Vista, CA 92083

ORGANIC HERB FARMS
Pacific Botanicals
360 Stephen Way
Williams, OR 97544

Trout Lake Herb Farm
Rt. 1, Box 355
Trout Lake, WA 98650

WILDCRAFTERS
Blessed Herbs
Michael Volchok
Rt. 5, Box 191A
Ava, MO 85020

Mike and Debby Minear
Rt. 1, Box 60
Little Hocking, OH 45742

Reevis Mountain School of Survival
HC02 Box 1543
Roosevelt, AZ 85545

Bibliography

Books

Balch, Phyllis, C.N.C., and James Balch, M.D. *Rx Prescription for Cooking.* Greenfield, IN: PAB Books Publishing, Inc., 1991.

Beijing, Shanghai, and Nanjing Colleges of Traditional Chinese Medicine and the Acupuncture Institute of the Academy of Traditional Chinese Medicine (Compiled by). *Essentials of Chinese Acupuncture.* Beijing, China: Foreign Languages Press, 1980.

Beinfield, Harriet, L.Ac., and Efrem Korngold, L.Ac., O.M.D. *Between Heaven and Earth—A Guide to Chinese Medicine.* New York: Ballantine Books, 1991.

Benedict, Ruth. *Patterns of Culture.* Boston, MA: Houghton Mifflin Company, 1934.

Bensky, Dan, and Andrew Gamble (translators). *Chinese Herbal Medicine Materia Medica.* Seattle, WA: Eastland Press, 1993.

Bensky, Dan, and Randall Barolet (translators). *Chinese Herbal Medicine Formulas and Strategies.* Seattle, WA: Eastland Press, 1990.

Berkow, Robert, M.D. (editor-in-chief). *The Merck Manual of Diagnosis and Therapy.* Rathway, NJ: Merck Research Laboratories, 1992.

Binford, Lewis R. *In Pursuit of the Past.* New York: Thames and Hudson, 1983.

Bown, Deni. *The Herb Society of America Encyclopedia of Herbs and Their Uses.* New York: Dorling Kindersley Publishing Inc., 1995.

Carper, Jean. *Total Nutrition Guide.* New York: Bantam Books, 1987.

Chin, Wee Yeow, and Hsuan Keng. *An Illustrated Dictionary of Chinese Medicinal Herbs.* Sebastopol, CA: CRCS Publications, 1992.

Chopra, Deepak, M.D. *Perfect Health—The Complete Mind/Body Guide.* New York: Crown Publishers, Inc., 1991.

___. *Quantum Healing—Exploring the Frontiers of Mind/Body Medicine.* New York: Bantam Doubleday Dell Publishing Group, Inc., 1989.

___. *Unconditional Life.* New York: Bantam Books, 1991.

Cowan, C. Wesley, and Patty Jo Watson (editors). *The Origins of Agriculture.* Washington, D.C.: Smithsonian Institution Press, 1992.

D'Adamo, Peter J., *Eat Right for Your Type*. New York, New York: G.P. Putnam's Sons, 1996.

Dufty, William. *Sugar Blues*. New York: Warner Books, 1976.

Erasmus, Udo. *Fats that Heal—Fats that Kill*. Burnaby, BC, Canada: Alive Books, 1986.

Flaws, Bob. *The Book of Jook—Chinese Medicinal Porridges*. Boulder, CO: Blue Poppy Press, 1995.

Flaws, Bob, and Honora Wolfe. *Prince Wen Hui's Cook—Chinese Dietary Therapy*. Brookline, MA: Paradigm Publications, 1983.

Fox, Stuart Ira. *Human Physiology*. Dubuque, IA: Wm. C. Brown Publishers, 1987.

Fratkin, Jake. *Chinese Herbal Patent Formulas—A Practical Guide*. Boulder, CO: SHYA Publications, 1993.

Geertz, Clifford. *The Interpretation of Cultures*. New York: Basic Books, 1973.

Gittleman, Ann Louise, M.S. *Your Body Knows Best*. New York: Simon & Schuster, Inc., 1996.

Glanze, Walter D. (managing editor). *Mosby's Medical, Nursing, and Allied Health Dictionary*. St. Louis, MI: The D.V. Mosby Company, 1990.

Haas, Elson M., M.D. *Staying Healthy with the Seasons*. Berkeley, CA: Celestial Arts, 1981.

____. *Staying Healthy with Nutrition*. Berkeley, CA: Celestial Arts, 1992.

Hammer, Leon, M.D. *Dragon Rises—Red Bird Flies (Psychology and Chinese Medicine)*. Barrytown, NY: Station Hill Press, 1990.

Hay, John. *Kernels of Energy, Bones of Earth*. New York: Eastern Press, Inc., 1985.

Heiser, Charles B. *Seed to Civilization (The Story of Food)*. Cambridge, MA: Harvard University Press, 1973.

Heller, Rachael F., Ph.D., and Richard F. Heller, Ph.D. *The Carbohydrate Addict's Diet*. New York: Penguin Books, 1993.

Hobbs, Christopher. *The Ginsengs—A User's Guide*. Santa Cruz, CA: Botanica Press, 1996.

____. *Handbook for Herbal Healing*. Santa Cruz, CA: Botanica Press, 1990.

Hsu, Hong-Yen, Ph.D., and Chau-Shin Hsu, Ph.D. *Commonly Used Chinese Herb Formulas*. Long Beach, CA: Oriental Healing Arts Institute, 1980.

Kaptchuk, Ted. *The Web that Has No Weaver*. New York: Cogndon & Weded, 1983.

Kunz, Jeffrey, M.D., and Asher Finkel, M.D. *The American Medical Association Family Medical Guide.* New York: Random House, 1987.

Kushi, Aveline. *Aveline Kushi's Complete Guide to Macrobiotic Cooking.* New York: Warner Books, 1985.

Kushi, Aveline, and Wendy Esko. *The Changing Seasons Macrobiotic Cookbook.* Wayne, NJ: Avery Publishing Group, Inc., 1985.

Kushi, Michio. *Book of Macrobiotics.* New York: Japan Publications, 1977.

___. *Macrobiotic Home Remedies.* New York: Japan Publications, 1985.

Lad, Vasant. *Ayurveda—The Science of Self-Healing.* Santa Fe, NM: Lotus Press, 1984.

___. *The Yoga of Herbs.* Santa Fe, NM: 1986.

Li, Cheng-Yu, C.M.D. (editor). *Fundamentals of Chinese Medicine.* Brookline, MA: Paradigm Publications, 1985.

Long, James W., M.D. *The Essential Guide to Prescription Drugs.* New York: Harper Perennial, 1992.

Lu, Henry C. *Chinese System of Food Cures—Prevention and Remedies.* New York: Sterling Publishing Company, 1986.

___. *Chinese Foods for Longevity.* New York: Sterling Publishing Company, 1986.

Lucas, Richard. *Secrets of the Chinese Herbalists.* West Nyack, NY: Parker Publishing Company, Inc., 1987.

Maciocia, Giovanni, *The Foundations of Chinese Medicine.* New York: Churchill Livingstone, 1989.

___. *The Practice of Chinese Medicine.* New York: Churchill Livingstone, 1994.

McDougall, John, M.D. *The McDougall Program.* New York: Penguin Books, 1991.

McElroy, Ann, and Patricia K. Townsend. *Medical Anthropology in Ecological Perspective.* Boulder, CO: Westview Press, Inc., 1985.

Monod, Jacques. *Chance and Necessity.* New York: Vantage Books, 1972.

Munakata, Kiyohiko. *Sacred Mountains in Chinese Art.* Springfield, IL: University of Illinois Press, 1991.

Muramoto, Naboru. *Healing Ourselves.* New York: Swan House Publishing Company, 1973.

Ni, Maoshing, Ph.D., CA, with Cathy McNease. *The Tao of Nutrition.* Santa Monica, CA: Seven Star Communications Group, 1987.

Ody, Penelope. *The Complete Medicinal Herbal.* New York: DK Publishing, 1993.

Ornish, Dean, M.D. *Dr. Dean Ornish's Program for Reversing Heart Disease.* New York: Random House, 1990.

Pennington, Jean, Ph.D., R.D. (revised by). *Bowes and Church's Food Values of Portions Commonly Used.* New York: HarperPerennial, 1989.

Pitchford, Paul. *Healing with Whole Foods—Oriental Traditions and Modern Nutrition.* Berkeley, CA: North Atlantic Books, 1993.

Raven, Peter, Ray Evert, and Susan Eichhorn. *Biology of Plants.* New York: Worth Publishers, Inc., 1987.

Requena, Yves, M.D. *Terrains and Pathology in Acupuncture.* Brookline, MA: Paradigm Publications, 1986.

Robin, Eugene D., M.D. *Matters of Life and Death: Risks vs. Benefits of Medical Care.* Stanford, CA: Stanford Alumni Association, 1984.

Robbins, John. *Diet for a New America.* Walpole, NH: Stillpoint Publishing, 1987.

Sears, Barry, Ph.D. *Enter the Zone.* New York: HarperCollins Publishers, 1995.

_____. *Mastering the Zone.* New York: HarperCollins Publishers, 1997.

Soulié de Morant, George. *Chinese Acupuncture.* Brookline, MA: Paradigm Publications, 1994.

Thomas, Clayton, L., M.D. (editor). *Taber's Cyclopedic Medical Dictionary.* Philadelphia, PA: F.A. Davis Company, 1987.

Thomas, David Hurst. *Archaeology—Down to Earth.* Orlando, FL: Harcourt Brace Jovanovich College Publishers, 1991.

Tierra, Lesley, L.Ac. *The Herbs of Life—Health and Healing Using Western and Chinese Techniques.* Freedom, CA: The Crossing Press, 1992.

_____. *Healing with Chinese Herbs.* Freedom, CA: The Crossing Press, 1997.

Tierra, Michael, L.Ac., O.M.D. *Planetary Herbology.* Santa Fe, NM: Lotus Press, 1988.

_____. *The Way of Herbs.* New York: 1983.

Turner, Kristina. *The Self-Healing Cookbook.* Grass Valley, CA: Earthtones Press, 1987.

Werbach, Melvyn R., M.D. *Nutritional Influences on Illness.* New Canaan, CT: Keats Publishing, Inc., 1988.

Yen, Kun-Ying, Ph.D. *The Illustrated Chinese Materia Medica.* Taiwan, Republic of China: SMC Publishing Inc., 1992.

Zhang, Zhongjing (translated by Luo Xiwen, MA, Ph.D.). *Synopsis of Prescriptions of the Golden Chamber.* Beijing, China: New World Press, 1987.

Zihlman, Adrienne L. *The Human Evolution Coloring Book.* New York: HarperCollins Publishers, Inc., 1982.

Periodicals

Adebajo, A. O. (Letter) "Is Rheumatoid Arthritis an Infectious Disease? *British Medical Journal*, September 28, 1991; 6805/303:786.

Ebringer, Alan. (Letter) "Is Rheumatoid Arthritis an Infectious Disease?" *British Medical Journal*, August 31, 1991; 6801/303:524.

Ireland, Corydon. "The Politics of Nutrition." *Vegetarian Times*, October 1992; 55–60.

Kjeldsen-Kragh, Haugen, Borchgrevink, Laerum, Eek, Mowinkel, Hovi, Forre. "Controlled Trial of Fasting and One-Year Vegetarian Diet in Rheumatoid Arthritis. *The Lancet*, October 12, 1991; 8772/338:899.

Kleinman, Arthur, and Lilias H. Sung. "Why Do Indigenous Practitioners Successfully Heal? *Soc. Sci & Med.*, 1979; Vol. 13/7–26.

Robbins, John. "Realities 1989." Excerpts from: *Diet for a New America*. Felton, CA: EarthSave, 1989.

Samanta, A., S. Roy, and K. L. Woods. "Gold Therapy in Rheumatoid Arthritis." *The Lancet*, September 7, 1991; 8767/338:642.

Silman, Alan J. "Is Rheumatoid Arthritis an Infectious Disease?" *British Medical Journal*, July 17, 1991; 6796/303:200.

Sturrock, R.D. "'Second Line,'" Drugs for Rheumatoid Arthritis." *British Medical Journal*, July 27, 1991; 6796/303:201.

Audio Cassettes

Chopra, Deepak. American Holistic Medical Conference: The New Physics of Healing. Boulder, CO: Sounds True Recordings, 1990.

Index